Evaluation and Treatment of Mental Illnesses

Evaluation and Treatment of Mental Illnesses

Edited by **John Dalvi**

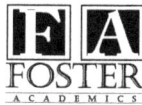

FOSTER
ACADEMICS

New Jersey

Published by Foster Academics,
61 Van Reypen Street,
Jersey City, NJ 07306, USA
www.fosteracademics.com

Evaluation and Treatment of Mental Illnesses
Edited by John Dalvi

International Standard Book Number: 978-1-63242-188-3 (Hardback)

Printed in the United States of America.

Contents

Preface

This book is a comprehensive compilation of works of different researchers from varied parts of the world. It includes valuable experiences of the researchers with the sole objective of providing the readers (learners) with a proper knowledge of the concerned field. This book will be beneficial in evoking inspiration and enhancing the knowledge of the interested readers.

It is important to assess mental illness seriously, to comprehend its nature, predict its long-term outcome and treat it with specific rather than generic treatment, such as pharmacotherapy. This book has three important sections, which cover introduction, evaluation and treatments methods of mental illness. Community-wide and cognitive-behavioral approaches are essential methods and should be incorporated to decrease the severity of symptoms of mental illness. Mental illness cannot be treated with one single kind of treatment method. Individual, community and socially-oriented treatments along with latest distance-writing technologies will allow a more effective and unified approach to fight mental illness world-wide.

In the end, I would like to extend my heartiest thanks to the authors who worked with great determination on their chapters. I also appreciate the publisher's support in the course of the book. I would also like to deeply acknowledge my family who stood by me as a source of inspiration during the project.

Editor

Part 1

Introduction

Psychopathology and Quality of Life in Children of Mentally Ill Parents

Silke Wiegand-Grefe, Susanne Halverscheid,
Franz Petermann and Angela Plass
University Medical Center Hamburg-Eppendorf
Center for Clinical Psychology and Rehabilitation at Bremen University
Germany

1. Introduction

Children of mentally ill parents are considered a high-risk population for the development of psychological disorders although the reported rates of affected children vary between studies. Whether or not a child will develop a mental illness himself depends on risk factors as well as protective factors. This chapter presents findings concerning the mental health status and the quality of life in children of mentally ill parents (N = 86). The results reveal an increased relative risk to develop psychopathological symptoms being 3 to 7 times higher than in children of the general population. At the same time, the quality of life in children with a mentally ill parent is substantially decreased. The psychological disturbances of the children are associated with the parents' perceived impairments caused by their mental illness. The results support the need for prevention programs for this special group of children.

2. Psychopathology in children of mentally ill parents

Children of mentally ill parents represent a high-risk population for the development of psychiatric disorders (Ramchandani & Psychogiou, 2009). The majority of studies examined the mental health status of children with a parent suffering from depression. The results reveal an increased symptomatology being 3 to 4 times higher compared to control samples (Weissman, Fendrich, Warner & Wickramaratne, 1992, 2005; Fergusson, Lynskey & Horwood, 1993; Gelfand & Teti, 1990). A study with children of parents suffering from diverse psychiatric disorders indicates a three- to sevenfold rate of psychopathology compared to the general population (Wiegand-Grefe, Geers, Plass, Petermann & Riedesser, 2009). Due to the psychiatric illness, psycho-social risk factors accumulate and determine each other (Mattejat, Lenz & Wiegand-Grefe 2011). Financial problems, resulting from an illness-related job loss, for example, constitute an additional burden on the family. In addition, the parent-child-interaction is often impaired, being highly associated with mental health problems in the children and a decreased quality of life. These risk configurations do not directly lead to developmental problems and psychiatric disturbances in the children, but rather interact with the children's vulnerability and resilience (Noeker & Petermann, 2008). The term resilience characterizes a hardiness against extreme stresses and straints that may emerge within the children's environments. Resilient children overcome the sometimes potential traumatic conditions in a compensatory manner that allows them to surmount the adversities, displaying a healthy psychological functioning in the long term. Resilient children exhibit a balanced temper, high self-esteem, active coping mechanisms, good problem solving skills and an effective and competent social behavior. They have a secure attachment to at least one attachment figure and exhibit a clear value orientation (Noeker & Petermann, 2008). Resilient children are also very capable of showing empathy and expressing their own emotional states (Lenz & Kuhn, 2011). Which moderating factors can foster the children's mental health despite adverse living conditions is a central question for the development of effective prevention programs. In families with a mentally ill parent, the parental style of coping with the illness as well as reliable family relations are considered to be crucial protective factors for the children's development (Wiegand-Grefe et al., 2010a; Wiegand-Grefe, Halverscheid & Plass, 2011).

3. Quality of life in children of mentally ill parents

To date, little research has been conducted to assess the quality of life in children of mentally ill parents (Wiegand-Grefe et al. 2010b; Bullinger, 2011). Research in this area focuses rather on children's and adolescents' own somatic or psychiatric illness (Ravens-Sieberer & Bullinger, 1998; Ravens-Sieberer et al. 2006, 2008; Bullinger et al., 2008; Mattejat et al. 2005). Studies have shown that mentally ill children have a lower health-related quality of life (HRQL) than healthy or somatically ill children (Mattejat & Remschmidt, 2003; Ravens-Sieberer et al., 2008). In several Australian cities, N = 3597 children at the age of 6-17 years were assessed in their quality of life (Sawyer et al., 2002). The sample consisted of three psychiatric subsamples (ADHD, major depression and conduct disorder), two groups of children with physical illnesses, and a healthy control group of children. All children were assessed through parental evaluations. Children with mental health problems had decreased levels of quality of life in comparison to healthy children. In four out of five scales, they also displayed poorer rates in quality of life compared to the children with physical illnesses.

In a study with depressive and healthy children, aged 7 to 15 years, HRQL proved to be higher in healthy children (N = 1695) than in children suffering from depression (N = 248) (Kiss et al., 2009). In relation to the children's self-evaluations, maternal ratings of HRQL in depressive children was lower than in the children's self-assessments, while mothers of healthy children came up with a higher estimation of HRQL than the children themselves. The children's age and gender had no influence on the agreement between self-assessments and maternal ratings, neither was the mother's level of education influential.

In the representative German BELLA study with N = 1843 children and adolescents, adolescents with eating disorders showed lower HRQL scores than adolescents with normal eating habits (Herpertz-Dahlmann et al., 2008).

In a Dutch study, therapists rated the quality of life of 310 children and adolescents, aged 6 to 18 years, who were either healthy or suffered from one of five different psychiatric disorders (ADHD, anxiety disorders, pervasive developmental disorders, affective disorders or other diagnoses). Overall, children with pervasive developmental disorders were assessed to have the lowest HRQL (Bastiaansen et al., 2004).

Another study conducted by the Dutch research group assessed how quality of life changes relative to fluctuations in psychopathology. It was hypothesized that HRQL can increase even when the severity of psychopathological symptoms does not change (Bastiaansen et al., 2005a). Thirty-three percent of the 126 children and adolescents aged 7 to 19 years showed improved rates in psychopathology as well as in their quality of life, 28 % improved in either one of the two areas, while 38 % of the children revealed no changes in both areas. However, 11 % of the children and adolescents showed increased rates in their HRQL within the given time frame, while the severity of their psychopathology did not change. Thus, psychotherapy should aim at improving patients' quality of life even though symptom reduction might not be possible.

In an outpatient-study, various factors besides psychopathology were assessed in their impact on the quality of life in 252 children and adolescents with mental health problems (Bastiaansen et al., 2005b). Within the examined child-related factors, decreased quality of life was associated with low self-esteem, poor social skills and comorbid somatic illnesses. Regarding the parent-related factors, maternal psychopathology and stress were linked with low HRQL in the children. In respect to environmental factors, a slight association between decreased quality of life was found in combination with a low socioeconomic status, little social support, poor family functioning, and stressful life events. The authors conclude that the treatment of psychological disturbances should be complemented by enhancing social competence, self-esteem, family functioning and social support.

Children who experience mental illnesses in their family are exposed to various stressors that are likely to influence their quality of life (Wiegand-Grefe et al., 2010b). Several studies of our work group document reduced levels of HRQL in affected children in contrast to comparative samples (Pollak et al., 2008; Jeske et al., 2009). Studies showed also relationships between children's HRQL and parental coping mechanisms (Jeske et al., 2009), family functioning (Pollak et al., 2008; Jeske et al., 2010) and parental attachment styles (Jeske et al., 2011).

This chapter presents the results of several studies examining psychopathology and quality of life in children of mentally ill parents. It is expected that the children are assessed by their parents to deal with more emotional and behavioral problems, the higher the parental subjective impairment is. It is also presumed that the quality of life in children of mentally ill parents is significantly lower than in children of the general population. Furthermore, it is expected that the HRQL is decreased with growing severity of parental symptomatology and that children's quality of life is reduced when the children suffer from emotional and behavioral problems themselves.

4. Study design

In a 9-month pilot study conducted within the project "CHIMPs – Children of mentally ill parents" at the University Medical Center Hamburg-Eppendorf, Germany, all patients referred to the Clinic of Psychiatry and Psychotherapy were registered from August 2005 to May 2006. For all patients, age, sex and diagnoses were recorded. Patients with minor children were examined further when they fulfilled the following inclusion criteria: aged 18-60 years, having at least one minor child between 0-18 years, receiving stationary treatment for at least five days, being sufficiently fluent in German language and giving informed consent for participating in the study. Exclusion criteria were: previous participation in the study in case of repeated hospitalization, a short duration of stationary treatment less than five days, and severe psychiatric or cognitive impairments. The patients were asked to answer questionnaires about their own mental health status and their children's situation.

When having several children, parents were asked to give only information on one randomly selected child in order to ensure the independence of observations.

5. Sample

Overall, 964 patients were registered. Among this sample, 167 (17%) patients had at least one minor child. Further 558 patients had no children (58 %), 104 patients had grown-up children above 18 years (11 %) and 135 patients were older than 60 years (14 %). Out of these 167 parents, 42 (25%) were not willing to participate in the study and further 39 parents (23 %) did not fulfill the inclusion criteria or had to be excluded from data analysis due to a large number of missing data. Overall, N = 86 parents answered the standardized questionnaires about the children's health-related quality of life, while a reduced number of N = 67 parents assessed the mental health status of their children.

The sample consists of 43 fathers and 43 mothers, aged between 23 and 59 years (M = 41 years, SD = 7.9). Forty-four patients are married (51 %), 19 parents are single or divorced (22 %), two parents are separated (2 %) and one patient is widowed (1 %). The most frequent school leaving certificate is a graduation from senior high-school (41 %), followed by graduations from intermediate secondary school (31%) and secondary general school (20%). Two parents are without school degree, 2 parents have another school leaving certificate. Regarding the qualifications, vocational trainings (39%) and University degrees (24%) are the most prevalent qualifications, 15% of the parents have no further qualification, 7 % hold another qualification. Thirty-one percent are white-collar employees, 20 % blue-collar workers, 16 % homemakers, 12 % self-employed, 3 % retired, and 2 % each are students or trainees.

Fifty-five parents (63 %) live together with their child, the remaining 31 patients (36 %) do not live with their children but have frequent contact to them (at least every two weeks). Here, a striking gender-specific effect can be observed: while 88% of the psychiatrically ill mothers live together with their children, only 53% of the fathers do so (χ^2=9.46, p=.002). The children who are not living with their mentally ill parent live either with the other parent (N = 21, 68 %), with relatives (N = 2, 6 %), in foster- or adoption families (N = 2, 6 %), in institutional care (N = 3, 10 %) or in their own apartment. The examined children are aged between 4 to 18 years (M = 11 years, SD = 4.49), the distribution of boys and girls is equally balanced (50 % each).

As primary diagnosis according ICD-10 (WHO, 2000), 27 patients (32 %) are diagnosed with an affective disorder, 23 parents (26 %) suffer from either anxiety disorders, an obsessive-compulsive disorder or PTSD, further 20 parents (23 %) engage in substance abuse (mostly alcohol) and 14 patients (16 %) are affected by schizophrenia. Two parents have a personality disorder (PD), namely a Borderline PD and an emotional-instable PD. Overall, 61% of the here examined parents have a comorbid psychiatric diagnosis.

6. Measurements

The mentally ill parents were asked to which extent they feel impaired by their illness through the German version of the Symptom-Checklist-14-R (SCL-14-R, Prinz et al., 2008). This self-report constitutes a short version of the SCL-90-R (Franke, 1995) and is used as a measure of general psychiatric symptomatology. It comprises 14 items on a 5-point Likert Scale, indicating the degree of symptomatology in the last seven days (not at all (0), a little bit (1), moderately (2), quite a bit (3), extremely (4)). The SCL-14-R includes three subscales: Depressiveness, Somatoform Complaints and Phobic Anxiety. The total score is measured with the Global Severity Index (GSI). The GSI has proven to be a good indicator for the actual symptom severity.

The psychiatric diagnoses of the parents were given by the attending psychiatrists in accordance with the diagnostic criteria of the ICD-10 (WHO, 2005).

For the assessment of emotional and behavioral problems in the children and adolescents, parents were administered the Child Behavior Checklist/4-18 (Working Group German Child Behavior Checklist, 1994). On the CBCL, parents rate their children on 113 specific problem items using a 3-point scale (not true (0), somewhat/sometimes true (1), very/often true (2)). The resulting scales comprise a total problem score, two broadband scores (internalizing and externalizing problems) and eight syndrome scales (social withdrawal, somatic complaints, anxious/depressed, social problems, thought problems, attention problems, delinquent behavior, aggressive behavior).

The health-related quality of life of the children and adolescents was assessed by their parents with the KINDL[R] questionnaire (Ravens-Sieberer & Bullinger, 2000). The KINDL[R] comprehends 24 items on a 5-point Likert scale. The resulting subscales are: physical well-being, emotional well-being, self-esteem, family, friends, and everyday functioning (school or nursery/kindergarten). Psychometric results revealed a high degree of reliability (Cronbach's a ≥ 0.70 for most of the sub-scales and samples) and a satisfactory convergent validity.

7. Results

7.1 Parents' subjective impairment by the mental illness

All parents indicate to feel at least "a little bit" impaired by their illness. The Global Severity Index (GSI) lies around M = 1.7 (SD = 0.79). While "depressiveness" represents the greatest impact for the patients, phobic anxiety influences the here examined parents to a lesser degree. In comparison to the clinical norm sample (Prinz et al., 2008), the mentally ill parents display higher mean values on all scales, reaching significant differences in t-tests on the GSI, "depressiveness" and "phobic anxiety". On the scale "somatization", the parents differ only in comparison to the general population (Geers, 2006).

	Study Sample		Comparative clinical sample		General population	
SCL-14-R Scales	M	SD	M	SD	M	SD
Global Symptom Severity Index (GSI)	1.66	0.79	1.15	0.77	#	#
Depressiveness	2.26	1.05	1.49	1.05	0.45	0.58
Somatoform Complaints	1.38	1.07	1.20	1.01	0.46	0.63
Phobic Anxiety	1.05	1.13	0.59	0.88	0.17	0.39

Table 1. SCL-14-R values of the study sample (N=62), a comparative clinical sample and a representative sample of the general population (from Wiegand-Grefe, Geers, Plass, Petermann & Riedesser, 2009).
Annotation: M = mean value, SD = standard deviation, # = not specified.

7.2 Psychopathology in children of mentally ill parents

The children's emotional and behavioral problems, assessed through the CBCL scales, are listed in table 2 as T-values, taking age- and gender-specific aspects of emotional and behavioral development into account.

CBCL Scales	M	SD	Minimum	Maximum	N
Social Withdrawal	58.11	9.08	50	88	61
Somatic Complaints	57.62	9.32	50	81	60
Anxious/Depressed	58.90	9.17	50	83	60
Social Problems	58.00	8.29	50	84	58
Thought Problems	56.37	9.36	50	80	60
Attention Problems	58.90	8.98	50	83	60
Delinquent Behavior	57.33	6.95	50	75	61
Aggressive Behavior	59.31	9.68	50	95	62
Internalizing Problems	57.33	11.83	38	82	61
Externalizing Problems	57.58	10.42	35	84	62
Total	58.92	11.47	38	86	61

Table 2. Distribution of T-Values of the CBCL subscales and main scales (N=62) (from Wiegand-Grefe et al., 2009). Annotation: M = mean value, SD = standard deviation, N = sample size.

In order to assess how many children display psychological problems in the clinical ($T \geq 64$), subclinical (T between 60-63) or normal range ($T \leq 59$), the T-scores have been categorized accordingly. On the syndrome scales, 14 % of the children and adolescents are seen to have somatic complaints, 13 % suffer from clinical or subclinical levels of anxiety and depression. On the main CBCL scales, 31 % of the parents report internalizing problems and further 9 % see subclinical internalizing problems. Regarding externalizing problems, 29 % of the parents report behavioral problems in the clinical range, another 16 % see externalizing symptomatology in the subclinical range. Overall, 40 % of the parents report at least subclinical problems in the internalizing domain, and 45 % of the parents see externalizing behavior to an at least subclinical degree. Considering the total problem score, 52 % of the children are rated to lie within the normal range of emotional and behavioral difficulties, while 32 % are seen to display subclinical symptoms and 14 % to exhibit clinically relevant symptomatology. Sixty-six percent of the examined children are reported not to display any clinically relevant symptoms on the syndrome scales. The remaining 32 % of children and adolescents suffer from clinically relevant symptoms on at least one dimension measured by the CBCL.

When comparing the relative frequencies of children of mentally ill parents, lying in the subclinical or clinical range on the CBCL syndrome scales, with those of the general child population (with the top 5 % constituting the subclinical range, and the top 2 % defining the clinical range), it can be stated that on all syndrome scales, children of mentally ill parents display 1.5- to 7-times heightened rates of clinically relevant symptomatology (table 3). It is striking that the children are especially prone to suffer from somatic symptoms (relative risk, RR = 7.26). Besides, they have a 6-fold risk to display thought and attention problems (RR = 6.45) and are five times more likely to engage in social withdrawal in comparison to the general child population (RR = 5.65).

	Subclinical and clinical range Reference value in the general population: 5 %		Clinical range Reference value in the general population: 2 %	
CBCL Subscales	%	relative risk	%	relative risk
Social Withdrawal	16.13	3.23	11.29	5.65
Somatic Complaints	19.35	3.87	14.52	7.26
Anxious/Depressed	24.19	4.84	12.90	6.45
Social Problems	17.74	3.55	6.45	3.23
Thought Problems	20.97	4.19	12.90	6.45
Attention Problems	17.74	3.55	12.90	6.45
Delinquent Behavior	14.52	2.90	3.23	1.61
Aggressive Behavior	24.19	4.84	9.68	4.84

Table 3. Relative frequencies and relative risk in children of mentally ill parents (N = 62) displaying CBCL scores in the subclinical or clinical range in comparison with children of the general population lying in the clinical range (top 2 %) and subclinical/clinical range (top 5 %) (from Wiegand-Grefe et al., 2009).

7.3 Parents' subjective impairments and the psychological difficulties of their children

Since a positive linear association is expected between the parents' subjective impairments and the children's psychopathology, SCL-14-R and CBCL scale values are correlated (table 4). Significant positive correlations exist between the parent's global severity index (GSI), the SCL-14-R dimensions somatization and phobic anxiety, and all main scales of the CBCL. The correlative association between parental "somatization" and the children's "internalizing problems" represents the highest association with r = .302 indicating a small to medium sized linkage between the variables. No association has been found between parental "depressiveness" and psychopathology in children.

Mean Values of SCL-14-R-Scales		Internalizing CBCL-Scale (T-values)		Externalizing CBCL-Scale (T-values)		CBCL Total Score (T-values)	
Global Symptom Severity Index (GSI)	r	.297	*	.275	*	.287	*
	p	.010		.015		.012	
	N	61		62		61	
Depressiveness	r	.204		.176		.182	
	p	.06		.09		.08	
	N	61		62		61	
Somatoform Complaints	r	.302	**	.233	*	.264	*
	p	.009		.03		.02	
	N	61		62		61	
Phobic Anxiety	ρ	.221	*	.279	*	.299	**
	p	.043		.014		.010	
	N	61		62		61	

Table 4. Correlative association between the SCL-14-R-Scales and the main CBCL-Scales (N=62) (from Wiegand-Grefe et al., 2009). Annotation: r = Pearson product-moment correlation coefficient; ρ = Spearman rank correlation coefficient; p= level of significance; * p <.05; ** p <.01; N = sample size.

7.4 Health-related quality of life in the children

The total score of the KINDL[R] was transformed with "0" indicating the poorest and "100" indicating the maximum value of health-related quality of life (HRQL). In the examined population of children of mentally ill parents, the total score of HRQL lies by 70.91 (SD = 12.88). The children's overall score on the dimension physical well-being lies by 71.01 (SD = 18.64), the "emotional well-being" lies around 71.28 (SD = 18.55). The KINDL[R] subscales range between 67.50 on the lowest end (self-esteem, SD = 17.22) and 74.26 constituting the maximum value (friends, SD = 13.77). The scales family (M = 68.51, SD = 19.33) and school (M = 70.00, SD = 18.24) rank in between. In comparison to the reference sample of the general population, the here examined children of mentally ill parents display low values in the total HRQL-score that can be explained and specified by poor results on the scales emotional well-being, family and school (Jeske et al., 2010, Wiegand-Grefe et al., 2010). When comparing the ratings of mentally ill mothers and fathers, it can be stated that no differences were found in their assessment of the HRQL in their children.

7.5 Subjective parental impairment and quality of life in the children

Slight negative associations have been found between the subjective parental impairment, as measured by the SCL-14-R, and the children's HRQL dimensions emotional well-being, self-esteem, family, school and the overall total score (table 5).

Mean Values of SCL-14-R-Scales		KINDL[R] Total Score	Physical well-being	Emotio-nal well-being	Self-esteem	Family	Friends	School
Global	r	-.274		-.189		-.267		-.253
Symptom	ρ		-.149		-.259		-.038	
Severity Index	p	.008**	.094	.048*	.012*	.009**	.373	.017*
(GSI)	N	77	80	79	75	78	76	70
Depressive-	r	-.288		-.216		-.289		-.305
ness	ρ		-.179		-.160		-.027	
	p	.006**	.059	.028*	.086	.005**	.408	.005**
	N	77	80	79	75	75	76	70
Somatoform	r	-.261		-.157		-.248		-.207
Complaints	ρ		-.169		-.325		.049	
	p	.011*	.068	.084	.002**	.014*	.337	.043*
	N	77	80	79	75	75	76	70
Phobic	r							
Anxiety	ρ	-.081	.010	-.055	-.164	-.047	-.040	-.133
	p	.243	.465	.315	.080	.340	.365	.137
	N	77	80	79	75	78	76	70

Table 5. Correlative association between SCL-14-R and KINDL[R] (N=62) (from Wiegand-Grefe et al. 2010). Annotation: r = Pearson product-moment correlation coefficient, ρ = Spearman rank correlation coefficient; p= level of significance; * p <.05; ** p <.01 (1-sided); N = sample size.

Further significant correlations exist between parental „depressiveness" and the children's HRQL in the total score and the areas of school functioning, family, and emotional well-being. Somatoform complaints of the parents are associated with poor "self-esteem" and decreased values on the dimensions school, family and the total score. No linear association was found between the HRQL in children and parental "phobic anxiety".

7.6 Psychopathology and health-related quality of life in the children

When regarding the association between the children's psychopathology and their health-related quality of life, considerable negative associations can be found between the main CBCL scales and all KINDL[R] dimensions. According to the results, parents see substantial losses in their children's HRQL with increasing emotional and behavioral problems (table 6).

CBCL Scales (T-values)		KINDL[R] Total Score	Physical Well-being	Emotion al Well-being	Self-esteem	Family	Friends	School
Total Problem Score	r	-.611		-.522		-.347		-.442
	ρ		-.405		-.597		-.291	
	p	.000***	.000***	.000***	.000***	.002**	.009**	.000***
	N	67	67	66	64	66	66	65
Externalizing Problems	r	-.492		-.445		-.396		-.295
	ρ		-.320		-.453		-.216	
	p	.000***	.004**	.000***	.000***	.000***	.040*	.008**
	N	66	67	66	64	66	66	65
Internalizing Problems	r	-.694		-.667		-.272		-.561
	ρ		-.561		-.744		-.278	
	p	.000***	.000***	.000***	.000***	.014*	.012*	.000***
	N	66	66	66	64	65	65	66

Table 6. Correlative association between CBCL and KINDL[R] (N=67) (from Wiegand-Grefe et al., 2010) Annotation: r = Pearson product-moment correlation coefficient, ρ = Spearman rank correlation coefficient; p = level of significance; * p <.05; ** p <.01; N = sample size

8. Discussion

In comparison to the general population, children of mentally ill parents have a substantial risk to develop psychopathological symptomatology. On the main scales and the syndrome scales of the CBCL, the children's relative risk to develop clinically relevant symptomatologies is three- to sevenfold. In the existing literature, children of mentally ill parents are reported to be assessed up to five times more likely to exhibit psychological difficulties (Kölch, Schielke, Becker, Fegert & Schmid, 2008). In the study at hand, 32 % of the parents see clinically relevant symptoms in their children. When including the cases of subclinical symptomatology, even 47 % of the examined children are regarded to be somehow affected by emotional and behavioral problems. This rate goes along with reported frequencies in comparable studies (Beidel & Turner, 1997; Hill, Locke, Lowers & Connolly, 1999; Kelley & Fals-Stewart, 2004; Lapalme, Hodgins & La Roche, 1997; Merikangas, Dierker & Szatmari, 1998). It may be argued that the percentage of affected children might even be higher considering the fact that many parents undergo feelings of guild and shame and therefore tend to minimize difficulties in clinical evaluations. It is striking, for example, that adolescents often report more difficulties in self-reports than the parents indicate in the according ratings (Najman et al., 2000). Thus, it might be expected that adolescents with a mentally ill parent might even exhibit higher rates of symptomatology than in the examined parental assessments.

In respect to the characteristics of the parental illness, positive associations were found between the severity of the illness, parental anxiety and somatic complaints and children's psychopathology. This result is analogous to other studies showing that the severity of parental symptomatology goes along with increased psychopathology in the children (Brennan et al., 2000; Hammen, Burge, Burney & Adrian, 1990; Keller et al., 1986; Weissman et al., 2005). It is rather astonishing that, contrary to other studies (Mattejat et al., 2000), no association was found between depressive symptoms in parents and emotional and behavioral difficulties in the here examined population of children. It can be assumed that parents with phobic anxieties and somatic complaints are especially sensitive for their children's difficulties. It is interesting that parental somatization is related to psychological problems in children on all CBCL main scales. This finding underlines that somatic complaints and illnesses in parents stand in a close relationship with children's mental health (Romer & Hagen), although somatizations have to be distinguished from severe somatic illnesses. Since patients with somatizations and anxieties tend to be over-sensitive towards potential difficulties, the results, indicating increased symptomatology in the children, should be cautiously interpreted.

In the present study, children with a mentally ill parent display a decreased quality of life in comparison to the general population. The overall quality of life in children is especially associated with the global severity of parental symptomatology, as well as parental somatization and depressiveness in specific. With increasing degree of perceived impairment, parents rated their children's HRQL to be poorer. In a previous study, it was found that children, who were exposed to a parental mental illness for a longer time frame, exhibited higher quality of life scores on the KINDL[R] scale "friends". Presumably, these children might have mastered their situation by compensating their familial difficulties with peer group activities.

The psychopathology of the examined children is substantially linked to the quality of life, as indicated by high correlations between the KINDL[R] and the CBCL scales.

In respect to methodological constrictions, it has to be underlined that the assessment of the children's psychopathology and quality of life is solely based on the parents' view. The informative validity of assessments by mentally ill parents has not yet been explored sufficiently. Hitherto, studies have examined response patterns in parents with depression and anxiety disorders. Overall, the findings do not allow drawing specific conclusions in respect to potential response biases. In general, the most credible source for internalizing disorders are self-assessments of children and adolescents, while externalizing problems are best assessed by parents (Fombonne, 2002). In the consequent CHIMPs project, families will be examined as a whole, which will allow contrasting the evaluations of mentally ill parents and partners with the children's self-reports. The suggestion to include teacher reports (Thiels & Schmitz, 2008) would certainly be promising and beneficial, but forms an obstacle in the shame-related area of parental mental illness.

9. Implications for clinical practice

The present chapter deals with the mental health status and the quality of life of children with a mentally ill parent. The impairments resulting from the mental illness are associated with the children's mental health and their quality of life. The heightened rates of psychopathology in the children underline the need to implement appropriate prevention programs. In the development of such preventive measures, the improvement of the children's quality of life should constitute a central component next to the reduction of psychopathological symptoms.

10. References

Achenbach, T. M. (1991). Manual for the Child Behavior Checklist / 4-18 and 1991 Profile. Burlington: University of Vermont, Department of Psychiatry.

Arbeitsgruppe Deutsche Child Behavior Checklist (1994). CBCL/4-18. Elternfragebogen über das Verhalten von Kindern und Jugendlichen. Deutsche Bearbeitung der Child Behavior Checklist. Köln: Arbeitsgruppe Kinder-, Jugend- und Familiendiagnostik (KJFD).

Bastiaansen, D., Koot, H.M., Ferdinand, R.F. & Verhulst, F.C. (2004). Quality of life in children with psychiatric disorders: Self-, parent and clinician report. American Academy of Child and Adolescent Psychiatry, 43, 221-230.

Bastiaansen, D., Koot, H.M. & Ferdinand, R.F. (2005a). Psychopathology in children: Improvement of quality of life without psychiatric symptom reduction? European Child and Adolescent Psychiatry, 14, 364-370.

Bastiaansen, D., Koot, H.M. & Ferdinand, R.F. (2005b). Determinants of quality of life in children with psychiatric disorders. Quality of Life Research,14, 1599-1612.

Beidel, D.C. & Turner, S.M. (1997). At risk for anxiety. I. Psychopathology in the offspring of anxious parents. Journal of the American Academy of Child and Adolescent Psychiatry, 36, 918-924.

Brennan, P.A., Hammen, C., Andersen, M.J., Bor, W., Najman, J.M. & Williams, G.M. (2000). Chronicity, severity and timing of maternal depressive symptoms: Relationship with child outcomes at age 5. Developmental Psychology, 36, 759-766.

Bullinger, M. (2011) Lebensqualität von Kindern und Jugendlichen im Kontext der Gesundheit ihrer Eltern. In: S. Wiegand-Grefe, F. Mattejat & A. Lenz (Hrsg.). Kinder mit psychisch kranken Eltern. Klinik und Forschung. (S. 401-415). Göttingen: Vandenhoeck & Ruprecht.

Fergusson, M., Lynskey, M.T. & Horwood, L.J. (1993). The effect of maternal depression on maternal ratings of child behavior. Journal of Abnormal Child Psychology, 21, 245-269.

Fombonne, E. (2002). Case identification in a epidemiological context. In M. Rutter & E. Taylor (Eds.), Child and adolescent psychiatry (4th ed., pp. 52-86). Oxford: Blackwell.

Franke, G. H. (1995). SCL-90-R. Die Symptomcheckliste von Derogatis – Deutsche Version – Manual. Göttingen: Hogrefe

Geers, P. (2006). Psychische Gesundheit der Kinder von Eltern mit psychischen Störungen. Bremen: Unveröffentlichte Diplomarbeit, Studiengang Psychologie, Universität Bremen.

Gelfand, D.M. & Teti, D.M. (1990). The effects of maternal depression on children. Clinical Psychology Review, 10, 329-353.

Goodman, S.H. & Gotlib, I.H. (1999). Risk for psychopathology in the children of depressed mothers. A developmental model for understanding mechanisms of transmission. Psychological Review, 106, 458-490.

Hammen, C., Burge, D., Burney, E. & Adrian, C. (1990). Longitudinal study of diagnoses in children of woman with unipolar and bipolar affective disorder. Archives of General Psychiatry, 47, 1112-1117.

Herpertz-Dahlmann, B., Wille, N., Hölling, H., Vloet, T.D., Ravens-Sieberer, U. & BELLA study group (2008). Disordered eating behavior and attitudes, associated psychopathology and health-related quality of life: results of the BELLA study. European Child and Adolescent Psychiatry, 17, 82-91.

Hill, S.Y., Locke, J., Lowers, L. & Connolly, J. (1999). Psychopathology and Achievement in children at high risk for developing alcoholism. Journal of the American Academy of Child and Adolescent Psychiatry, 38, 883-891.

ICD-10-GM Version (2005) Internationale statistische Klassifikation der Krankheiten und verwandter Gesundheitsprobleme (ICD)- German Modification. Band 1: Systematisches Verzeichnis. Kooperationsausgabe. Stuttgart: Kohlhammer. Deutsche Krankenhaus Verlagsgesellschaft mbH

Jeske, J., Bullinger, M., Plass, A., Petermann, F. & Wiegand- Grefe, S. (2009). Risikofaktor Krankheitsverarbeitung. Zusammenhänge zwischen der Krankheitsverarbeitung einer elterlichen psychischen Erkrankung und der gesundheitsbezogenen Lebensqualität der Kinder. Zeitschrift für Psychiatrie, Psychologie und Psychotherapie, 57, 207-213

Jeske, J., Bullinger, M. & Wiegand-Grefe, S. (2010). Familien mit psychisch kranken Eltern. Zusammenhang von Familienfunktionalität und gesundheitsbezogener Lebensqualität der Kinder. Familiendynamik 35: 338-347.

Jeske, J., Bullinger, M. & Wiegand-Grefe, S. (2011). Do attachment patterns of parents with a mental illness have an impact upon how they view the quality of life of their children? Vulnerable Children and Youth Studies 6, 39-50.

Keller, M.B., Beardslee, W.R., Dorer, D.J., Lavori, P.W., Samuelson, H. & Klerman, G.R. (1986). Impact of severity and chronicity of parental affective illness on adaptive functioning and psychopathology in children. Archives of General Psychiatry, 43, 930-937.

Kelley, M.L. & Fals-Stewart, W. (2004). Psychiatric disorders of children living with drug-abusing, alcohol-abusing, and non-substance-abusing fathers. Journal of the American Academy of Child and Adolescent Psychiatry, 43, 621-628.

Kiss, E., Kapornai, K., Baji, I., Mayer, L. & Vetró, Á. (2009). Assessing quality of life: mother-child agreement in depressed Hungarian. European Child and Adolescent Psychiatry, 18, 265-273.

Kölch, M., Schielke, A., Becker, T. Fegert, J.M. & Schmid, M. (2008). Belastung Minderjähriger aus Sicht der psychisch kranken Eltern. Ergebnisse einer Befragung stationär behandelter Patienten mit dem SDQ. Nervenheilkunde, 27, 527-532.

Lapalme, M., Hodgins, S. & La Roche, C. (1997). Children of parents with bipolar disorder : A metaanalysis of risk for mental disorders. Canadian Journal of Psychiatry, 42, 623-631.

Lee, C. & Gotlib, I.H. (1991). Adjustment of Children of depressed mothers: A 10-month follow-up. Journal of Abnormal Psychology, 100, 473-477.

Lenz, A., Kuhn, J. (2011). Was stärkt Kinder psychisch kranker Eltern und fördert ihre Entwicklung? Überblick über Ergebnisse der Resilienz- und Copingforschung. In: S. Wiegand-Grefe, F. Mattejat& A. Lenz (Hrsg.). Kinder mit psychisch kranken Eltern. Klinik und Forschung. (S. 269-298). Göttingen: Vandenhoeck & Ruprecht.

Mattejat, F., Remschmidt, H. (2003) Zur Erfassung der Lebensqualität bei psychisch gestörten Kindern und Jugendlichen- Eine Übersicht. (Online), 30/07/2011, Available from http://www.kjp.uni-marburg.de/lq/index.php?include=publikat

Mattejat, F., Wüthrich, C. & Remschmidt, H. (2000). Kinder psychisch kranker Eltern. Forschungsperspektiven am Beispiel von Kindern depressiver Eltern. Nervenarzt, 71, 164-172.

Mattejat, F., Lenz, A. & Wiegand-Grefe, S. (2011). Kinder psychisch kranker Eltern – Eine Einführung in die Thematik. In: S. Wiegand-Grefe, A- Lenz& F. Mattejat(Hrsg.) Kinder mit psychisch kranken Eltern. Klinik und Forschung. (S. 13-24). Göttingen: Vandenhoeck und Ruprecht.

Mattejat, F., Koenig, U., Barchewitz, C., Felbel, D., Herpertz-Dahlmann, B., Hoehne, D.,Janthur, B., Jungmann, J., Katzenski, B., Kirchner, J., Naumann, A., Nölkel, P., Schaff, C.,Schulz, E., Warnke, A., Wienand, F. & Remschmidt, H. (2005). Zur Lebensqualität von psychisch kranken Kindern und ihren Eltern: Ergebnisse der ersten multizentrischen Studie mit der Elternversion des Inventars zur Erfassung der Lebensqualität bei Kindern und Jugendlichen (ILK). Kindheit und Entwicklung, 14, 39-47

Merikangas, K.R., Dierker, L.C. & Szatmari, P. (1998). Psychopathology among offspring of parents with substance abuse and/or anxiety disorders: A high-risk study. The Journal of Child Psychology and Psychiatry, 39, 711-720.

Najman, J.M., Williams, G.M., Nikles, J., Spence, S., Bor, W., O'Callaghan, M., LeBroque, R. & Andersen, M.J. (2000). Mothers' mental illness and child behavior problems: cause-effect association or observation bias? Journal of the American Academy of Child and Adolescent Psychiatry, 39, 592-602.

Noeker, M. & Petermann, F. (2008). Resilienz: Funktionale Adaptation an widrige Umgebungsbedingungen. Zeitschrift für Psychiatrie, Psychologie und Psychotherapie, 56, 255-263.

Pollak, E., Bullinger, M. Jeske, J. Wiegand-Grefe, S (2008): How do mentally ill parents evaluate their childrens quality of life? Associations with the parent's illness and family functioning. Praxis der Kinderpsychologie und Kinderpsychiatrie, 57, 301-314.

Prinz, U., Nutzinger, D.O., Schulz, H., Petermann, F. Braukhaus, C. & Andreas, S. (2008). Die Symptom-Checkliste-90-R und ihre Kurzversion: Psychometrische Analysen bei Patienten mit psychischen Krankheiten. Physikalische Medizin, Rehabilitationsmedizin, Kurortmedizin, 18, 337-343.

Ramchandani, P. & Psychogiou, L. (2009). Paternal psychiatric disorders and children's psychosocial development. Lancet Journal, 374, 646-653

Ravens-Sieberer, U. & Bullinger, M. (1998). Assessing health-related quality of life in chronically ill children with the German KINDL: first psychometric and content analytical results. Quality of Life Research, 7, 399-407

Ravens-Sieberer, U. & Bullinger, M. (2000). KINDL-R. Fragebogen zur Erfassung der gesundheitsbezogenen Lebensqualität bei Kindern und Jugendlichen. Revidierte Form. Manual. (Online), 30/07/2011, Available from http://www.kindl.org/daten/ pdf/ManGerman.pdf

Ravens-Sieberer, U., Erhart, M., Wille, N., Wetzel, R., Nickel, J. & Bullinger, M. (2006). Generic Health-Related Quality-of-Life Assessment in Children and Adolescents. Pharmacoeconomics, 24, 1199-1220

Ravens-Sieberer, U., Erhart, M., Wille, N., Bullinger, M. & BELLA study group (2008). Health-related quality of life in children and adolescents in germany: results of the BELLA study. European Child and Adolescent Psychiatry,17, 148-156.

Romer, G. & Haagen, M. (2007). Kinder körperlich kranker Eltern. Göttingen: Hogrefe.

Sawyer, M.G., Whaites, L., Rey, J.M., Hazell, P.L., Graetz, B.W. & Baghurst, P. (2002). Health-related quality of life of children and adolescents with mental disorders. Journal of the American Academy of Child and Adolescent Psychiatry,41, 530-537.

Thiels, C. & Schmitz, G.S. (2008). Selbst- und Fremdbeurteilung von Verhaltensauffälligkeiten bei Kindern und Jugendlichen. Zur Validität von Eltern- und Lehrerurteilen. Kindheit und Entwicklung, 17, 118-125.

Weissman M.M., Leckman, J.F., Merikangas, K.R., Gammon, G.D. & Prusoff, B.A. (1984). Depression and Anxiety Disorders in Parents and Children. Results From the Yale Family Study. Archives of General Psychiatry, 41, 845-852.

Weissman, M.M., Wickramaratne, P., Nomura, Y., Warner, V., Verdeli, H., Pilowsky, D.J., Grillon, C. & Bruder, G. (2005). Families at high and low risk for depression. A 3-Generation Study. Archives of General Psychiatry, 62, 29-36.

Wiegand-Grefe, S., Geers, P., Halverscheid, S., Petermann, F. & Plass, A. (2010a). Kinder psychisch kranker Eltern. Zusammenhänge zwischen der Krankheitsbewältigung einer elterlichen psychischen Erkrankung und der Gesundheit der Kinder. Zeitschrift für Klinische Psychologie und Psychotherapie, 39, 13-23.

Wiegand-Grefe, S., Geers, P., Petermann, F. & Plass, A. (2011). Kinder psychisch kranker Eltern: Merkmale elterlicher psychiatrischer Erkrankung und Gesundheit der Kinder aus Elternsicht. Fortschritte der Neurologie und Psychiatrie, 79, 32-40.

Wiegand-Grefe, S., Geers, P., Plass, A., Petermann, F. & Riedesser, P. (2009). Kinder psychisch kranker Eltern. Zusammenhänge zwischen subjektiver elterlicher Beeinträchtigung und psychischer Auffälligkeit der Kinder aus Elternsicht. Kindheit und Entwicklung, 18, 111-121.

Wiegand-Grefe, S., Halverscheid, S. & Plass, A. (2011). Kinder und ihre psychisch kranken Eltern. Familienorientierte Prävention – Der CHIMPs-Beratungsansatz. Göttingen: Hogrefe.

Wiegand-Grefe, S., Jeske, J., Bullinger, M., Plass, A. & Petermann, F. (2010b). Lebensqualität von Kindern psychisch kranker Eltern. Zusammenhänge zwischen Merkmalen elterlicher Erkrankung und gesundheitsbezogener Lebensqualität der Kinder aus Elternsicht. Zeitschrift für Psychiatrie, Psychologie, und Psychotherapie, 58, 315-322.

Wolke, D. (2008). Von Null bis Drei: Entwicklungsrisiken und Entwicklungsabweichungen. In F. Petermann (Hrsg.), Lehrbuch der Klinischen Kinderpsychologie (6., völlig veränd. Aufl., S.65-80. Göttingen: Hogrefe.

Ziegenhain, U., Derksen, B. & Dreisörner, R. (2004). Frühe Förderung von Resilienz bei jungen Müttern und ihren Säuglingen. Kindheit und Entwicklung, 13, 226-234.

Understanding the Psychosocial Processes of Physical Activity for Individuals with Severe Mental Illness: A Meta-Ethnography

Andrew Soundy[1], Thomas Kingstone[2] and Pete Coffee[3]
[1]University of Birmingham, Birmingham,
[2]Freshwinds Charity, Birmingham,
[3]School of Sport, University of Stirling
[1,2]England
[3]Scotland

1. Introduction

Physical activity can benefit individuals with severe mental illness (SMI) (Richardson et al., 2005). The benefits of physical activity for individuals with SMI are threefold: psychological, social and physical. Psychologically, patients can experience mood elevating effects, reduced anxiety, improved concentration, increased self-esteem and reduced psychiatric symptoms like voices (Faulkner & Biddle, 1999). Socially, co-patients in the physical activity setting can motivate, support and encourage interaction (Fogarty & Happell, 2005), facilitating the development of a positive social identity. Physically, patients can combat a significant side effect of anti-psychotic medication such as weight loss (Faulkner et al., 2003).

Despite individuals with SMI understanding that there are benefits from engaging in physical activity, many have limited confidence in their ability to exercise and often perceptual biases (e.g., concerns generated from self-presentation, negative interpretaion of an interaction) can act as barriers in new and unknown settings (Soundy et al., 2007). A perceived inability to exercise, coupled with a lack of social support can lead to a further reduction in exercise participation and, potentially, permanent withdrawal from exercise (Ussher et al., 2007). Thus, there are (a) barriers that affect the initiation of exercise, as well as (b) barriers that prevent the adoption of a more physically active lifestyle. In support, a recent Cochrane review (Gorcyznski & Faulkner, 2011) has called for research to develop further understanding into how best to help patients with SMI begin and continue to exercise.

Whilst some initial understanding has been provided regarding the initial engagement in physical activity, further information is needed to illustrate how experiences of physical activity vary. To this end, research is needed to consider and illustrate the psychosocial barriers and facilitators to activity in the adoption of exercise, but also in the long term maintenance of activity. This has been illustrated, although not comprehensivly evaluated, in previous research: In some research this is explicitly adressed, for example, Carless (2007) considers physical activity as phases requiring support when beginning (awareness raising) and during (engagement and practical facilitation) activity. Other research implicitly addresses this; for example, Raine et al., (2002) consider the engagement of exercise in community and illustrate the experience of inititating and maintaining activity. It is clear, however, that barriers and facilitators to activity are likely to change across the lifespan of engagement in physical activity. In order to generate a greater understanding of this topic and of the processes involved, considerable detail of the experience of patients with SMI is required. Previous studies that detail the experience of community based activities provide this information. A qualitative approach that explores and reports on individual experiences across physical activity interventions may be best placed to forge this understanding. The process, phases and current understanding of introducing physical activity has been gauged by a number of well considered qualitative studies (Carter-Morris & Faulkner, 2003; Carless, 2008; Carless & Douglas, 2004;2008a;2008b; Carless and Sparkes, 2008; Crone, 2007; Faulkner and Sparkes, 1999; Shiner et al., 2008; Soundy, 2007). However, to the best of the authors' knowledge there is currently no review that synthesises and proposes advancements based upon this important and valuable information.

2. Purpose

Exercise and physical activity have a clear role in alleviating the secondary symptoms of SMI, such as low self-esteem and social withdrawal (Faulkner, 2005). This chapter provides some suggestions of the underpinning mechanisms by considering psychosocial factors (e.g. a sense of autonomy, self-efficacy, social support, task competency and distraction) that change as a result of participation (Mutire, 2003). Barriers and facilitators to activity are present both during the initiation phase of activity and within a maintenance phase of activity. This chapter will consider how psychosocial factors impact on barriers and facilitators to activity when patients with SMI (a) initially engage in physical activity and (b) seek to develop and sustain a physically active lifestyle.

3. Methods

We used a meta-ethnographic approach, as defined by Noblit and Hare (1988), and more recently Campbell et al (2003) and Weed (2008). The approach involves selecting relevant empirical studies to be synthesised, reading them repeatedly and noting down key concepts. These key concepts become the raw data for the synthesis. The synthesis of the results and discussion of empirical research studies is conducted with the purpose of identifying a unique vision and interpretation of literature. But as Weed (2008) notes, the purpose of the review is not to find the truth; rather, it is to find 'a truth'.

Traditionally, the method of a meta-ethnography involves a seven stage process (Campbell et al., 2003; Noblit & Hare, 1988; Weed, 2008). Stages 1 and 2 involve getting started and sampling: This meant obtaining qualitative studies that consider the psycho-social processes involved with initiating and developing a physically active lifestyle. A search of the literature was conducted by the primary author. The author undertook an electronic search in December 2010 of CINAHL, AMED, EMBASE and MEDLINE databases using key words related to physical activity (EXERCISE, SPORT, PHYSICAL ACTIVTY), mental health (SEVERE MENTAL ILLNESS, SCHIZOPHRENIA), and the type of methodology used in each study (QUALITATIVE, IN DEPTH, UNSTRUCTURED OR SEMI STRUCTURED INTERVIEWS). Key authors in the area were contacted and several journals that related to this area were also searched including: *Journal of Mental Health, Psychiatric Services, & British Journal of Psychiatry*. In addition to this one key author (Dr D Carless) was contacted by email for details of his current research.

Following this search, thirteen studies were identified. This is in line with similar types of review articles (e.g., Campbell et al (2003) used 7, Malpass et al (2009) used 16, Soundy et al (2011) used 10). In order to create a range of studies that would be most comparable, appropriate for the aims of the research and useful within this analysis, a set of screening questions and standards were applied during the initial reading of the articles. Three key screening questions were employed: 'Does this paper report empirical findings from qualitative research and did that work involve both qualitative methods of data collection and an inductive method of analysis?', 'Is this research relevant to the synthesis topic?' and 'Does this work provide a distinct contribution to the analysis above and beyond the collective findings?' The inclusion criteria included the following: Each study needed to be reported in a peer review journal and written in english. The findings from each study needed to be generated from a specific sport or exercise intervention. The exercise or physical activity had to be undertaken outside the patient's mental health day centre. Data from each study had to be generated using empirical qualitative data that was non-fiction. Finally, each study had to present separate results and discussion sections so the correct meta-ethnographic analysis could be undertaken; without both sections the review could not be completed.

This meant the following studies were excluded: Carless and Douglas (2008a) because a deductive approach was used in their analysis; Carless and Sparkes (2008) because a lack of a discussion meant that second order interpretations could not be undertaken and this may have also limited third order interpretations; Carless (2008) because the study referred to a life history rather than a specific sport or exercise process or intervention; Carless and Douglas (2008b) because the study presented case studies and lacked an analytical consideration of the literature; Douglas and Carless (2010) because the study was a fictional tale; and, Soundy (2007) because it formed part of a PhD thesis and was not published. Eight studies were selected to be used within the meta-ethnography and included: Carless (2007), Shiner et al. (2008), Crone (2007), Fogarty and Happell (2005), Faulkner and Sparkes (1999), Carter-Morris and Faulkner (2003), Carless and Douglas (2004), and Crone and Guy (2008). Our exclusion criteria should not be interpreted as suggesting any devaluation of the excluded research; in fact, we have used our discussion to take account of their findings.

Similar to Campbell et al. (2003), we used stages 3 and 4 to read the selected relevant empirical studies repeatedly and note down key concepts as they began to emerge. The key concepts generated from individual studies were examined in relation to other studies. We used tables and grids to help in this and to display themes and concepts (Atkins et al., 2008; Campbell et al., 2003). In other words, we summarised and wrote commentary on the results and discussion sections of each article. The first order constructs considered the results of the studies and the second order constructs considered the discussion section of the studies (these tables can be obtained from the first author upon request).

During stage 5 we examined the reciprocal and refutational relationships between studies and examined how we could further existing knowledge found in any individual study (Britten et al., 2002; Van Manning et al., 1988). Noblit and Hare (1988) refer to this as a line of argument synthesis. In essence, we conducted a thematic analysis on our findings through summarising the first and second order concepts. This approach allowed us to maintain the language used in each study while creating new metaphors within the synthesis (Doyle, 2003). During stage 6 we created synthesised translations or third order constructs. We achieved this by examining our key themes generated from the first and second order interpretations along with the idiomatic interpretation and considered how the themes, ideas, metaphors and comments illustrated a process of activity from the onset. This included two issues as discussed above: (1)

increasing uptake/initial engagement in exercise, and (2) how to successfully maintain long-term engagement in exercise. Stage 7 involved presenting the results.

4. Results

Three primary themes are presented within the first and second order interpretations: (1) psychological attributes, (2) barriers, and (3) facilitators. Finally, we consider the process of activity involvement, this is represented by two third order themes (1) the uptake of exercise (2) the prolonged engagement in exercise. The purpose of this was to allow the analysis to clearly represent the primary aims of our research.

4.1 Psychological attributes
The psychological attributes theme included aspects of the physical activity or exercise setting that influenced the experience of participants. The sub-themes generated included *identity*, and *dependency, control and autonomy*.

4.1.1 Identity
Establishing a new identity (such as a footballer; Carter-Morris and Faulkner, 2003) or recreating an identity (restarting a previous interest; Carless and Douglas, 2004) were integral aspects of participating in a new sport or activity. Intially, this is something that could draw patients towards the activities, because it allowed them to consider or project their future self. Through activity, patients could consider and be associated with positive identities, possibly past selves (Carless, 2007). This gave patients a sense that they could get back to their old self (Forgarty & Happell, 2005) and obtain previously lost feelings, experiences and interactions. This represented a resumption of being 'normal', obtaining normality, or being restored to a past identity (Carless, 2007). This was important in drawing the patients towards the exercise.

Patients were inspired by the nature, motivation and knowledge of other patients within the activity or sports setting (Crone, 2007). The group activity provided a time for sharing personal experiences and this helped provide a sense of unity with others in the group (Crone, 2007). In addition to this the new relationships formed within the activity setting helped develop patients' identities (Shiner et al., 2008): Belonging to an exercise or sports activity provided opportunity for patients to develop a sporting or exercise identity, since most discussions within the setting focused towards this (Carter-Morris & Faulkner, 2003). This process of sharing and engaging with others in turn influenced patients' attitudes towards fitness and motivation for activity (Fogarty & Happell, 2005).

A patient's identity would best be maintained following positive and successful activity or exercise experiences. These experiences helped develop a patient's identity within the group and this also helped challenge their identity as a service user (Carter-Morris & Faulkner, 2003). The patient's identity could extend to a particular identity within the group and a meaningful social role (Carless, 2007; Carter-Morris & Faulkner, 2003). This included patients who were given responsibility for a group (e.g., a person who organised travel arrangements) or a specific role in the activity (e.g., the captain of a team). Following regular or maintained engagement the patient's athletic identity could be transferred from the group setting into other situations such as their day centre and this in turn could influence other users at these locations (Fogarty & Happell, 2005). Often this occurred because the activity provided a positive topic of conversation when reflecting on their day's achievements (Carless & Douglas, 2004).

4.1.2 Dependency, control and autonomy

Activity developed autonomy (Carless, 2007) through providing a sense of achievement, satisfaction (Crone & Guy, 2008), empowerment and perceived confidence (Fogarty & Happell, 2005; Sparkes & Faulkner 1999). In regard to initial engagement in exercise, prior knowledge, including benefits, joy or contentment of activity was instrumental to decisions (Crone, 2007). The interventions in themselves gave the service user opportunity to think about future activities (Fogarty & Happell, 2005). Goals towards activities varied from becoming independent and autonomous in the community (Shiner et al., 2008) to undertaking a normalising activity (Carter-Morris & Faulkner, 2003). For others, activity provided a chance to change environments (Faulkner & Sparkes, 1999). Being associated with an athletic identity gave patients a sense of certainty and an idea of who they could become. This in itself provided a great reason for attending, but also provided a sense of empowerment and autonomy to the service users.

Autonomy was assisted by the patients being able to associate themselves with the activity and taking responsbility for the achievement gained (Carless, 2007; Carless & Douglass, 2004). Thus, through actvity, patients could become less dependent on others and perceive greater control in social settings, such as community sport or exercise environments (Carless, 2007). Autonomy was also created within the activity session through support from others. This was achieved because patients were able to choose when and if they revealed information about themselves (Faulkner & Sparkes, 1999). The exercise group provided a stable and non intrusive topic of conversation that was a natural part of the activity. Thus, they didn't have to talk about aspects of themselves that they did not want to disclose. The sense of having a choice to disclose information in a non pressured or judging environment helped the possibility of a patient returning to the setting and maintaining exercise.

4.2 Barriers

The barriers theme included aspects related to preventing successful uptake and maintenance of activity. The sub-themes generated included *location, access and finances, medication and symptom change, social support* and *cognitive.*

4.2.1 Location, access and finances

Patients were prevented from engaging in activity if the location of the activity was too far away or inaccessible (Shiner et al., 2008). However, some patients found that other activities 'got in the way' of the physical activity program; for example, daily chores (Crone, 2007). Thus, both the location of activity and the timing of the activity may prevent patients with SMI from taking-up exercise. Almost unanimously across the studies activity was prevented by financial cost (Carless, 2007; Carless & Douglas, 2004; Crone, 2007; Crone & Guy, 2008; Shiner et al., 2008). Activities such as walking could be recommended as a low cost alternative (Fogarty & Happell, 2005). If the tangible, emotional or esteem support following the completion of research was not continued then the possibility of patients maintaining activity long-term could be severely diminished (Faulkner & Sparkes, 1999).

4.2.2 Medication and symptom change

Medication had an influence on all patients (Crone & Guy, 2008); it often influenced their level of drowsiness, motivation and could slow patients down, taking the 'shine' off their ability to undertake exercise or physical activity (Carter Morris & Faulkner, 2003). One of the biggest factors that influenced participation was changes in symptoms (Carless, 2007) or a fluctuating medical status (Shiner et al., 2008). One consequence of this was the *need* to allow patients to withdraw (Crone, 2007), even though withdrawal is generally considered undesirable (Carless & Douglas, 2004). In other words, patients' medication and symptoms interacted to cause a universal barrier against the uptake and maintenance of activity; this meant consistent and sustained engagement in exercise was unlikely.

4.2.3 Social support

In order for patients to initiate activity, social support was essential. However, the wrong type of support contributed to increased resistance towards activity engagement. For example, resistance to exercise increased when little support or empathy was expressed by health care professionals in regard to the negative side effects of medication (Carter-Morris & Faulkner 2003), or when health care professionals had low expectations (Carless & Douglas, 2004). If patients are not encouraged by friends and family (Crone, 2007) they are unlikely to initiate or maintain exercise. A lack of consistency of support through the physical activity process (Carless, 2007) can act as a barrier to maintaining activity. This may be because of the feelings of being isolated. Social support can become problematic if support is dependent on one or few people involved with activity or at the end of the activity program where no further provision for support has been accounted for (Faulkner & Sparkes, 1999).

4.2.4 Cognitive

The patient's cognitions during activity had an important influence on activity attendance. These cognitions often occurred in new situations where patients experienced a lack of personal control (Carless, 2007) due to the unknown or uncertainty of a situation (Crone, 2007). Barriers could be created within settings (Carless & Douglas, 2004); for example, the confidence of the patients could be tested in a 'new' situation that might be perceived as threatening (Faulkner & Sparkes, 1999) or could be lower as a result of the illness (Shiner et al., 2008). Additionally, some patients did not like competitive circumstances (Carless & Douglas, 2004). If patients did not want to participate they could experience an increase in their symptoms for example, voices multiplying (Faulkner & Sparkes, 1999). Alternatively, the patients' symptoms, moods or emotions could prevent them from exercising (Shiner et al., 2008). As such, changes to a patient's identity, mood and emotions, and motivation for activity can take a long time to be developed. Carless (2007) suggests such a process can take years. Thus, experiencing or reflecting negative experiences may be a consistent barrier to patients initiating and maintaining activity.

4.3 Facilitators

The facilitators theme included aspects related to successful uptake and maintenance of the activity. The sub-themes generated included *location, positive experience, physical and psychological benefits,* and *social support.*

4.3.1 Location

The location provided a patient with a new situation and a chance to grow and express themselves. Patients valued the chance to leave their normal residence (Faulkner & Sparkes, 1999) and engage in the wider community (Carter-Morris & Faulkner, 2003). Patients suggested that there was a sense of excitement in trying a new activity or in seeing new places (Crone, 2007). For some patients, the travel and scenery provided enjoyment and the activity could represent something to look forward to and be associated with (Carless, 2007). Successful experiences were required in order to maintain activity.

4.3.2 Positive experience

Various conditions impacted on a patient's ability to initiate exercise. Patients suggested that motivation comes from actually doing something (Carless, 2007) or breaking from a stagnant routine (Faulkner & Sparkes, 1999); at the most basic level, doing something was better than doing nothing (Crone & Guy, 2008). Some patients like to start slowly when engaging with exercise (Carless & Douglas, 2004); on the other hand, some wanted a chance to push themselves (Forgarty & Happell, 2005). This 'choice' aided their confidence and competence (Carless, 2007) and it meant patients created memorable experiences (Crone, 2007). Thus, the patients could be excited and hopeful about a new experience, but required a choice of how to engage with the process from the uptake activity.

The key process required for the maintenance of activity was if the patient found the experience of undertaking physical activity to be rewarding. Patients experienced a valued sense of achievement in being able to reflect on an activity and in being associated with it (Carless, 2007; Crone & Guy, 2008). Exercise provided a distraction from voices, or something that provided assistance in controlling voices (Faulkner & Sparkes, 1999), together with helping to prevent social withdrawal (Carter-Morris & Faulkner, 2003). The physical activity provided patients with some form of comfort towards a goal and sense of control (Faulkner & Sparkes, 1999) or responsibility about an activity (Carless & Douglas, 2004). Simply put, exercise engagement helped patients progress from not feeling able to respond or challenge their illness to feeling more able to incorporate physical activity alongside it (Crone, 2007).Thus, a goal that can be established by and through activity is for a patient to become more autonomous and independent.

4.3.3 Physical and psychological benefits

Following activity consistent psychological changes were reported by many studies, including mood elevating effects, anxiety reducing effects, improved concentration, increased self esteem and social competence (Faulkner & Sparkes, 1999; Crone & Guy, 2008). Exercise and sport also provided an opportunity to unwind, reducing stress levels and promoting a sense of calmness (Faulkner and Sparkes, 1999; Carless & Douglas, 2004), leading to greater motivation and enjoyment (Fogarty & Happell, 2005). Patients also had a better body image (Faulkner & Sparkes, 1999). Exercise may also benefit a patient's psychotic symptoms and delusional belief systems, and also reinforce a more positive version of reality (Faulkner & Sparkes, 1999; Carter-Morris & Faulkner, 2003). With more exposure to activity, patients could also benefit from a decrease in anxiety towards community involvement (Shiner et al., 2008).

Physiological changes were also reported, including positive bodily change (Carless, 2007), better sleep (Crone, 2007; Faulkner & Sparkes, 1999), better health and well-being, increased fitness and weight loss (Forgarty & Happell, 2005), and increased energy levels (Crone & Guy, 2008; Faulkner & Sparkes, 1999). There were also changes in other aspects of well being such as better hygiene, seeking out opportunities for counselling, and taking the initiative to acquire information for themselves to engage further in community activities (Faulkner & Sparkes, 1999). Patients that can experience even some of these psychological or physiological changes will clearly have a greater chance of maintaining activity

4.3.4 Social support

Social support is central to the uptake and prolonged engagement in physical activity. Before the physical activity has been initiated the social needs of patients have to be considered. To ensure the most productive uptake of physical activity all staff are required to provide individualised and structured support for a patient (Forgarty & Happell, 2005); for instance, informing a patient of who was leading the activity session (Crone & Guy, 2008). It was important that staff did not place expectations on patients, particularly if a patient was unfit (Fogarty & Happell, 2005). Therapists were required to encourage patients in overcoming motivational barriers, be knowledgeable about sport, as well as being sensitive and supportive through the activity process (Crone, 2007; Crone & Guy, 2008; Shiner et al., 2008). All interaction with patients had to be initiated in a safe and comfortable way (Faulkner & Sparkes, 1999). There was no need or request for staff at the activity or sports setting to discuss a patient's mental illness, symptoms or problems. Support revolved around encouraging engagement and creating positive experiences for patients. It was important to be with others and share experiences (Crone, 2007). Health care professionals that supported the program acted as gatekeepers of it (Crone, 2007; Crone & Guy, 2008). In essence, to ensure uptake of exercise patients needed to feel they were entering a known, safe and supporting environment.

During the physical activity experience social support acted as a foundation for prolonged engagement. Social time had to be a part of any physical activity setting for service users (Carless & Douglas, 2004; Faulkner & Sparkes, 1999). Known and trusted friendships developed between staff and patients (Carless, 2007; Carter-Morris & Faulkner, 2003) and in other studies a training partner provided support and encouragement (Forgarty & Happell, 2005). These friendships could be associated with changes in the patient's symptoms (Shiner et al., 2008; Faulkner & Sparkes, 1999). The cohesive nature of the exercise group helped to encourage a patient's interest and ongoing activity (Fogarty & Happell, 2005); friendships facilitated positive cognitions and attitudes towards exercise (Faulkner & Sparkes, 1999), and enhanced the possibility of further and prolonged engagement.

Following successful activity participation, exercise or sport became an avenue for conversation and interaction (Carter-Morris & Faulkner, 2003), and there was enjoyment in spreading the word about participation in an activity (Carless & Douglas, 2004). The social interaction helped increase social confidence (Crone, 2007; Crone & Guy, 2008) and provided initiation for life improvements (Faulkner & Sparkes, 1999). Thus, the development of patient's social skills can be seen as part of a productive process that helps reinforce and maintain a sporting identity, and this in turn indicates a desire to maintain and develop activity and exercise engagement.

4.4 Considering the process of activity involvement

This theme illustrates how identity can change with physical activity involvement. Two sub-themes make up this theme: (1) phases of activity, and (2) evolving identity.

4.4.1 Phases of activity

Physical activity involvement was established through phases. Three primary phases were identified during the patients involvement with physical actvitity. *Pre activity* – considered the time before activity is initated. During this time patients are dependent on staff and others to inform them of the activity, including potential benefits. In thinking about the future activity, they could be faced with uncertainty about what could happen and worries from past experiences. For those who took part previously, they may have different associations or more confidence. *Within activity* – this stage is associated with time when particpants are engaged with the physical activity setting from the moment when they enter the activity environment to the moment they exited the environment. *Post activity* – this considers times following activity and includes reflecting on the experiences of activity. Table 1 details how participants' autonomy and identity is influenced and changed, and how patients may come to exit from the experience and the need for support during this phase.

Phase	Evolving autonomy	Evolving Identity	Exiting activity	External Phases of Support
Pre-activity	*Dependency* Patients depend on support, encouragement and information from others. *Uncertainty* Patients have informing worries about situation, who will be there, what will or could happen and what to expect from activity.	*Existing identity* The patients are defined by their current condition, their current preoccupation (illness, passivity). *Projected identity* They may have anticipation about who they could become, or re-establishing who they were.	*Limited interest* Don't enjoy sport or physical activity *No support* Not enough information, motivation or assistance from others. *Uncertainty* Not enough known about the activity. *Too greater change* change attempted or required is too much. *Past experience* Negative experiences may predetermine perception.	*The value of support* A known environment becomes a more certain environment, important of knowing the people and the facility. *Primary Role of HCPs* Encouraging, motivating, educating and directing patients.
Within Activity	*Achievement* Going through the process provides a sense of achievement and perceived control. *Being heard* From taking part, being heard and listened to there is value in a patient being able to	*Distraction* Enabling activity through removing concerns. Sport identity engulfs existing identity. Distraction can enable or disable identity change. *Positive Experience* Enthusiasm and	*Bad interaction or experience* Existing from getting to location, within location or following location *Uncertain environment –* Experiences become negative, participation	*Distracting* Support within sessions helps provide a distraction to experiences *Listening –* SMI user control content of conversation. *Reflective*

Phase	Evolving autonomy	Evolving Identity	Exiting activity	External Phases of Support
	express themselves. Opportunity to be heard. *Expression of self* Activity provides a context to express feelings through movement.	Enjoyment of activity draws patient away from existing identity. *Group Interaction* Identity of others impacts on patients.	ceases.	*questioning -* Provide change for reflection and evolving phase. *Social* Increasing network of support and known environment.
Post activity	*Considering experiences* Positive experiences, valued friendships. Developing autonomy confidence to do more activity *Developing independence* Through seeing achievement, acknowledging possibilities Development of motivation towards more activity and other global activities. *Reflecting* Modifying existing knowledge of environment, interaction and ability. Challenging uncertainty and unreliability of new situations	*Reflections* Reflection within self and with others through interaction. Projected identity is enforced. Past identity is remembered. *Reflective processes* Acceleration and evolution of identity. *Expanding identity* Identity impacts on patients outside the exercise setting. *Becoming* Part of the identity is incorporate into self.	*Bad experiences* Experience or interaction, reaction to experience (increasing voices) was negative. *Limited control* Was present and process becomes unsafe and uncertain.	*Monitoring experience* Evolving and encouraging activities and transferring and supporting other engagement. *Listening and valuing* Patient expressions of their experiences are important as they

Table 1. Illustrating three phases of physical activity involvement

4.4.2 The evolving identity

From the above sub-theme it can be established that one primary goal of physical activity is to develop a patient's identity through physical activity and sport. Thus, physical activity can help the patient transfer from being someone who may consider community activities passively towards someone who is proactive towards activities. Alongside this the patient's existing identity is challenged through a number of key processes to become an evolved identity. Figure 1 provides an idea of how activity challenges a patient's existing identity and facilitates the evolution of identity.

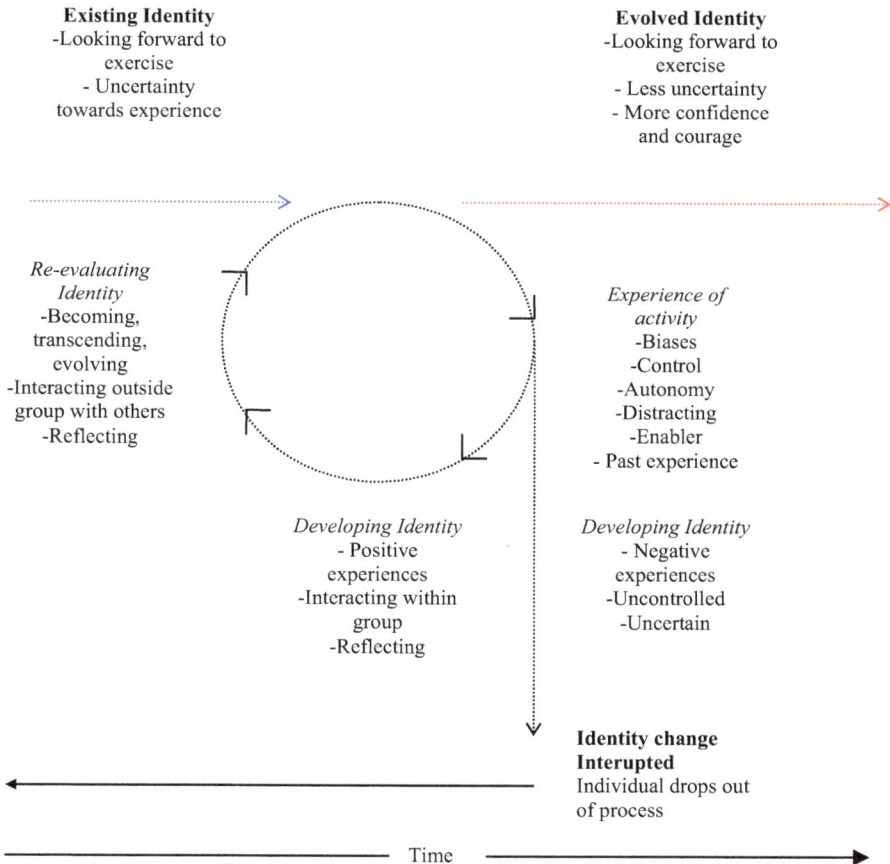

Existing Identity
-Looking forward to
exercise
- Uncertainty
towards experience

Evolved Identity
-Looking forward to
exercise
- Less uncertainty
- More confidence
and courage

*Re-evaluating
Identity*
-Becoming,
transcending,
evolving
-Interacting outside
group with others
-Reflecting

*Experience of
activity*
-Biases
-Control
-Autonomy
-Distracting
-Enabler
- Past experience

Developing Identity
- Positive
experiences
-Interacting within
group
-Reflecting

Developing Identity
- Negative
experiences
-Uncontrolled
-Uncertain

**Identity change
Interupted**
Individual drops out
of process

Time

Fig. 1. The evolving identity cycle

The evolving identity cycle shows that the perception or experience of activity is vital in helping develop the patient's identity. The cycle demonstrates the challenges to identity that can exist before the activity has begun and during the activity. These challenges are illustrated by the barriers mentioned in section 4.2 and are clearly more significant in regard to the uptake of physical activity. Barriers are generated by worry, caused by an unknown or uncertain experience, and then again during activity where perceptual biases, ambiguous or negative interactions and inadequate support may act to prevent the patient embracing the experience. Following a negative experience the ability to change, evolve and adapt the patient's identity is likely to fail. Conversely, following a positive experience a patient is able to use interaction and reflection to transform their identity. A more positive cycle exists once the patient is able to consider the activity as more of a certain, safe and supported experience. This positive cycle is essential in supporting the maintenance of activity.

5. Discussion

Engagement in physical activity for patients with SMI requires careful consideration. Exploring the psychosocial experience of physical activity and exercise for patients with SMI has provided a useful understanding of the processes involved in initiating and maintaining activity, as well as establishing barriers and facilitators of activity. This information is well placed to inform both patients with SMI as well as those who have a support role such as health care professionals, carers, and family members. This discussion will look to summarise the barriers and facilitators of activity before turning attention to both psychosocial phases of activity and the evolution of a patient's identity.

5.1 Initiating activity

Two of the biggest physical barriers for patients with SMI included being too tired to exercise or being unable to exercise because of their illness (Ussher et al., 2007). Stability in symptoms of illness is a good precursor to initating activity (Carless, 2007). Part of this was a direct result of their medication and its side effects (Gorczynski & Faulkner, 2011; Roberts & Bailey, 2011). Another consistent and challenging barrier to activity participation was the location of the activity and the costs involved with the activity. The problem of finances is compounded by the problem of frequent unemployment and dependence on benefits (Hodgson et al., 2011). Carless and Douglass (2008a) suggest that tangible support is required for patients to address these barriers.

There are difficulties patients with SMI can initially experience that are not experienced long term, such as an unknown setting, experiences and interactions. These aspects of engaging in physical activity challenge the patients self-esteem, courage, autonomy and motivation (Butterly et al., 2006; Soundy, 2007). Being able to attend activity sessions provides an opportunity to become more independent (Shiner et al., 2008). However, beginning activity can be difficult as patients may have a lack of initiative (Roberts & Bailey, 2011). Patients need to perceive what the experience will involve because not being sure of what is required of them during exercise, being self-conscious, feeling unsafe, and being afraid to get injured are common barriers to activity (Gorczynski & Faulkner, 2011; Ussher et al., 2007). In addition, problems can be created in new and uncertain social environments where patients may be more sensitive to interactions and experiences (Soundy, 2007).

The benefit of activity can be simply undertaking a new situation, creating a sense of meaning or purpose and an opportunity to break old routines. Positive experiences before the activity (achievement, positive memories) help provide more enthausiasm (Carless, 2007). The structure of programs before delivery should consider certain aspects, such as being informative (Carless & Douglas, 2008a), providing users with a program that meets their own pace (Gorczynski & Faulkner, 2011), and has in place a good motivational leader

(Richardson, 2005). Aspects such as the journey to the new environment can be something to be received positively (Crone, 2007). Being able to do something that can add to or change their lifestyle and routine was highly valuable to patients with SMI. Physical benefits were also present and included the general effects of participating in activity like weight loss (Fogarty & Happell, 2005; Chiverton et al., 2007) or indeed just having knowledge of the benefits of a more healthy lifestyle (Tetlie et al., 2009; McDevitt et al., 2006).

Before activity is initiated, feelings of isolation can prevent activity engagement (Hodgson et al., 2011; Roberts & Bailey, 2011). A good support network is required to combat the experience many users have of social isolation, marginalisation and stigmatisation (Ellis et al., 2007; Gorczynski & Faulkner, 2011). Patients must be carefully supported from the initial interaction with services. The right kind of individualised support service that acknowledges patients' preferences and experiences is required to achieve a more successful adoption of exercise. Support is needed in different ways including encouragement, finances and listening (Carless & Douglas, 2008a). It should also be provided by known mental health professionals (Hodgson et al., 2011).

5.2 Maintaining activity

Autonomy for the activity was slowly provided for users as they took responsibility for attendance (Carless & Douglas, 2004). A sense of autonomy and achievement and purpose is obtained from activity (Crone, 2007). Prolonged engagement is enhanced once a sense of acheivement, purpose and enjoyment is obtained.

Psychologically being able to experience achievement, to realise goals, to experience a sense of control, to have a distraction from negative aspects of the illness provides a basis for enjoying activity. The exercise group provides a setting that empowered the patient to share information about them self (Faulkner & Sparkes, 1999). A postive and enjoyable experience can provide an important part of conversation within and outside the exercise settings (Carless & Douglas, 2004).

Much of the appreciation from patients who undertake an activity can focus on the routine nature of the activity; this enhances rapport and relationships and the enjoyment of a meaningful activity (Marzolini et al., 2009). Support is required once activity begins: one-to-one support (from staff and by other users or patients) can provide an important distraction and encouragement for patients (Carless & Douglas, 2008a; Crone & Stembrige, 2007; Roberts & Bailey, 2011; Soundy, 2007). There is an important role for instructors within this to provide appropriate support, as Richardson et al., (2005) state *"Enthusiastic, knowledgeable, and supportive exercise leaders are as important as the actual exercise prescription itself"* (page 327). Accordingly, social support provides certainty and confidence when engaging in new environments. However, it is still possible for patients to experience or percieve threats or problems with the environment such as anxiety attacks (Carless, 2008). Providing a safe, welcoming and friendly environment is needed to acheive adherence over the long term, where some inconsistency in attendence can be expected (Soundy, 2007). Indeed a caring and relaxed environment can help patients enjoy the experience (Carless & Douglass, 2004).

A chain of supportive networks is needed from identifying a program of activity to maintaining that program of activity. Some of the most positive results of physical activity are achieved in inpatient settings where there are greater levels of day-to-day support (Ellis et al., 2007). The attributes of those supporting the intervention are essential as a faciliator to continued activity (Chiverton et al., 2007; Soundy, 2007); conversely, the stigma associated with mental illness from patients working in exercise settings may be a barrier (Crone & Stembrigdge, 2007). Group based activities are often associated with higher levels of adherence than patient programs. One of the reasons given for this is because group activities that are supervised can eliminate the avoidable barriers to exercise (Marzolini et al., 2009). In addition, group activities promote social interaction and contribute to a more enjoyable experience (Fogarty and Happell, 2005; Holley et al., 2011). One role of activity is to create and maintain supportive social relationships (McDevitt et al., 2006). Thus, being able to provide and maintain a social network within the activity setting is important for prolonged engagement. The utilization of social networking devices may be a way to encourage and develop patient's social expression, unity, support and identity (Killackey et al., 2011). Conversely, a limited network or isolated support can create reliance and dependency on health care professionals which can have negative effects (Faulkner & Sparkes, 1999; Soundy, 2007).

5.3 The creation and evolution of a social identity

One of the biggest challenges when working with patients with SMI is how to maintain the users engagement with an activity program (Hodgson et al., 2011). Programs that use behaviour modification principle, like social support or goal setting are more effective than more simple programs (Richardson et al., 2005). Following the support that is gained early in promoting activity further development of different and sustainable relationships are required and obtained in the group setting. This greater range of relationships means patients have less reliance on a smaller support network (Soundy, 2007). Successful achievement within the exercise setting helps provide patients with an increased sense of self-efficacy (Richardson et al., 2005). Indeed, engagement in exercise increases a participant's confidence in social settings and provides them with a sense of a social identity which enables them to further engage with fellow exercise participants.

Belonging to a group and attending physical activity sessions provides users with a sense of purpose and creates a social confidence that can then be transferred to new settings (Hodgson et al., 2011). A sense of belonging also influences how patients redefine their self-identity (Shea, 2009). Exercise and physical activity in a community setting provides a setting that can help promote a sense of belonging and therefore provides an excellent opportunity for refining their self identity (Shea, 2009). For some users this may be a sense of returning to who they used to be and or towards normality (Carless & Douglass, 2008b).

6. Implications for health care professionals

A network of supportive relationships that are sustainable is required in order for successful participation in exercise. Health care professionals need to consider the provision of support from introducing the patient to the idea of becoming more physically active through to introducing patients into a new setting. Clearly, there is also a need for health care professionals to be able to recognise the different dimensions (informational, tangible, emotional and esteem) of socal support (Carless & Douglas, 2008a).

It is essential that patients feel able to talk to others about negative experiences and interactions; this provision within the mental health setting and community setting is needed to address the identified barriers to activity. We urge HCPs to invest time in listening to and sharing in patients' experiences. Capturing changes in social support that occurs through engagement in exercise and physical activity may be best achieved by using existing inventories; for example, Sarason et al., (1987) provide a short form inventory that considers the social support that others provide in an individual's environment.

The psychological changes during exercise may be best captured by considering how patients confidence, self-efficacy and self-identity is challenged and shaped through the process of exercise, from intial to sustained engagement in exercise. The means of assessing these may be made through observations, informal conversation or through non-taxing inventories; for example, Bandura (1997) proposes a way to develop an inventory tool for self-efficacy. Improvement in any of these psychological domains will have a clear impact on the patients lifestyle and well-being.

7. Future recommendations

There is a need for research to consider assessing how interventions can influence confidence, self-identity, self-efficacy and social support following physical activity interventions. It is important that further research is able to distingush the best tools that can be used to assess such effects. More specifically, we suggest there is a need for future research to consider each of these psychosocial variables in greater detail. For example, in regards to social support, reseach could explore the most effective ways to capture change in the network and structure of patients' support. In addition to this, research could establish whether perceived availability of support and/or enacted (received) support exerts positive effects upon outcomes.

8. Conclusion

The development of a social identity is a natural and very beneficial aspect of undertaking a physical activity or sports based group. There are barriers that prevent initiation to activity as well as barriers that exist once activity has begun. Physical activity and sport has the potential to break down the barriers and help create a new social identity for the user. Undertaking activity helps develop the user's confidence and courage and through realising a new and changed identity users appear more able to engage with community based physical activity.

9. Acknowledgments

Thanks to Dr D Carless for providing references for supporting the search for articles and for his extensive work within this field of research.

10. References

Atkins, S., Lewin, S., Smith, H., Engel, M., Fretheim, A., Volmink, J. (2008). Conducting a meta-ethnography of qualitative literature: Lessons learnt. *BMC Medical Research Methodology*, 8, pp. (1-10).

Bandura, A. (1997). *Self-efficacy: The exercise of control.* New York: Freeman.

Britten, N., Campbell, R., Pope, C., Donovan, J., Morgan, M., Pill, R. (2002). Using meta ethnography to synthesise qualitative research: A worked example. *Journal of Health Services Research Policy*, 7, pp. (209-215).

Campbell, R., Pound, P., Pope, C., Britten, N., Pill, R., Morgan, M., Donovan, J. (2003). Evaluating meta-ethnography: A synthesis of qualitative research on lay experiences of diabetes and diabetes care. *Social Science & Medicine*, 56, pp. (671-684).

Carless, D. (2008). Narrative, identity and recovery from serious mental illness: A life history of a runner. *Qualitative Research in Psychology*, 5, pp. (233-248).

Carless, D. (2007). Phases in physical activity initiation and maintenance among men with serious mental illness. *International Journal of Mental Health Promotion*, 9, pp. (17-27).

Carless, D., Douglas, K. (2004). A gold programme for people with severe and enduring mental health problems. *Journal of Mental Health Promotion*, 3, pp. (23-39).

Carless, D., Douglas, K. (2008a). Social support for and through exercise and sport in a sample of men with serious mental illness. *Issues in Mental Health Nursing*, 29, pp. (1179-1199).

Carless, D., Douglass, K. (2008b). The role of sport and exercise in recovery from serious mental illness: Two case studies. *International Journal of Men's Health*, 7, pp. (137-156).

Carless, D., Sparkes, A. C. (2008). The physical activity experiences of men with serious mental illness: three short stories. *Psychology of Sport and Exercise*, 9, pp. (191-210).

Carter-Morris, P., Faulkner, G. (2003). A football project for mental health service users. *Journal of Mental Health Promotion*, 2, pp. (24-30).

Crone, D. (2007). Walking back to health: A qualitative investigation into service users' experiences of a walking project. *Issues in Mental Health Nursing*, 28, pp. (167-183).

Crone, D., & Stembridge, L. (2007). Getting a move on. *Mental Health Today*, April, pp (30-32).

Doyle, L. H. (2003). Synthesis through meta-ethnography: Paradoxes, enhancements and possibilities. *Qualitative Research*, 3, pp. (321-344).

Ellis, N., Crone, D., Davey, R., & Grogan, S. (2007). Exercise interventions as an adjunct therapy for psychosis: a critical review. *British Journal of Clinical Psychology*, 46, pp. (95-111).

Hodgson, M. H., McCulloch, H. P., Fox, K. R. (2011). The experiences of people with severe and enduring metnal illness engaged in a physical activity programme integrated into the mental health service. *Mental Health and Physical Activity*, 4, pp. (23-29).

Holley, J., Crone, D., Tyson, P., & Lovell, G. (2011). The effects of physical activity on psycholgoicla well-being for those with schizophrenia: A systematic review. *Biritsh Journal of Clinical Psychology*, 50: pp. (84-105).

Killackey, E., Anda, A. L., Gibs, M., Alvarez-Jimenez, M., Thompson, A., Sun, P., & Baksheev, G. N. (2011). Using internet enabled mobile devices and soical networking techniolgies to promote execise as an inervention for young first episode psychosis patietns. *BMC Psychiatry*,11, pp. (80).

Malpass, A., Shaw, A., Sharp, D., Walter, F., Feder, G., Ridd, M., & Kessler, D. (2009). "Medication Career" or "Moral Career"? The two sides of managing antidepressants: A meta-ethnography of patients' experience of antidepressants. *Social Science and Medicine*, 68, pp. (154-168).

McDevitt, J., Snyder, M., Miller, A., & Wilbur, J. (2006). Perceptions of barriers and benefits to physical activity among outpatients in psychiatric rehabiliation. *Journal of Nursing Scholarship*, 38, pp. (50-55).

Noblit, G.W., Hare, R.D. (1988). *Meta-ethnography: Synthesising qualitative studies*. New York: Sage

Faulkner, G and Biddle, S. (1999) Exercise as an adjunct treatment for schizophrenia: A review of the literature. *Journal of Mental Health*, 8, pp. (441-457).

Faulkner, G., Soundy, A. A., & Lloyd, K. (2003). Schizophrenia and weight management: a systematic review of interventions to control weight. *Acta Psychiatrica Scandinavica*, 108, pp. (324-332).

Faulkner, G., and Sparkes, A. (1999). Exercise as therapy for schizophrenia: an ethnographic study. *Journal of Sport and Exercise Psychology*, 21, pp. (52-69).

Gorczynski, P., & Faulkner, G. (2009). Exercise therapy for schizophrenia. *Cochrane database of systematic reviews*, 2010. Issue 5. Art. No. CD004412.
DOI: 10.1002/14651858.CD004412.pub2.

Raine, P., Truman, C., Southerst, A. (2002). The development of a community gym for people with mental health problems: influences on psychological accessibility. *Journal of Mental Health*, 11, pp. (43-53).

Richardson, C. R., Faulkner, G., McDevitt, J., Skrinar, G. S., Hutchinson, D. S., Piette, J. D. (2005). Integrating physical activity into mental health services for persons with serious mental illness. *Psychiatric Services*, 56, pp. (324-331).

Roberts, S. H., & Bailey, J. E. (2010). Incentives and barriers to lifestyle interventions for poele with severe mental illness; a nrrative sytnthesis of quantitative, qulaitative and mixed methods studies. *Journal of Advanced Nursing*, 67, pp. (690-708).

Sarason, I. G., Sarason, B. R., Shearin, E. N., Pierce, G. R. (1987). A brief measure of soical support: practical and theoretical implications. *Journal of Soical and Personal Relationships*, 4, pp. (497-510).

Shea, J. M. (2009). Coming back to normal: the process of self-recovery in those with schizophrenia. *Journal of the American Psychiatric Nurses Assoication*, 16, pp. (43-51).

Shiner, B., Whitley, R., Van Citters, A. D., Pratt, S. I., Bartels, S. J. (2008). Learning what matters for patients: qualitative evaluation of a health promotion program for those with serious mental illness. *Health Promotion International*, 23, pp. (275-282).

Soundy, A. (2007). *Understanding physical activity in individuals with severe mental illness*. A doctoral thesis. University of Exeter.

Soundy, A., Faulkner, G., Taylor, A. (2007). Exploring Variability and Perceptions of Lifestyle Physical Activity Among Individuals with Severe and Enduring Mental Health Problems: *A Qualitative Study. Journal of Mental Health*, 16, pp. (493-503).

Soundy, A., Smith, B., Dawes, H., Pall, H., Gimbrere, K., Ramsay, J. (2011). Patient's expression of hope in three neurogloical conditions; a meta-ethnography. *Health Psychology Review*, ifirst, 1-25. DOI: 10.1080/17437199.2011.568856.

Tetlie, T., Heimsnes, M., & Almvi, R. (2009). Using exercise to treat patients with severe mental illness: how and why? *Journal of Psychsocal Nursing and Mental Health Services*, 47, pp. (32-40).

Ussher, M., Stanbury, L., Cheeseman, V., Faulkner, G. (2007). Physicl activity preferences and perceived barriers to activity among persons with severe mental illness in the united kingdom. *Psychiatric Services*, 58, pp. (405-408).

Van Mannen, J., Manning, P.K., & Miller, M.L. (1988). Series editors' introduction. In G.W. Noblit & R.D. Hare (Eds.), *Meta-ethnography: Synthesising qualitative studies* pp. (5-6). London: Sage

Weed, M. (2008). A potential method for the interpretive synthesis of qualitative research: Issues in the development of meta-interpretation. *International Journal of Social Research Methodology*, 11, pp. (13-28).

Part 2

Evaluation

3

Temporal Stability of Repeated Assessments of Problematic Internet Use Among Adolescents: A Prospective Cohort Study

Lawrence T. Lam[1,2]
[1]*The School of Medicine Sydney, The University of Notre Dame Australia*
[2]*Disciple of Paediatrics and Child Health,*
Sydney Medical School, The University of Sydney,
Australia

1. Introduction

The growth of Internet usage has been phenomenal in the last decade. According to the latest statistics on worldwide usage of the Internet, there has been a 4-times increase in the number of users.[1] In terms of regional distributions by geographic locations, Asia is the area with the highest number of Internet users in the world in 2009 with more than 764.4 millions.[1] With such a large population of Internet users, misuse and loss of control in the use of the Internet should not be expected rare events.

Problematic Internet use has been identified as a potential mental health issue that exhibits some signs and symptoms similar to other established additions since the mid-90s.[2-5] Since then the term "Internet Addiction" has been proposed and different opinions have been put forward as to whether problematic Internet use should be considered as a psychiatric disorder or a mental illness similar to other well established addictive disorders.[6-11] Until now, "Internet Addiction" is not included as a disorder in the latest version of the Diagnostic and Statistical Manual of Mental Disorders-IV Text Revision (DSM-IV-TR) as well as in the International Classification of Diseases-10 (ICD-10).[12-13]

The major contention of whether the problematic use of the Internet should be considered as an addiction in the conventional sense, such as in the case of substance dependent disorder, is how well Internet addiction can fulfil the validation criteria as a psychiatric disorder.[14] Robins and Guze, who first proposed a set of formal criteria for establishing the validity of psychiatric diagnoses, suggested five criteria.[15] These include: a clear clinical description of the disorder; evidence from laboratory studies; exclusion of other disorders; follow-up studies; and family studies.[15] In terms of the first criterion, a volume of work by many researchers has provided an informative debate.[6-11] Evidence from laboratory studies implies the possibility of bio-markers and validated psychiatric and psychological assessments. Recent studies using imaging techniques have provided some results for supporting differences in brain activities between problematic and normal Internet users.[16-18] Studies on the co-morbidities of problematic Internet use have been paving the way for the establishment of a clear picture for differential diagnoses of "Internet Addiction".[19] Follow-up studies, as suggested by George, reflect the ability of demonstrating temporal stability of the diagnosis and family studies suggest the possibility of a genetic basis for the disorder.[14] These criteria are most difficult to satisfy and there is a lack of evidence in the area of problematic Internet use. To be able to demonstrate the temporal stability of a diagnosis of "Internet Addiction", distinct clinical profiles of symptoms are to be maintained overtime and not evolved into a different disorder. In order to demonstrate the temporal stability of a diagnosis of "Internet Addiction", cohort studies with repeated assessments using a validated instrument are necessary. So far, no such report has been identified in the literature.

The primary aim of this study is to bridge the knowledge gap in providing information on the temporal stability in the assessment of problematic Internet use, or the lack of it, across different time points among a cohort of young people recruited in a prospective longitudinal study. Individuals who were identified as problematic Internet users repeatedly across all time points were considered as "temporal stable" cases.

2. Materials and methods

This prospective cohort study was conducted in Guangzhou city of the Guangdong Province in Southeast China in July 2008. Guangzhou is the capital city of the Guangdong Province which is the most populous province in China. It was estimated that the population size of the city was nearly 10 million in 2006. Institute ethics approval for the study was granted by the Department of Psychological Education of Elementary and Secondary Schools of the Province Administration.

The methodologies of the baseline phase of the study were described in previous reports.[20] In brief, the sample was generated from the total student population of adolescents who attended high schools within the region and were registered with the Guangzhou city secondary school registry. A stratified random sampling method with stratification according to the proportion of students in metropolitan and rural areas was used for sample generation. The sample consisted of adolescents aged between 13 and 18 years.

The cohort study was conducted on campus at different schools with baseline data collected via a health survey carried out within the same week. Selected students from different schools were recruited with informed consent, either granted by students' parents or students themselves depending on their ages, to participate in the survey. Students were invited to fill in a self-reported questionnaire designed specifically for the study. The cohort was then followed for 9 months with resurvey conducted on problematic Internet use at 3 months and 9 months after the baseline survey.

Problematic use of the Internet was assessed by the Internet Addiction Test (IAT) also known as the Young's Internet Addiction Scale (YIAS) designed by Young.[21] The IAT is a 20 item self-reported scale based on the DSM-IV diagnostic criteria for pathological gambling. It includes questions that reflect typical behaviours of addiction. An example question is: "How often do you feel depressed, moody, or nervous when you are off-line, which goes away once you are back on-line?" Respondents were asked to indicate the propensity of their responses on a Likert scale ranging from 1 (rarely) to 5 (always). Total scores were calculated with possible scores ranging from a minimum of 20 to a maximum of 100. The severity of addiction was then classified according to the suggested cut-off scores with 20-49 points as "normal", 50-79 points as "moderate", and 80-100 points as "severe".[21] As only a few students scored 80 points or higher in this study, the exposure variable was dichotomised into two categories: "Severe/moderate" and "normal" for ease of data analysis.

Other information collected in the baseline survey included demographics, metropolitan or
rural schools, location of family residence, whether the respondent was a single child, and
parental education levels. Psychosocial information was also collected on drinking status,
depression, and satisfaction with family relationships. Depression was assessed using the
Zung Self-rating Depression Scale (SDS) and family relationships were assessed using the
Family satisfaction subscale of the Multidimensional Student's Life Satisfaction Scale
(MSLSS) at baseline.[22-23]
Data were analysed using the Stata V10.0 statistical software program.[24] As this study was
descriptive in nature, variables were summarised with frequencies and percentages.
Temporal stability in the assessment of problematic Internet users, or the lack of it, was
reported as estimated proportions of problematic users identified across different points in
time. The 95% confidence intervals for these estimated proportions were also calculated.
Comparisons of the mean IAT scores between the "temporal stable" and "temporal
unstable" cases at baseline, 3 month and 9 month follow-ups were conducted using
independent Student's t-tests.

3. Results

A total of 1618 students were recruited and responded to the baseline survey providing
usable information. Of these 1293 students responded to the follow-up questionnaires at the
3 and 9 month follow-ups. This represented a follow-up rate of 79.9%. Comparisons
between the respondents and non-respondents indicated no statistically significant
differences in terms of age, sex, and whether attending city or rural schools. The
characteristics and outcome measures of the respondents were summarised in Table 1.
Slightly less than half of the sample were aged below 15 years (n=619, 47.9%) with a mean
age of 15.0 years (s.d.=1.8). There were slightly more females (n=722, 55.8%) than males, and
about half were studying in a city school (n=650, 50.3%). In terms of demographics, the
majority of the families resided in the city (n=923, 71.4%) and slightly more than half were
the only child in the family (n=735, 57.1%). The majority of their parents attained at least a
level of secondary education, with about 15% of fathers and 11% of mothers receiving post
secondary education levels including university and post graduate education. One hundred
and seventy one (13.2%) students scored moderate to severe on the Zung's Depression Scale
and about 10 percent (n=132) of respondents reported drinking 3-4 times within a month
prior to the baseline survey. More than a quarter of students indicated that they were very
dissatisfied with their family relationships (n=280, 21.7%) at baseline.
In terms of assessment for problematic Internet use, 11.1% (n=143) of the sample could be
classified as having a high risk of problematic Internet use at baseline, 8.3% (n=107) at the 3
month follow-up, and 5.6% (n=72) at the 9 month follow-up.
Table 2 and 3 summarised the number of students assessed to be problematic Internet users
across different time points throughout the entire follow-up period. As shown, only 25
students were classified as problematic Internet users at all three time points at baseline, 3
months, and 9 months. These represented less than 2% (1.9%, 95%C.I.=1.3%-3.8%) of the
entire cohort, and 17.5% (95%C.I.=11.6%-24.7%) of the 143 assessed as problematic Internet
users at baseline. Only 32 students (2.5%, 95%C.I.=1.7%-3.5%) were classified as problematic
Internet users consecutively at baseline and at 3 months follow-up, and 13 students (1.0%,

Variables	Frequency (%)
Problematic use of the Internet at baseline	
Moderate/Severe	143 (11.1)
Normal	1250 (88.9)
Problematic use of the Internet at 3 months follow-up	
Moderate/Severe	107 (8.3)
Normal	1186 (91.7)
Problematic use of the Internet at 9 months follow-up	
Moderate/Severe	72 (5.6)
Normal	1221 (94.4)
Demographics	
Age group	
<15 yrs	619 (47.9)
≥15 yrs	674 (52.1)
Sex	
Male	571 (44.2)
Female	722 (55.8)
City school	
Yes	650 (50.3)
No	643 (49.7)
Family located at	
Rural	182 (14.1)
Semi-rural	188 (14.5)
City	923 (71.4)
Single child	
Yes	735 (57.1)
No	552 (42.9)
Father's education level	
Lower than senior high school	433 (34.8)
Senior high/technical	616 (49.5)
University of higher	196 (15.7)
Mother's education level	
Lower than senior high school	570 (44.5)
Senior high/technical	565 (44.1)
University of higher	146 (11.4)
Depression symptom	
Moderate/severe	171 (13.2)
Normal	1121 (86.8)
Dissatisfaction with family relationship	
Very dissatisfied	280 (21.7)
Others	1013 (78.3)
Drinking in the last month	
3-4 times	132 (10.3)
1-2 times or none	1153 (89.7)

Table 1. Frequency distributions of problematic Internet use across time, demographics, and other variables of adolescents in the study sample (N=1293)

Baseline survey	3 months resurvey				Total
	Yes		No		
	9 months resurvey		9 months resurvey		
	Yes	No	Yes	No	
Yes	**25**	32	19	67	143
No	13	37	15	1085	1150
Total	38	69	34	1152	
Grand Total	107		1186		1293

Table 2. Proportions of problematic Internet user identified by different times of survey

Problematic Internet user identified at different time points	Frequency	Percentage (95%C.I.)
Normal user across all surveys	1085	83.8 (81.6-85.7)
Identified only at baseline	67	5.2 (4.0-6.5)
Identified only at 3 months resurvey	37	2.9 (2.0-3.9)
Identified only at 9 months resurvey	15	1.2 (0.7-1.9)
Identified at baseline and 3 months resurveys	32	2.5 (1.7-3.5)
Identified at baseline and 9 months resurveys	19	1.5 (0.9-2.3)
Identified at 3 months and 9 months resurveys	13	1.0 (0.5-1.7)
Identified at all 3 surveys	25	1.9 (1.3-2.8)

Table 3. Frequency and percentages (95%C.I.) of problem Internet users by time categories (N=1293)

95%C.I.=0.5%-1.7%) at 3 month as well as at 9 month follow-up. Comparisons of the mean IAT scores between "temporal stable" and "temporal unstable" cases indicated significant differences between groups across all three time points with the "temporal stable" group scoring higher by 18.0 (95%C.I=12.5-23.4), 15.9 (95%C.I.=10.4-21.4), and 20.7 (95%C.I.=14.8-26.6) at baseline, 3 month and 9 month follow-up respectively.

4. Discussion

This study aims to examine the assessment profile of problematic Internet usage across time in a cohort of young people in Southeast China. The main reason for the study is to provide information on temporal stability in the assessment of problematic Internet usage in response to one of the requirements of Robins and Guze's criteria for the validity of a psychiatric diagnosis for "Internet Addiction". The results of the study indicated that of the 143 students identified as problematic Internet users at baseline, only 25 (17%) were re-identified as problematic users in the two follow-up surveys. If a criterion that a larger proportion of individuals assessed to be problematic Internet users were re-identified repeatedly at all three time points indicated temporal stability, then the results of the study did not provide strong evidence for temporal stability in the assessment of problematic Internet use. In terms of the temporal stability of the diagnosis, to the knowledge of the authors this is the first attempt of the diagnostic validity of "Internet Addiction" as a potential psychiatric disorder. Due to the lack of a similar study on the same topic, a comparison of results would be difficult.

There could be three possible interpretations of the results. First, is that temporal stability in the assessment of problematic Internet use is difficult to achieve, as it has been noted in other established psychiatric disorders.[14] This may be due to transient characteristics of problematic Internet use. Results from a longitudinal study on risk factors for "Internet Addiction" among adolescents suggested that mood state, particularly depression, is predictive of Internet use.[26] Since mood state in adolescents is highly sensitive to circumstantial as well as their internal physical conditions, mood fluctuations occur frequently. The transient characteristics of problematic Internet use may just be a behavioural manifestation of their mood changes. The second interpretation of the results is that the lack of temporal stability in the assessment of problematic Internet use is because of a lack of validity and reliability of the assessment instrument. One major criticism on the proposal of a clinical diagnosis of "Internet Addiction" is that the psychometric properties of most assessment instruments designed for measuring "Internet Addiction" as a psychological construct are unsupported by rigorous examinations.[27] Of the few reports on the validation of the IAT published in the international literature, factor structural and convergent validity were the main focus.[28,29] However, no information on test-retest reliability was provided, thus the temporal validity of the construct that the IAT is designed to assess is unknown. The results of this study suggest a general lack of temporal validity. Third, temporal stability can only be achieved for those who are at very high risk of problematic usage, but not for users with moderate risk. Results of this study render some support to the notion that "temporal stable" cases scored significantly higher on the IAT than "temporal unstable" cases consistently across time. The possible explanation of the results obtained from the study could be anyone one, or a combination, of the above interpretations.

As in all studies, there are strengths and weaknesses in this study. This is a population-based study that includes a random sample of students. No significant differences have been found between respondents and non-respondents suggesting a representative sample. A potential limitation has been identified in this study. Information on problematic Internet use is collected via self-reporting. Hence this will constitute a report bias in the outcome variable. To improve the study quality, in future studies informants should be used in conjunction with information collected from respondents.

In conclusion, it is important to have a general consensus on the definition of "Internet Addiction" within the psychiatric and psychological community in order to design and develop an appropriate assessing instrument that is based on well-framed theoretical models and is supported by empirical data. Once the appropriate instrument has been adopted, the temporal stability in the assessment is also an important aspect in establishing a proper clinical diagnosis for a psychiatric disorder. In the area of problematic Internet use, given the vast growing population of Internet users, there is an urgent need for researchers and clinicians to develop a general consensus on the issue as well as to work towards a proper evidence-based diagnosis and potential treatment strategies for the problem.

5. Acknowledgements

The authors would like to acknowledge the Ministry of Education, Guangdong Province, PR China in providing financial support for the study.

6. Declaration

All authors ensure that there is no conflict of interest of any kind that involved in the production of this manuscript nor is the study associated with any commercial bodies. No competing financial interests exist.

7. References

[1] Miniwatts marketing Group. Internet usage statistics. Bogota, Colombia. Available on:http:\\www.internetworldstatistics.com/stats.htm (last accessed 05/05/2010)

[2] Young KS. Psychology of computer use: XL. Addictive use of the Internet: a case that breaks the stereotype. Psychology Report 1996; 79:899-902.

[3] Young KS. (1998) *Caught in the net.* NY, John Wiley & Sons.

[4] Oreilly M. Internet addiction: a new disorder enters the medical lexicon. Canadian Medical Association Journal 1996; 154:1882-3.

[5] Shapira NA, Lessig MC, Goldsmith TD, et al. Problematic internet use: proposed classification and diagnostic criteria. Depression and Anxiety 2003; 17:207-16.

[6] Young KS. Internet addiction: The emergence of a new clinical disorder. Cyberpsychology & Behavior 1998; 1:237-44.

[7] Shaffer HJ, Kall MN, Vander BJ. "Computer addiction": a critical consideration. American Journal of Orthopsychiatry 2000; 70:162-8.

[8] Ko CH, Yen JY, Chen CC, Chen SH, Yen CF. Proposed diagnostic criteria of Internet Addiction for adolescents. J Nerv Ment Dis 2005; 193:728-33.

[9] Block JJ. Issues for DSM-V: Internet Addiction. Am J Psychi 2008; 165:3.

[10] Pies R. Should DSM-V Designate "Internet Addiction" a mental disorder? Psychiatry [Edgmont] 2009; 6:31-7.

[11] Lenihan F. Computer addiction- a sceptical view: Invited commentary on: Lost Online. Advances in Psychiatric Treatment 2007; 13:31.

[12] American Psychiatric Association. Diagnostic and Statistical Manual of Mental Disorders, Fourth Edition, Text Revision (DSM-IV-TR). Arlington, VA: American Psychiatric Publishing Inc. 2000.

[13] World Health Organisation. The ICD-10 Classification of mental and behavioural disorder: diagnostic criteria for research. Geneva: World Health Organisation, 2003.

[14] George S, Lenihan F. Is Internet addiction a valid psychiatric disorder? Available on: http://priory.com/psychiatry/Internet_Addiction.htm. (last accessed 06/05/2010)

[15] Robins E, Guze SB. Establishment of psychiatric validity in psychiatric illness: its application to schizophrenia. American Journal of Psychiatry 1970; 126:983-7.

[16] Ko CH, Liu GC, Hslao S. Yen JY, Yang MJ, Lin WC, et al. Brain activities associated with gaming urge of online gaming addiction. J Psychiatric Research 2008; 43:739-47.

[17] Zhou Y, Lin FC, Du YS, Qin LD, Zhao ZM, Xu JR. et al. Gray matter abnormalities in Internet addiction: A voxel-based morphometry study. Eur J Radiol 2009; 17. [Epub ahead of print]

[18] Park HS, Kim SH, Bang SA, Yoon EJ, Cho SS, Kim SE. Altered regional cerebral glucose metabolism in internet game overusers: a 18F-fluorodeoxyglucose positron emission tomography study. CNS Spectr 2010; 15:159-66.

[19] Ko CH, Yen JY, Yen CF, Chen CS, Chen CC. The psychiatric comorbidity of Internet addiction: a review of the literature. European Psychiatry in press.

[20] Lam LT, Peng ZW, Mai JC, Jing J. Factors associated with Internet addiction among adolescents. Cyberpsycology and Behaviour 2009; 12:551-5.

[21] Young KS. The Internet Addiction Test. Center for On-Line Addictions. Bradford, USA. Available at:
http://www.netaddiction.com/resources/Internet_addiction_test.htm.
(last accessed 30th Nov. 2008).

[22] Widyanto L., McMurran M. The psychometric properties of the Internet Addiction Test. Cyberpsychol Behav 2004; 7:443-50.

[23] Zung W. A self-rating depression scale. Archives of General Psychiatry 1965; 12:63-70.

[24] Huebner ES, Laughlin J E, Ash C, Gilman R. Further validation of the Multidimensional Students' Life Satisfaction Scale. Journal of Psychological Assessment 1998; 16:118-134.

[25] StataCorp (2007). Stata Statistical Software: Release 10.0. College Station, TX: Stata Corporation.

[26] Ko CH, Yen JY, Chen CS, Yeh YC, Yen CF. Predictive values of psychiatric symptoms for Internet Addiction in adolescents: A 2-year prospective study. Arch Pediatric Adolesc Med 2009; 163:937-43.

[27] Beard KW. Internet addiction: a review of current assessment techniques and potential assessment questions. CyberPsycho Behav 2005; 8:7-14.

[28] Widyanto L., McMurran M. The psychometric properties of the Pathological use of the Internet Test. Cyberpsychol Behav 2004; 7:443-50.

[29] Khazaal Y, Billeux J, Thorens G, Khan R, Louati Y, Scarlatti E, et al. French validation of the Internet Addiction Test. CyberPsychol Behav 2008; 11:703-6.

4

The Youth Comprehensive Risk Assessment (YCRA) as a Treatment Guidance Tool for Adolescents with Behavioral and Developmental Challenges

Kenneth M. Coll[1], Brenda J. Freeman[2], John Butgereit[1],
Patti Thobro[3] and Robin Haas[3]
[1]Boise State University,
[2]Northwest Nazarene University,
[3]Cathedral Home for Children,
USA

1. Introduction

This chapter describes the evolution of the Youth Comprehensive Risk Assessment (YCRA) by first describing the need, then the evolution of the assessment tool, and finally studies that provide validation.

2. The need: Risk factors associated with troubled adolescents

Much has been written about the factors that contribute to troubled adolescence. Hawkins, et al. (1992) and Hawkins, et al. (2000) found mounting evidence that adolescents who are most at risk for committing serious and violent crimes tend to display high levels of risk factors such as alcohol and other drug (AOD) abuse or addiction, lack of parent-child closeness, family conflict, beliefs and attitudes favorable to criminality, early childhood aggressiveness, antisocial behavior, and poor peer acceptance. Additionally, juvenile delinquency has long been associated with certain societal ills, such as easy access to alcohol and other drugs and family splintering (Hawkins, et al., 2000). Huizinga, et al. (2000) noted serious delinquency with co-occurring AOD abuse and mental health problems. However, common clinical practice is to provide broad-based assessment, with heavy reliance on clinical judgment without a self report component. This is now deemed a major limitation to distinguishing higher and lower risk youth (Huizinga, et al., 2000).

It is not uncommon for troubled youth who commit serious and violent crime to find themselves in therapeutic communities (TC) and/or residential treatment facilities (Coll, et al., 2004; LeCroy & Ashford, 1992: Lyons, Kisiel, Dulcan, Cohen, & Chesler, 1997). Indeed, MacKenzie (1999) found that out-of-home placements for delinquent adolescents grew 51% between 1987 and 1996. Not surprisingly, adolescents treated via out-of-home placements were more likely to report higher levels of AOD abuse and more severe behavioral problems than adolescents treated via outpatient programs (Coll et al., 2003). Despite the severity of initial problems, youth in out-of home placements typically reported significantly reduced drug use and criminal activities and improved psychosocial development and interpersonal functioning outcomes after at least six months of treatment (Coll, et al., 2003; Hanson, 2002). Indeed, the professional literature is replete with reports of beneficial outcomes of residential treatment for adolescents and society in general including reduction in recidivism (re-offending), cost-benefit savings for communities and society, and increases in academic performance, and psychological adjustment (French, McCollister, Sacks, McKendrick, & De Leon, 2002; Grietens & Hellinckx, 2003). Consistent with recommendations by Huizinga, et al., (2000) and Hawkins, et al., (2000), Lyons, et al. (1998) noted that to successfully determine the appropriateness of care for those in residential settings, the needs of youth must be assessed in a systematic, reliable, and clinically-relevant manner. Child welfare funding sources are now demanding such information, recommending a thorough assessment process that covers a number of known risk areas (Mordock, 2000). Other studies with residential youth offenders have also indicated that carefully assessing major risk behaviors and promoting intensive, individualized treatment should become the preferred practices for working with youth in residential treatment (Burdsal, Force, & Klingsporn, 1990; Grimley, Williams, Miree, Baichoo, Greene, & Hook, 2000). Individualized comprehensive assessment processes are considered paramount for producing positive outcomes, as is the need to provide information to counselors and other staff members (e.g., teachers, youth workers) in order to enhance the intentionality of their treatment and to increase their ability to appropriately customize treatment plans.

2.1 Site
The adolescent residential treatment site is a Joint Commission for the Accreditation of Healthcare Organizations [JCAHO- now called The Joint Commission (TJC)], accredited 80-bed facility with an on-site accredited school located in the Rocky Mountain Region of the United States. The facility received court-referred adolescents, most of who are involved in criminal activity. Often these referrals are perceived by officers of the court, parents, and the adolescent themselves as their "last chance" treatment before being placed in long term and highly restricted juvenile detention. The residents, ages 11 -18, are court mandated for a variety of offenses ranging from running away to homicide. Treatment at the facility typically consists of a full school day; recreational, outdoor, and equine therapy; and individual, group, and family counseling. Residents average per week one hour of individual counseling, four hours of group counseling, and thirty minutes of family counseling. Although efforts to provide objective evidence of treatment efficacy have always been made by professional staff, pursuit of JCAHO (TJC) accreditation has made this imperative. Case reviews of residents who did not succeed in the program suggested prominent factors of substance abuse, aggression, and running away. Based on these early findings and professional literature reviews, more formal assessment procedures were instituted by professional staff, which ultimately led to the development of a comprehensive risk assessment process, now called the YCRA.

2.2 Population
The population typically is 45 to 50% female and 50 to 55% male. The ethnic composition tends to be about 90% Caucasian, 5% Hispanic, and 5% African-American. The average age is typically about 14.5 years (range was 12-17). The adolescents are assessed during the first month of their stay by a team of licensed professional counselors, psychologists, and social workers.

2.3 Development of a comprehensive risk assessment process and instrumentation called the YCRA

Efforts of the staff at the adolescent treatment facility to respond to the aforementioned trends and recommendations began approximately fifteen years ago. Specifically, professional staff investigated the presence of common factors among adolescent and child clients who failed to successfully complete their residential treatment programs. Case reviews suggested that the most prominent prediction factors for program failure included high run-away risks, multiple prior placements, aggression, substance use, and poor family resources.

On the basis of these early findings and literature recommendations for individualized comprehensive assessment (Lyons, et al., 1997), more formal assessment procedures were instituted as part of the treatment process. Increased early assessment efforts at admission were designed to ascertain those areas around which youth were the most troubled, needed longer treatment, required greater supervision, and posed a higher risk to self and others. Additionally, it was hypothesized that these efforts would help predict which youth would improve better and/or faster in treatment, and what additional information might be needed about each youth to further enhance treatment efficacy. Treatment staff in residential treatment have historically disagreed on whom was "more troubled or less troubled," creating clinical discrepancies and inconsistencies. Thus, consistent with suggestions from the professional literature to discern frequency and intensity of risk factors, an identification process was developed to contrast those residents who scored high or "yes" in chemical abuse, conduct-disorder behaviors, criminal thinking, and low family bonding and those who did not. This identification process was deemed important because staff often disagreed on treatment approaches, as well as which residents were at higher risk, needed more help, or functioned most poorly.

To this end, standardized self-report instruments were selected, including the SASSI-A2 (Substance Abuse Subtle Screening Inventory for Adolescents, second edition, Miller, 2001), and the FACES-III (Family Adaptability and Cohesion Scales, Olson, 1985). Additional clinical judgment information was gathered at admission and included the presence of any conduct-disorder behaviors (APA, 1994) and the extent of criminal thinking patterns, which was based on Samenow's (1998) 17 errors of criminal thinking behavior. Instruments used in this investigation adhered to Mordock's (2000) recommendations that child and youth assessment processes include both sound clinician-rated measures and standardized client-completed measures. A discussion of the measures used in this study is included below.

2.4 Standardized client-completed measures

To measure chemical addiction/abuse, the SASSI-A2 (Miller, 2001) was utilized. The SASSI-A2 has been shown to be useful in a broad array of contexts, including court systems and mental health settings (F. Miller, 2001). According to Miller, the adolescent form of the SASSI was developed for ages 12 to 18. The SASSI-A2 consists of 52 true/false questions and 26 items with a 0 to 3 scoring format. This allows for self-report of negative consequences of use of alcohol and other drugs. Through research and clinical trials carried out over 16 years (Miller), the test has exhibited greater than 90% accuracy in identifying those with chemical dependency. Miller indicates that items on the SASSI-A2 touch a broad spectrum of topics seemingly unrelated to chemical abuse, which makes the instrument less threatening to abusers. Other studies have validated such findings (see Coll et al., 2003).

Olson's (1985) FACES III was utilized to measure family functioning and specifically family bonding. FACES III is intended for members of families across the life cycle. The 20 items with a 1-4 Likert scale were developed to be readable and understandable to adolescents as young as 12 years old. For the purpose of this study, the cohesion scale, defined by Olson as the emotional bonding that family members have toward one another, was used. According to Olson, internal reliability for the cohesion scale is .77 and test-retest reliability is .83. Content validity is reported to be very good (Olson, 1985).

2.5 Clinician-rated measures

Behaviors symptomatic of conduct disorder were assessed by the staff counselors (all holding master's degrees in counseling or social work and holding state licenses) using previous records and a DSM-IV-TR (APA, 2000) conduct disorder checklist. These interviews were conducted after the adolescent was on-site for at least two weeks. A conduct disorder checklist using the DSM-IV criteria has been recommended in the literature as an effective way for assessment and monitoring conduct disorder behaviors (Miller, Trapani, Fejes-Mendoza, & Eggleston, 1995; Zoccolillo & Rogers, 1992).

Criminal thinking was also rated by staff counselors using a scale based upon Samenow's (1984; 1998) 17 errors in thinking. On two occasions, Samenow visited the facility and trained staff in using his criminal thinking assessment process. Sample inquiries include "For each of the following characteristics, please rate (the youth) on the extent to which he demonstrates these tendencies or thinking patterns:" pride (e.g., refusal to back down, even on little points), victim stance (e.g., conveying a sense of the "poor me" attitude), and anger (e.g., using anger to try and control people). A Likert scale was used to assess each thinking error (1=almost not at all, 2=some, 3=half the time, 4=frequent, and 5=almost all the time). Assessing criminal thinking patterns and errors using Samenow's (1998) approach has been in clinical use for many years (Coll, Juhnke, Thobro, & Haas, 2003; Coll, Thobro, & Haas, 2004). Examples of such thinking errors include power tactics, refusing to accept responsibility, and lack of empathy (Samenow, 1984, 1998).

3. The youth comprehensive risk assessment

These assessments were initially piloted and reported under an "umbrella" assessment that was employed as a comprehensive risk factor summary based on the six factors developed from the professional literature (listed below). This summary is now used to make level-of-care decisions (i.e. residential, group home, outpatient care). In the piloting phase, scores from the SASSI-A2 and FACES-III, as well as historical and anecdotal information from the client's record, were included. Additionally, the staff assessments of clients' criminal thinking patterns and history of conduct-disordered behaviors were also included in the risk assessment. This group of assessments and the protocol followed in the administration and interpretation of the total package became a comprehensive risk factor and social functioning summary called the YCRA (Coll et al., 2004).

The YCRA was submitted and approved as a performance measurement system with the Joint Commission for the Accreditation of Health Organizations (JCAHO, now TJC) (1998). Per the JCAHO approved definition, the YCRA is specifically defined as a clinical assessment process utilized by trained mental health professionals to systematically gather information and make clinical judgments related to six risk areas: (a) risk to self (including risk for suicide, self-harm, becoming a victim, and risk-taking); (b) risk to others (including aggression, sexually inappropriate behavior, and destruction of property); (c) social and adaptive functioning (including developmental disorders, handicaps, cognitive disorganization, and social skills); (d) substance abuse/dependency; (e) family resources; and (f) degree of structure needed (frequency of out-of-home placements and need for supervision). Subscales and individual items from the MPD, SASSI-A2, the conduct disorder checklist, and the criminal thinking assessment, as well as historical and anecdotal information, are used to determine scores in five of the six areas (risk to self, risk to others, social and adaptive functioning, substance abuse/dependency, and degree of structure needed). The FACES III and historical/anecdotal information are used to measure the level of family resources.

The YCRA has met the rigorous criteria necessary for inclusion on JCAHO's list of approved performance measurement systems. The YCRA has met or exceeded system adherence to all of the JCAHO quality principles, including sampling, standardization, monitoring, documentation, feedback, education, and accountability (JCAHO, 1998). The YCRA used a non-equal interval Likert scale of 1 to 4x2 (8) based on the recommendations of child welfare experts (CWLA roundtable, 1999), with 1 being slight, 2 being mild, 3 being moderate and four times two (8) being severe and requiring immediate treatment interventions. The distinction between three and eight (4x2) was deemed very important to bring immediate treatment foci to these severe areas. An initial research investigation found that the YCRA predicted adolescent offenders' struggles with poor social skill development and life meaning (Coll, Thobro, & Haas, 2004). Currently, clinicians at the adolescent treatment facility where the YCRA was developed systematically gather information from these assessments and develop treatment goals and interventions related to the six risk areas. At 6-month intervals, the residents undergo a re-evaluation, which is designed to make adjustments in treatment planning and decisions about discharge (including timeframe and placement options). Two additional research studies are summarized here to provide further validation to the robust utility of the YCRA for assessment and effective treatment planning and implementation.

3.1 The YCRA distinguishes higher and lower risk youth
In using the YCRA, 13 residents indicated none of the risk factors present at high levels, 19 residents indicated one indicator present at a high level, and 18 indicated two indicators present at high levels. These 50 residents were categorized as "lower risk". Twenty-seven of the residents indicated three indicators present at high levels, and 20 indicated all factors present at a high level. As clinical and other professional staff (e.g., teachers, administrators) strongly agreed that this warranted 'high risk' status, these 47 residents were categorized as "higher risk". These two groups were used in the following analyses.

The "higher risk" residents were compared with the "lower risk" residents. T-test analyses and effect size calculations (Cohen, 1988; Dunlop, Cortina, Vaslow, & Burke, 1996) ascertained statistically significant differences and the magnitude of the differences between the two groups on clinical perceptions from professional staff on the six YCRA areas.

The higher risk residents were reported by staff to have significantly more problems with social functioning ($t = 2.95$, $df = 95$, $p = .004$; $d = .70$), substance abuse ($t = 2.12$, $df = 95$, $p = .037$; $d = .44$), and needed a significantly higher degree of structure in treatment ($t = 2.94$, $df = 95$, $p = .005$; $d = .74$). They also exhibited a significantly higher risk to self ($t = 2.20$, $df = 95$, $p = .03$; $d = .48$), and to others ($t = 3.98$, $df = 95$, $p = .000$; $d = .93$). Analyses indicated that higher and lower risk youth were not significantly different in family resources available, with both groups reporting high need for such resources.

Cohen (1988) suggested that effect sizes (d) of .20, .50, and .80 be considered small, medium, and large, respectively. Based on these criteria, effect sizes fell in the medium to large range. The conclusion can thus be made that these results have not only statistical significance but also practical significance. Another way to interpret effect sizes is by transforming them into percentiles (Gall, Borg, & Gall, 1996). The range of reported effect sizes equates to percentile differences ranging from 17 to 42 percentile points. The large percentile point differences between the groups support the practical significance of these findings.

In terms of specific treatment strategies for higher risk to self, Coll, Thobro, and Haas (2004) noted that depressed adolescents show very different symptomology than adults, typically with fewer verbal expressions of depression, and with much more disruptive behaviors. As Capuzzi and Gross (1996) indicated, depressive behavior in adolescents is commonly found in irritable mood rather than depressed mood, and in somatic complaints and social withdrawal. Interventions now being implemented for helping depressed adolescents include asset building, focusing on increasing sense of self-worth and reducing isolation, teaching stress management, encouraging better communication and problem solving skills, helping promote inner directedness (e.g., through journaling), and providing appropriate psychotropic medications (Jongsma, Peterson, & McInnis, 1996).

The results of this study also reveal poor family resources (including low bonding) as a major treatment issue for all youth investigated. Bowlby's (1988) therapeutic tasks for building better attachment and healthy human development are currently being infused into family, group, and individual interactions at this facility. Two key therapeutic tasks identified for building a secure base include exploring various unhappy and painful aspects of life with a trusted facilitator and consistent encouragement, sympathy, and, on occasion, guidance.

In terms of the risk factors of social and adaptive functioning and need for supervision, the facility staff is currently integrating social skill feedback and intensive supervision (e.g., on-on-one supervision) within the context of 'Life Space Intervention' (Brentro, et. al., 1998). Life Space Intervention is a humanistic, developmental approach that accents on-on-one interactions at 'teachable moments' (e.g., when processing recent antisocial behaviors) by getting the youth's perspective, clarifying perceptions, and helping youth develop strategies to succeed. Challenge is inherent in delivering effective treatment strategies for youth offenders. Progress can be a slow process and the aforementioned interventions require consistent and compassionate involvement.

The agency is also exploring stepped-care treatment to increase efficiency and effectiveness (e.g., focusing on less expensive, intrusive writing therapies in combination with more expensive, intrusive face-to-face counseling). For example, writing therapy and especially distance writing (between youth and family members, school counselors, et al.) has proven to be quite powerful (L'Abate, 2011). L'Abate (2011) recently indicated that especially with impulsive, acting out adolescents, distance writing (with properly targeted workbooks) greatly helps these adolescents to learn to think before acting.

3.2 The YCRA distinguishes treatment strategies for more 'disengaged' youth

The second research study investigated what significant YCRA differences existed between more family disengaged youth and less disengaged (Per FACES III assessment) and what were the treatment implications.

For comparison purposes, youths were grouped into "disengaged" (n = 155) and "nondisengaged" (n = 143), that is, separated, connected, and enmeshed per the FACES-III cut off scores (Olson 1986). The t-test analysis indicated significant differences between the groups scoring significantly higher in behaviors related to destruction of property (p = .05, ES = .25), deceitfulness or theft (p = .002, effect size [ES] = .36), and serious violation of the rules (p < .000, ES = .56). There was no significant difference between the groups for aggression to people and animals (p = .578).

The t-test analysis also indicated significant differences between the groups for   other at-risk behaviors, per the YCRA, with the disengaged group scoring significantly higher in risk to self ($p < .000$, ES = .46) and substance abuse ($p = .006$, ES = .33) and significantly lower in family resources ($p < .000$, ES = .52).

Further supporting the statistical and practical significance of this study, based on effect sizes, are Gall, Borg, and Gall's (1996) criteria. These researchers noted that another effective way to interpret small, medium, and large effect sizes is by transforming them into percentiles. The range of reported effect sizes equates to percentile differences between the groups, ranging from 17% for smaller effect size differences to 42% for larger effect size differences. The large percentile point (effect size) differences. Again, the large percentile point (effect size) differences between the groups in this study support the practical significance of these findings. (For example, differences between the groups for risk to self would be at least 25 %.)

A family intervention program to address these and other questions is currently being piloted at this treatment facility. Components of the intervention include ongoing discussion and specific goal setting with families based on the FACES-III Cohesion Scale items (e.g., spending time together and asking each other for help) and thorough asset searching to reinforce strengths and adoptable functioning of the youths and family. As Olson (2000) recommended, counselors are being active in structuring and monitoring family interaction to block or interrupt disruptive family interactions. The youth offender counselors at this agency are also striving to set modest concrete objectives to be reached through small increments of change to reduce anxiety and help families maintain change over time, per Olson's suggestions.

In addition, systemic interventions agency-wide are currently being discussed and have been inspired by the "Bridge Program" (Crowley & Bishop, 2008). New practices and policies under review include introducing families to staff members who are involved with their children, creating a calendar of events to keep families better informed, and inviting family members to go along on field trips and to attend special activities. Also, as previously mentioned, distance writing is also being implemented as a less intrusive strategy to increase family bonding (L'Abate, 2011).

This emerging comprehensive program certainly needs to be empirically tested. Yet, intentional individual, family, and agency-wide systemic interventions for adolescents and their families are being developed on the basis of these results. The uses of the FACES-III, Conduct Disorder Checklist, and YCRA have added needed consistency. The FACES-III, Conduct Disorder Checklist, and YCRA assessment processes are also reducing subjectivity. The results of this investigation are being used in more effective policies and practices and in providing more intentional training of caregivers, clinicians, teachers, families, and others to understand and help develop youths and their families' strengths.

4. Discussion

The goal of this chapter was to provide information to the counselors and other staff (e.g., teachers, youth workers) so that they could increase the intentionality of treatment and customize their treatment plans appropriately. Whereas this assessment tool was developed to improve services at one facility, it also may inform treatment procedures beyond as indicated by the identification of key mental health risk factors. Based on the YCRA additional studies explored here, treatment strategies at the facility have been implemented to assure and improve quality. The following includes an overview of the treatment provided.

Most of the referrals to the facility from the county court systems do not indicate a high need for substance abuse assessment and treatment (typically only about 20% to 30% of the referrals indicated a possible chemical dependency problem). Through the use of the YCRA, the facility now has changed its policy of comprehensive chemical abuse assessment from "when indicated" to "mandatory". Facility professionals have found Prochaska and DeClemente's (1992) stages-of-change model particularly helpful in conceptualizing youth as related to the YCRA, particularly the five stages of change: precontemplation, contemplation, preparation, action, and maintenance. Some youth are now more clearly identified in the "precontemplator" stage of motivation for change, defined as not considering change in problem behaviors, and lacking significant awareness related to these behaviors, even though such behaviors have brought a great deal of trouble. Such conceptualization has assisted staff in providing consistent interventions based upon Motivational Enhancement Therapy (e.g., Change Plan Worksheet, rolling with resistance) as well as reducing personal frustration and impatience (Miller & Rollnick, 2002).

YCRA factors such as higher risk to others (e.g. assault, sexual aggression, destruction of property) and poor social and adaptive functioning are common. Facility professionals are reporting benefits from YCRA information provided about conduct disorder and criminal thinking as social interactive dysfunctions that continue across generations and have severe consequences for others. This social-historical context within which the youth has functioned is often overlooked, frequently leading to failed treatment (Kazdin, 1993). Richters and Cicchetti (1993) emphasized the importance of early identification and treatment of conduct disordered behavior, which occurs when using the YCRA. Some effective strategies for reducing such risk according to Hawkins, et al. (2000) are being incorporated at the facility through YCRA assessment, including encouraging youth involvement in active classroom instruction; emphasizing interactive teaching and cooperative learning; using tutoring of the socially rejected youth; and providing assertiveness training. Solution focused counseling and Glasser's WDEP (wants, doing, evaluation, plan) approach are also being implemented as sound practices to promote insight and behavior change (Corey, 2001).

4.1 YCRA limitations and future research

The population is drawn from a single institution. Future YCRA research should include a larger number of participants from a diversity of residential youth settings. Future research should follow participants longitudinally to measure treatment outcomes.

5. Conclusion

This chapter provided evidence for the value of using the YCRA to formally assess risk factors, via clinical observation and self-reports. This emerging process needs to continue to be empirically tested. Yet, it can be argued that a more efficient system of care is developing for adolescents at this particular facility. The use of the YCRA has added consistency at this treatment facility. Lyons, et al. (1997) noted that the current youth offender assessment procedures rely too heavily on subjective ratings that are strongly influenced by clinician's idiosyncratic approaches. The assessment process described here reduces such subjectivity. The results are now being used in more effective training of caregivers, clinicians, teachers, families, and others to understand youths' individual needs and strengths.

For more information visit www.youthriskassessment.com

6. References

American Psychiatric Association (2000). *Diagnostic and Statistical Manual of Mental Disorders* (4th ed., rev.). Washington, DC: Author.

Bowlby, J. (1988). *A Secure Base.* London: Basic Books.

Brendtro, L.K., Brokenleg, M., & Van Bockern, S. (1998). *Reclaiming youth at risk.* Bloomington, Indiana: NES.

Burdsal, C., Force, R., & Klingsporn, M. J. (1990). Treatment effectiveness in young male offenders. *Residential Treatment for Children and Youth, 7,* 75-88.

Capuzzi, D., & Gross, D. R. (1996). *Youth at Risk* (2nd ed.). Alexandria, VA.: ACA

Child Welfare League of America (2000). Roundtable, personal communication, June 7, 2000, Denver, Colorado.

Cohen, J. (1988). *Statistical power analysis for the behavioral sciences* (2nd ed.). Hillsdale, NJ: Erlbaum.

Coll, K. M., Juhnke, G. A., Thobro, P., & Haas, R. (2003). A preliminary study using the Substance Abuse Subtle Screening Inventory – Adolescent Form (SASSI-A2) as an outcome measure with youth offenders. *Journal of Addictions and Offender Counseling, 24,* 11-22.

Coll, K.M., Thobro, P., & Haas, R. (2004). Relational and purpose development in youth offenders. Journal of Humanistic Counseling, Education and Development, 43, 41-49.

Corey, G. (2001). *Theory and practice of counseling and psychotherapy (6th ed.).* Belmont, CA: Wadsworth/Thompson Learning.

Dunlop, W., Cortina, J., Vaslow, J., & Burke, M. (1996). Meta-analysis of experiments with matched groups or repeated measures designs. *Psychological Methods, 1,* 170–177.

French, M.T., McCollister, K/E., Sacks, S., McKendrick, K., & De Leon (2002). Benefit-cost analysis of a modified therapeutic community for mentally ill chemical abusers. *Evaluation and Program Planning, 25,* 137-148.

Gall, M. D., Borg, W. R., & Gall, J. P. (1996). *Educational research: An introduction* (6th ed.). White Plains, NY: Longman.

Grietens, H., & Hellinckx, W. (2003). Evaluating effects of residential treatment for juvenile offenders by statistical metaanalisis: A review. *Aggression and Violent Behavior, 9,* 401-415.

Grimley, D., Williams, C.D., Miree, L.L., Baichoo, S., Greene, S., & Hook, E., (2000). Stages of readiness for changing multiple risk behaviors among incarcerated male adolescents. *American Journal of Health Behavior, 24,* 361-369.

Hanson, G. R. (2002). Therapeutic community: What is a therapeutic community? *National Institute of Drug Abuse Research Report* (NIH Publication Number 02-4877).

Hawkins, J.D., Catalano, R.F., & Miller, J. Y. (1992) Risk and protective factors for alcohol and other drug problems in adolescence and early adulthood: Implications for substance abuse prevention. *Psychological Bulletin, 112,* 54-105.

Hawkins, J.D., Herrenkohl, T. I.., Farrington, D. B., Brewer, F., Catalano, R.F., Harachi, T.W., & Cothern, L. (2000). Predictors of youth violence. Juvenile Justice Bulletin, April, 2000, 1-11.

Huizinga, D., Loeber, R., Thornberry, T.P., & Cothern, L. (2000). Co-occurrence of delinquency and other problem behaviors. *Juvenile Justice Bulletin,* November, 2000, 1-7.

Jongsma, A. E., Peterson, L.M., & McInnis, W.P. (1996). *The child and adolescent psychotherapy treatment planner.* New York, NY; Wiley.

Joint Commission on Accreditation of Healthcare Organizations (1998). *Technical Implementation Guide.* JCAHO.

Kazdin, A. E. (1993). Treatment of conduct disorder: Progress and directions in psychotherapy research. *Development and Psychopathology,* 5, 277-310.

L'Abate, L. (2011). With L. S. Sweeney (Eds). *Research on writing approaches in mental health,* Birney, UK: Emerald group Publications Limites

LeCroy, C. W., & Ashford, J. B., (1992). Children's mental health: Current findings and research directions. *Southwest Research and Abstracts,* 28, (1) 13-20.

Lyons, J. S., Kisiel, C. L., Dulcan, M., Cohen, R., & Chesler, P. (1997). Crisis assessment and psychiatric hospitalization of children and adolescents in state custody. *Journal of Child and Family Studies,* 6 (2), 2-18.

Lyons-Ruth, K. (1999). The two-person unconscious: Intersubjective dialogue, enactive relational representation and the emergence of new forms of relational organization. *Psychoanalytic Inquiry, 19,* 576-617.

MacKenzie, L.R., (1999). Residential placement of adjudicated youth, 1987-1996. *Office of Juvenile Justice Fact Sheet,* September, 1999, 117.

Miller, D., Trapani, C., Fejes-Mendoza, K., Eggleston, C. (1995). Adolescent female offenders: Unique considerations. *Adolescence,* 30, 429-435.

Miller, F. (2001). *Substance Abuse Subtle Screening Inventory (SASSI) manual, second edition.* FL: SASSI Institute.

Miller, W. R. & Rollnick, S. (2002). *Motivational interviewing: Preparing people to change.* NY: Guilford Press.

Mordock, J.B. (2000). Outcome assessment: Suggestions of agency practice. *Child Welfare League of America Journal,* 57, 689-710.

Olson, D. (1985). *Family Inventories.* University of Minnesota: author.

Prochaska, J. O., & DeClemente, C. C. (1992). Stages of change in the modification of problem behavior. In Hersen, M., Eisler, R., & Miller, P. M. *Progress in behavior modification,* 28. Sycamore, IL: Sycamore Publishing.

Richters, J. E., & Cicchetti, D. (1993). Mark Twain meets DSM-III-R: conduct disorder, development and the concept of harmful dysfunction. *Development and Psychopathology,* 5, pp. 5-29.

Samenow, S.E. (1998). *Before it's too late.* New York: Times Books.

Samenow, S. (1984). *Inside the Criminal Mind.* New York: Times Books.

Zoccolillo, M., & Rogers, K. (1992). Characteristics and outcome of hospitalized adolescent girls with conduct disorder. *Journal of the American Academy of Child and Adolescent Psychiatry,* 30, 973-981.

5

Applications of 3D Simulation in Mental Health: Utilities and New Developments

José A. Carmona Torres, Adolfo J. Cangas Díaz
and Álvaro I. Langer Herrera
University of Almería
Spain

1. Introduction

During the last two decades, there has been growing interest in psychology and psychiatry in the use and possible applications of Virtual Reality and, in general, procedures using 3D simulation environments as a tool applied to both evaluation and treatment of psychopathological disorders. It is well known that the enormous advances in recent years in development of 3D simulation environments have made them increasingly similar to real life, and the flexibility in creating new and ever more complex Virtual Reality programs has made it easier to apply this type of procedure as a supporting tool for intervention in the study, treatment and evaluation of a wide variety of mental disorders.

It should be mentioned that the use of this type of technology is not proposed as a replacement for traditional intervention procedures and evaluation methods, but as a tool to be used within the framework of treatment or evaluation used, whether cognitive-behavioral or other. Therefore, it should be emphasized that the use of 3D simulation environments in clinical practice be understood exclusively in the context of the psychotherapeutic orientation used, where this technique would make senses along with the rest of the practices included in each intervention framework. Its use is therefore not considered alone or as a replacement for other evaluation and treatment procedures used.

As many other researchers in the field of Virtual Reality have mentioned, the use of this type of technology has numerous advantages over traditional treatment and evaluation systems. Some of the main advantages of its use are (Scozzary & Gamberini, 2011; Adams et al., 2009; Botella et al., 2007; Perpiñá et al., 2003):

1. *Experiences similar to real life.* The main characteristic of this technology is that it allows a person to experience something similar to what he might in the real world if he were in that context. Thus VR can cause the same emotions, thoughts, and behavioral responses in general, as if the person were exposed to the real context that is being simulated by VR.
2. *Safety of the Virtual World.* VR environments are presented as a safe context where the person is not exposed to the risks that he would be in the real world. In this sense, the person immersed in the virtual world can experience emotions, thoughts and react knowing that nothing in the virtual environment that really frightens him in the real world can cause him any harm, which allows the context of therapy to be perceived by the person as a safe environment where he can behave freely and without any risk.

3. *Simulation of real world situations.* As we all know, the use of 3D simulation allows any situation in the real world to be realistically recreated. This characteristic is especially relevant in both evaluation and intervention, since it allows the person to be submerged in a virtual world with characteristics similar to those in the real world, where their responses in certain conflictive contexts can be studied, and which could, in turn, improve the ecological validity of measures using VR instruments over the usual procedures.

4. *Presentation of situations at any time.* Another important characteristic of VR is that it enables the desired scene to be simulated at any time, and it is unnecessary to wait until the situation occurs in the real world. This characteristic would allow the patient to be exposed to clinically significant contexts as often as necessary, overcoming the limitation of the usual interventions in which you must wait for a certain event to occur to expose the person to that context.

5. *Control of scenes presented.* The use of VR systems allows the therapist greater control over the stimuli in situations presented. Certain parameters in the scene can be manipulated, for example the intensity of the stimuli presented. In fact it makes evaluation and treatment more flexible and adaptable to each person, as well as the demands of the therapist or researcher.

6. *Confidentiality.* Indeed, the fact that it is unnecessary to expose the person to real contexts, as VR environments make it possible to carry out exposure sessions right in the therapist's office, total confidentiality of participant responses and his treatment are guaranteed, since the use of 3D simulation environments allows the person to be exposed to any context similar to those in real life.

The use of 3D Simulation or Virtual Reality definitely makes it possible to overcome some of the limitations of the usual procedures in both evaluation and treatment of disorders. That is why, as seen in the following section, a growing number of studies have been directed at the application and evaluation of the usefulness and effectiveness of this type of technology applied to clinical psychology.

2. Applications of 3D Simulation in the field of mental disorders

As mentioned above, many studies have concentrated on the application and study of the possible usefulness of the use of 3D simulation environments or virtual reality to psychopathological disorders, and at present there are a large number of studies on it. Thus, as suggested by Gutiérrez Maldonado (2002), the study done by Schneider in the eighties in the last century with acrophobic patients, in which he used lenses that could be manipulated to alter the sensation of depth perceived by acrophobic patients, could be considered a first pioneering procedure in the field of VR (Schneider, 1982). Although this type of strategy did not yet use computers, since then there has been growing interest by researchers around the world in possible applications of VR in clinical psychology and psychiatry.

As it is not within the scope of this chapter to describe the many studies that have used VR in a diversity of fields related to mental disorders, we go on below to point out some of the most characteristic, as a sample of some of the main VR applications developed to date for evaluation, treatment and study of psychological disorders.

2.1 Treatment of anxiety disorders

The field of anxiety disorders has received the most attention by researchers, who have developed VR scenarios for a diversity of specific phobias, such as fear of spiders, fear of flying, agoraphobia, social phobia, claustrophobia, panic disorder with agoraphobia or for Post Traumatic Stress Disorder (PTSD), among other disorders (Scozzari & Gamberini, 2011).

The applications developed directed at treatment of anxiety disorders have focused on being able to submerge the person in a VR environment similar to real life where he is gradually exposed to those stimuli or situations which trigger phobic avoidance responses characteristic of persons who show some type of anxiety disorder. The purpose of this exposure is the elimination of the avoidance responses, as well as reduction of the associated emotional and physiological states by getting the person used to the threatening situations avoided until then. It is a way of getting the person used to phobic stimuli avoided to which, as we know, an intense initial response triggered by the situation feared would precede a gradual decrease in the intensity of these experiences, as well as associated avoidance responses. Intervention using a VR environment would therefore pose an alternative to the classic exposure *in vivo* used traditionally as the treatment of choice for phobias and other anxiety disorders at present, in which, as we will see, the use of VR has been shown to be at least equally effective as an exposure technique for treatment of such problems.

2.1.1 Fear of flying

The consequences of a phobic response related to fear of flying can become a significant problem causing important social problems and difficulties on the job for people who suffer from it. The huge expense and cost in human resources (buying a plane ticket, travel by therapist, time used outside of the office, etc.) that *in vivo* exposure can cause for the treatment of fear to flying have led researchers to be interested in VR applications to this disorder very early on.

Rothbaum, et al. (1996) evaluated the efficacy of virtual reality exposure therapy in a case study of a person suffering from fear and avoidance of flying diagnosed formally as a specific phobia. To do this, these authors developed a virtual environment that reproduced the interior of an airplane, where the person was seated, exposed to take off and landing as well as several different weather conditions during the flight (calm and storm). The patient, equipped with head-mounted display (HDM) and audio (which reproduced the typical sounds of a flight), was also able to hear the therapist's recommendations during each of the stages of exposure carried out. The results showed the effectiveness of virtual reality exposure therapy (VRET) in reducing fear of flying of the participant. Since then, other case studies have separately demonstrated the effectiveness of virtual reality exposure therapy, for example in a helicopter simulator (North et al., 1997). Furthermore, several controlled studies have demonstrated the effectiveness of this type of VR exposure compared to the usual treatment for this type of problems. Both VRET and *in vivo* exposure proved to be equally effective both in reducing the symptomology and in the number of participants that continued getting on a real plane after treatment. These results were maintained in a 12-month follow-up, and the majority of the participants said that if allowed to choose the type of treatment, they preferred virtual reality to real exposure (Rothbaum, et al., 2000; Rothbaum et al., 2002; Maltby et al., 2002; Mühlberger et al., 2003; Rothbaum et al, 2006; Botella et al., 2004).

2.1.2 Acrophobia and claustrophobia

In an attempt to expose people to contexts generated by anxiety, such as fear of closed spaces (claustrophobia) or heights (acrophobia), virtual simulation environments have also been developed to solve some of the problems exposure usually has, such as going outside the therapist's office. In a controlled study by Rothbaum et al. (1995), the efficacy of virtual reality graded exposure treatment was compared to a group with no treatment. The virtual environments simulated included a bridge or walk over water, balconies and a glass elevator. The results showed significantly better improvement in persons subjected to the VR environments than the group with no treatment. However, in this study, no comparison was made with a group that had undergone the classic *in vivo* exposure. Emmelkamp et al. (2002) developed VR environments for this similar to those used in *in vivo* exposure in order to compare the two treatments. The simulation environments created included a four-story shopping center with stairs and railings, the fire escape ladder of a building and a roof garden on a university building from which the plaza below could be seen. The results showed that VR exposure was as effective as *in vivo* exposure. Something else observed in other studies regarding the effectiveness of this type of treatment in people with acrophobia, is that these results are maintained in follow-ups after several months (Krijn et al., 2004).

The group of Botella and collaborators did a first case study focusing on exposure to enclosed spaces (claustrophobia), in which the patient was exposed to a total of three scenarios with graduating difficulty, recreating a balcony or small garden, a small room with doors and large window and, finally, an even smaller room than the one before with no furniture or windows in it. This exposure with VR reduced all the avoidance and fear measurements, providing evidence on the effectiveness of VR exposure (Botella et al., 1998). These results were confirmed by another controlled study, and after three months, the follow-up showed that exposure with VR was an effective treatment for fear and avoidance behaviors in people with claustrophobia (Botella et al., 2000).

2.1.3 Fear of spiders and fear of driving

Fears related to insects, and in particular, fear of spiders, have also received attention by researchers, who have developed Augmented Reality (AR) environments, which are a type of virtual simulation environment in which real-life images not computer-generated are combined with computer-generated images. It could be said that it is a combination of exposure *in vivo*, since the person is seeing the objects and real life events that surround him at all times, and VR images. For example, case studies have been performed in which the person is exposed to virtual spiders, with which the person is able to interact, for example, by picking them up or simply letting them pass over their hands. A first exposure in a case study proved to be successful in reducing fear of spiders, observing after treatment that the patient's dysfunctional behavior related to spiders was reduced considerably, as was, for example, the reduction observed in obsessive-compulsive rituals this person did before treatment (Carlin et al., 1997). García-Palacios et al. (2002) also did a controlled study in which VR treatment was compared to a group without treatment, observing here also the effectiveness of treatment with VR, in which 83% of the participants assigned to the VR group showed a clinically significant improvement compared to 0% observed in the group without treatment.

In a case study dealing with fear of driving, a virtual simulator consisting of six scenarios including different weather and driving conditions, such as snow, fog, rain, etc., was used. The 3D simulation equipment included a steering wheel, controls for accelerator and brake and virtual glasses. In general, persons subjected to these VR environments showed a decrease in their dysfunctional behavior in activities in daily life, showing reduced anxiety and avoidance, not only after treatment, but also throughout the sessions, and these results were maintained in a follow-up after seven months (Wald & Talor, 2000). Similar results have been observed in other studies, showing that this type of exposure is promising for treatment of people with this type of phobia (Wald & Taylor, 2003).

2.1.4 Social phobia and panic disorder

Many studies have concentrated on the study of applications and possible benefits of using VR environments for exposure to social contexts in persons diagnosed with social phobia and specifically, fear of public speaking. The use of VR environments improved some of the problems or limitations presented by *in vivo* exposure as the treatment of choice for this type of problems, given the difficulty of controlling the variables when a person is exposed to this type of social context. Therefore, the use of VR environments provides better control of stimuli, persons and scenarios presented, improves the confidentiality of the participant when exposed to public situations, etc. For example, a study by Anderson et al. (2005) evaluated the usefulness of cognitive-behavioral treatment for anxiety of public speaking with VR in ten persons diagnosed with social phobia or panic disorder with agoraphobia, where the main symptom was fear of public speaking. A scenario with a virtual podium was simulated from which the participant had to talk to an audience which varied in number, and that audience could also be controlled by the therapist, for example, showing them to be interested, bored, etc. After treatment, the participants showed significant improvement in the self-report measures, expressed satisfaction with the treatment and maintained these improvements in a three-month follow-up. The study done by Wallach et al. (2009), in which he carried out a randomized controlled trial in persons diagnosed with phobia of public speaking should also be mentioned. Again, the results showed similar results both for traditional cognitive-behavioral treatment and VR treatment, both showing significantly higher results than those in the group without treatment on the waiting list.

Several controlled studies on panic disorder have been carried out with promising results (Vincelli et al., 2003). For example, the VR program developed by Botella et al. (2007) enabled the perceptions and bodily states associated with a panic attack to be simulated. It was able to simulate palpitations and difficulty breathing, with three intensity or severity levels, visual sensations such as clouded vision, double or tunnel vision. The program consisted of 6 scenarios, a training room, a house, subway, bus, shopping mall and a tunnel. One of the most outstanding characteristics of this VR exposure program was the possibility of controlling the "difficulty" of each of the scenarios available, since it was possible to control the number of people in the scene, the duration of each scene, adversities such as an elevator getting stuck between floors, etc. This VR exposure treatment was then compared to the classic *in vivo* exposure, and to a group on the waiting list (no treatment). Just as in other studies which have compared both types of treatments, the results showed that the improvement observed after the VR treatment was similar to what was observed using *in vivo* exposure, and in turn, both were significantly more effective than the waiting list.

2.1.5 Post Traumatic Stress Disorder (PTSD)

Several themes have been used as simulated scenarios by different programs recently developed for the treatment of post traumatic stress disorder (PTSD). There are VR simulators for veterans of the wars in Vietnam, Afghanistan and Iraq, for victims of the attack on the World Trade Center in New York and traffic accidents (Rothbaum et al., 2001;

Difede & Hoffman, 2002; Wiederhold & Wiederhold, 2010). This type of program usually recreates the usual real contexts in this type of situation, for example, a convoy of vehicles going down a road in the desert of Afghanistan, where the convoy is attacked by guerillas who block the road, or a helicopter flying over the jungle in the Vietnam War. One example of these scenarios which has shown good results insofar as the efficacy of this type of technology for the treatment of PTSD is the one developed by Rizzo et al. (2010), which simulates a Middle Eastern city where a market place, devastated streets, checkpoints, ramshackle buildings, warehouses, mosques, shops and dirt lots strewn with junk can be seen. The buildings can be entered. Furthermore, in an attempt to generate as much realism as possible in the scenes simulated, moving vehicles and people walking down the street can be seen outside. Case studies have demonstrated the effectiveness such VR exposure in improving symptoms associated with this disorder (Rothbaum et al., 1999), and controlled studies done to date have also shown the effectiveness of VR exposure in reducing the associated symptoms (Gamito, et al., 2010; MacLay et al., 2011).

2.2 Substance abuse and addictive behaviors
An already classic procedure in the study and evaluation of addictive behavior is related to exposure to stimuli and use contexts (cue reactivity) in the field of substance abuse. What is pursued in such procedures is to evaluate the craving response that is triggered by exposure to stimuli and situations related to substance use. Traditionally, this exposure has used videos, photos or imagination. However, the results have not been very promising, both because of the lack of standardization of traditional procedures and little generalization of behavior in therapy with regard to what these persons do when they find themselves in a real drug use context (Bordnick et al. 2004).

VR procedures have been created that consist of presenting the client with different objects and persons related to drug use, by showing him the substances evaluated themselves, objects or "paraphernalia" related to their use, leisure places associated with use, etc., to produce and evaluate the craving response that is triggered by such stimuli. Then this information is used for the treatment, trying to lower the craving response through extinction, change of cognitions and other techniques that have been shown effective for treating these problems.

In the area of addictions, one of the fields that have received the most attention has been treatment of craving behavior and smoking. Bordnick et al. (2004) did a controlled pilot trial in which they compared the intensity of the craving response in 13 participants who were addicted to tobacco when exposed to an immersive VR environment with neutral stimuli and stimuli related to smoking, including an unanimated room where there were objects such as packs of cigarettes, an ashtray, a lighted cigarette, an electric coffee pot, etc. At the same time, in another room, a party is simulated, where other people are smoking and drinking, and they offer the participant a cigarette. The results show a significant effect in the intensity of the craving responses for those situations related to smoking. Based on these results, the authors underline that, in view of the capacity of VR environments for elicitation of craving responses in users, this type of technology is presented as a valid standardized method for the study of addictive behavior. At the present time, these results have been corroborated again by several studies in adult populations (Carter et al., 2008), in young adults aged 19 to 24 (Traylor, et al., 2008), and in teenagers in a case study (Bordnick et al., 2005). VR environments have also been designed for group viewing on a desk top computer monitor (Baumann & Sayette, 2006), as well as in an internet-based 3D simulation environment (Woodruff et al., 2007). In all the studies cited, results were similar with respect to the effectiveness of VR environments for eliciting craving responses in smokers.

VR environments have been used for alcoholics to diminish the craving response as part of cue-exposure therapy. A study by Lee et al. (2007) used different VR scenarios in which they recreated two types of bars (Western and Oriental), where different types of people (alone or accompanied) appear having a drink. Objects related to drinking, like bottles with alcoholic beverages (beer, whiskey), appetizers next to them, and a poster advertising liquor on the wall are also shown, along with the typical background noise of this kind of establishment. The results showed the effectiveness of the VR cue-exposure therapy in reducing craving. Other studies have concentrated on specifically evaluating whether, as occurs with other substances, exposure to stimuli related with alcoholic consumption trigger craving responses. To do this, Bordnick and his team developed a scene in a kitchen, a party and an office (during a conversation). Viewing these scenes was accompanied by smell and auditory stimuli, with significant results in eliciting craving (Bordnick, et al. 2008). This has been corroborated in other studies comparing the craving responses of drinkers and non-drinkers (Ryan et al., 2010).

Concerning the use of other substances, particularly stimulants, in a study in which a 3D simulation environment was developed for evaluation of craving responses in users of crack-cocaine, shows people using these substances. Again the results backed the effectiveness of this type of VR scenario in eliciting craving (Saladin et al., 2006). This was also found for use of methamphetamines on the Internet using the online platform Second Life (Culbertson, et al., 2010).

Finally, we just point out that these results have also been validated in VR situations for other types of substance, such as cannabis (Bordnick et al., 2009) or heroine (Kuntze et al., 2001). For example, the study on cannabis used two scenarios showing key objects associated with it use, in which one of them showed different objects or paraphernalia related to use of cannabis, while in the other situation, animated characters were observed consuming cannabis.

2.3 Food and body image disorders

Various groups of researchers have shown interest in studying the reactions of people with this type of disorder when immersed in VR contexts compared to other types of exposure, because of VR's possible therapeutic applications as a tool for evaluation and treatment of alterations in body image.

One of the groups that have shown the most interest in studying and in the possible applications of VR to this field has been Riva and collaborators. This group created a 3D simulation environment called Virtual Environment for Body Image Modification or VEBIM (Riva, 1999) which was directed at treating body image distortion and dissatisfaction with one's body which is usually associated with this type of disorder. This treatment, which has become known as Experiential Cognitive Therapy, combines traditional cognitive-behavioral intervention with the use of VR environments. Taking a look at the characteristics of 3D simulation environments designed, the first scene is used to weigh the person and find out his real weight. Then two scenes are shown, a kitchen and an office, which show different types of food and drink, where the participant can eat anything, and the program notes the calories in each one eaten. After that, a new scene is shown in which images of models (men and women) are posing like in advertisements for the purpose of breaking with associated emotions and beliefs. In the following scene, the participant is shown a mirror where he can see her own real image. Again, this exposure is used to apply several different cognitive intervention methods. The last scene consists of a corridor which ends in four rooms of different sizes where the person can only go through the door that coincides with the width of his body. Case studies have shown the effectiveness of this type of treatment in improving awareness of own body image and significantly reducing dissatisfaction with it, and as the authors point out, the person showed strong motivation to change after intervention (Riva et al., 1999). At the same time, these results have been confirmed by other studies with (Riva, et al. 2000) and without controls (Riva et al., 2002, 2003).

Perpiñá et al. (1999, 2002) also developed six VR environments for treating body image, which are very similar to those developed by Riva et al. (1999), recreating scenes similar to those described above, simulating a kitchen where food can be eaten, where the person has to say what his weight is after eating, and his subjective and desired weight. After that, there is a scene with different body constitutions. The following scene simulates two mirrors, where a 3D image of a body in one of them can be varied until the participant thinks it represents his own body. The second-to-the-last scene shows a door where the participant has to calculate the space for his to be able to get through. And in a last scene, different body parts have to be varied and the person is asked to model his subjective and desired body, and the shape that, according to his, a significant other would have of his. These authors compared the effectiveness of the VR treatment described above with cognitive-behavioral treatment for this type of disorder in a controlled study. The results showed significant improvement with both treatments. However, those who were exposed to VR environments showed a significant improvement in general psychopathology measures, measures specific to anxiety disorders, and also more satisfaction with their body in social situations, less negative thinking and attitudes about their own body, less fear of gaining weight, and less fear of reaching their healthy weight (Perpiñá et al., 1999). These results were maintained and even improved one year later (Perpiñá et al., 2004). Another study by these authors should also be mentioned (Perpiñá et al. 2003), this time on binge eating disorder. They developed a virtual environment comprised of a kitchen where different kinds of food with high calory content (pizza, hamburgers, etc.) were shown, and another with low calories, considered safe (apples, salad, etc.). In this scene, the participant had to choose something to eat, and was then asked how anxious he was, urge to binge, guilt and sense of reality of the experience. It was observed that eating in this virtual world triggered responses of anxiety, urge to binge and moderate to high levels of guilt. Furthermore, the participants indicated that it felt very real. These results definitely show the ability of VR to provoke the characteristic responses present in people with binge eating disorders (Perpiñá et al., 2003).

In another study to evaluate the type of responses triggered by VR environments in this type of problem, Letosa-Porta et al. (2005) developed a tool for perfecting some of the technical limitations of previous studies called Body Image Assessment Software (BIAS). BIAS provided greater freedom in modeling body proportions of the virtual person (avatar) to make it as similar as possible to the participant's measurements, and at the same time it allowed modification of specific body parts while maintaining a holistic vision of the avatar. Furthermore, this application was designed to be applied in any desktop computer, which facilitates its use and makes it available to large populations. The authors first evaluated the capacity of this program to produce responses related to exposure to these contexts, such as anxiety and depression, in people with eating disorders, with positive results (Gutiérrez-Maldonado et al., 2006, 2009). Furthermore, the psychometric characteristics of this VR program were evaluated, showing good reliability and validity (Ferrer-García & Gutiérrez-Maldonado, 2008).

2.4 Psychotic disorders

VR applications in the field of psychotic symptoms have focused mainly on the simulation and study of the experiences that these people have, that is, their psychotic symptoms, such as visual and auditory hallucinations, and also, for rehabilitation and evaluation of their cognitive and social skills.

Environments have been developed for evaluation of social skills of schizophrenic patients that are directed at specifically evaluating their social competence or behavior by simulating scenes in which the participant is involved in common conversations, such as being introduced to a stranger, making a date with a friend and talking about business with a person from work (Park et al., 2009). In this study, the usefulness of this virtual simulation program for differentiating significantly between persons with and without diagnosis of schizophrenia was observed in the measure of their functional skills. In another study, the usual treatment for training in social skills with role-playing was compared to VR role-playing. After this comparison, the VR group showed more interest in training in social skills and better generalization of the skills acquired, observing that the VR group acquired more conversational skills and assertiveness than the group with the usual treatment (Park et al., in press). At the same time, continuing with evaluation of activities in daily life, Josmann et al. (2009) used VR environments to simulate a supermarket. This program was designed for use in desktop computers. The main results showed the presence of statistically significantly differences in the action of schizophrenic subjects and those without any clinical diagnosis in this context. This again supports the use of VR systems in this type of population.

Freeman and collaborators have performed several studies on psychotic symptoms in the general population, assessing paranoid ideation in particular. They evaluated the effectiveness of VR environments for producing persecutory thinking in a non-clinical university population (Freeman et al., 2003), in which they simulated a library with different neutral avatars. Although most of the participants attributed positive attitudes to the characters, a few had referenced ideas and attributed ideas of persecution to the different characters that appeared. Later, in another study, the effect of virtual exposure in a scene in a subway car was evaluated in a clinical and non-clinical population (Fornells-Ambrojo et al. 2008), and in a non-clinical group alone (Freeman et al. 2008). The promising results showed that both populations had a high proportion of persecutory thinking and ideas related to the situation and the characters included in the 3D simulation of the subway car.

The Virtual Reality Apartment Medication Management Assessment (VRAMMA) was created for evaluating medication management skills in schizophrenic subjects. This VR program simulates an apartment in which the person is evaluated for the type and time of use of psychiatric drugs to find out how well he follows medication treatments, shown by the people in the VR context, and to validate the instrument used for such purposes. Results were significant insofar as it differentiated correctly between the actions of schizophrenic subjects and those with no diagnosis, observing more errors in those with schizophrenia in both the number of pills taken and the right time to take them (Kurtz, et al.2007).

Finally, programs have also been developed to simulate the type of visual and auditory hallucinations that schizophrenic persons may have. For example, a living room where voices are heard and different visual hallucinations, such as a picture frame in which the persons face or expression changes, the television turns on or off by itself, etc. In this same project, in a second stage to increase the realism of the hallucinations used, a psychiatric ward was recreated where the type of auditory and visual hallucination of a particular patient could be simulated. In this new scenario, an image of the Virgin Mary appears and speaks to the participant, and other animations, such as the word "death" in the headlines of a newspaper, or random flashes of light, which were included in this study, according to the patients themselves, were closer to the type of hallucinatory experiences that these people usually have. Finally, it should be mentioned that these scenes were developed for use in personal computers, thereby guaranteeing wider diffusion of this program among students and mental-health-care center workers (Banks, et al., 2004). Another study, by Yellowlees & Cook (2006) recreated a psychiatric ward which included self-critical voices, a television on which someone is criticizing the patient, and a mirror in which the person reflected seems to be dying. Among the participants in this study who used the program, 76% said that the simulated scenes improved their knowledge of auditory hallucinations and 69% of visual hallucinations.

2.5 Other disorders
Having reviewed the main disorders VR has been applied to, some of the most relevant studies concentrating on the possible utility of VR for application in other disorders are described below.

In first place, one field that has received much attention because of the possible advantages to be derived from the use of VR has been the evaluation of Attention Deficit Hyperactivity Disorder (ADHD). The main application of VR to this type of disorder has been directed at persons by adapting more commonly used computerized evaluation tools, such as the Continuous Performance Task (CPT), to evaluation of this type of behavior. The possibility of the therapist experimentally controlling the distracting stimuli that are presented in the 3D simulator enables these attention evaluation tasks to be perfected, and therefore to improve the ecological validity of the measures used. For example, Rizzo et al. (2001) developed a virtual classroom for evaluation of attention and the deficits associated with hyperactivity, in which the usual elements that appear in this context, like a teacher, desks, a window with a view outside, etc. are simulated. In this context, the child had to respond to certain auditory and visual stimuli, similar to traditional sustained attention tests, and also provides the evaluator with the possibility of using sounds, simulated objects or a combination of both distractions for the task. Later, other authors have evaluated the effectiveness of this program for evaluating children with this type of problem. The Continuous Performance Task Virtual Classroom has been demonstrated to be sensitive for discriminating between students with ADHD and those without, and could also have advantages for other similar measures insofar as its validity given the similarity of VR simulated scenarios to real life (Adams, et al., 2009).

In the field of cognitive rehabilitation, one of the applications that is awakening the most interest in researchers is the use of VR for improving the skills of patients with some disorder in the autistic spectrum. Several tools have been developed in which virtual worlds are created that are being used for training certain deficient skills in people with this type of diagnosis. The study by Strickland et al. (1996) marked the beginning of VR program development for evaluating functional skills in daily life, such as training how to cross a street with cars in it. In the last ten years, other more recent studies have pursued evaluating the potential usefulness of VR as a tool to develop social skills in children with autistic disorder. Several simulated scenarios have been developed for this, such as a bar where two people are sitting talking to see whether the participant avoids getting between them according to social conventions, or whether he steps on flowers and plants in a park, or in a typical social situation in a café. In general, good results have been found that show evidence of the usefulness of VR as a technique for study and improvement of social skills in persons with this type of disorder (Mitchell et al., 2007, Parsons et al., 2004, Parsons et al., 2005).

3. New developments in 3D simulation

After reviewing some studies that have used VR environments in their applications to different mental disorders, two new developments of this type of technology for addictions and other related mental problems are described below.

3.1 My-School: Detection of drug use and bullying in young people using 3D simulation environments

The group directed by Adolfo J. Cangas and collaborators from Spain has developed a three-dimensional simulation tool for evaluation called My-School (MS), which is specifically directed at detecting drug use and bullying in young people of school ages.

The MS program, which was designed to be used in personal computers (Windows), consists of 17 scenes through which participant reactions to conflictive situations are evaluated. MS recreates some of the most significant situations in which drug use and bullying problems usually appear to young people in educational, family and leisure contexts. The specific scenes recreated in MS take place in the school playground, in a classroom, in a park and at the participant's home. The participant finds himself immersed, in the style of contemporary video-games, in scenes where he is faced with different conflictive situations and has to say what he would do in each.

In general, scenes related to bullying show situations in which the participant is bullied by schoolmates, another in which he sees how another schoolmate is bullied and one in which it is the participant who is bullying another student. The substance use scenes evaluate use of alcohol, tobacco, cannabis, MDMA or "ecstasy" and cocaine. The My-School 3D program also evaluates family dynamics, and their relations with other students (Carmona et al., 2010a).

My-School has been shown to have good psychometric properties showing adequate reliability and construct validity, and above all, has shown its usefulness in early detection of substance use, particularly alcohol, tobacco and cannabis (Carmona et al., in press; Carmona et al., 2010), as well as for detection of cocaine and MDMA or "ecstasy" (Carmona, et al., 2010b). In conclusion, My-School is presented as a new 3D simulation application that has shown its usefulness for the detection of risk behaviors in young students. At present, this same group is improving the graphic engine of the original program to increase the realism of the scenes, the characters and interactions included in the first version in addition to developing new scenes related to behaviors associated with eating disorders. On the other hand, it is being adapted for direct application online over the Internet. In this sense, the MS program only needs an ordinary PC for its use, which would allow it to be applied to large populations, thus facilitating its diffusion and application.

3.2 The Playmancer Project: A video game for the treatment of addictive behaviors in adults

The main purpose of the European Playmancer Project is the creation, development and validation of a video game (serious game) directed at treatment of mental disorders and rehabilitation of people with chronic pain.

This research group has developed a video game for treatment of mental disorders specifically directed at persons with eating disorders and pathological gambling. The game scenario is an adventure game called Islands where the patient is confronted with various challenging situations, in which the affective state of the patient has a strong influence on the game. The aim is to change underlying attitudinal, cognitive-behavioral and emotional processes of patients in order to teach the patient to control his emotions, plan and learn to relax when he finds himself immersed in conflictive situations. These same scenes are used for rehabilitation of chronic pain, by attempting to improve physical functions, including inadaptive cognitions and emotions related to pain, for example, fear of moving (Moussa & Magnenant, 2009).

Although at present the Islands video game is still under evaluation and validation of its clinical efficacy, preliminary results with this 3D simulation tool have already shown that there is a relationship between playing the video game and the appearance of emotional and physiological reactions associated with its use (Jiménez-Murcia et al., 2009). It is therefore being shown to be a promising tool in the area of use of new technologies and, specifically in video games (serious games) for mental illnesses, given its capacity to provoke specific cognitive and emotional reactions.

4. Conclusion

This chapter has reviewed some of the main studies that concentrate on possible applications of virtual reality (VR) to the field of study, evaluation and treatment of mental disorders.

The main clinical studies that have used VR environments in their application to different mental disorders have focused on evaluating the usefulness of these scenarios for generating the behavioral, cognitive and emotional reactions in the person immersed in the virtual world that these same contexts would produce in real life, something which has been widely proven in the many applications studied (e.g., Bordnick et al., 2008; Ferrer-García et al., 2009; Culbertson et al., 2010). Moreover, a large number of studies have concentrated on comparing the effectiveness of this new type of treatment with VR with the usual interventions used, and to date, many case studies, non-systematic studies and controlled studies have shown the effectiveness of VR treatments in a wide range of disorders, such as anxiety, eating disorders, or in addictions, among other alterations (Gutiérrez-Maldonado, 2002). Specifically, in the studies reviewed in this chapter, Virtual Reality Exposure Therapy (VRET) has been shown to be at least equally effective as *in vivo* exposure in the framework of traditional cognitive-behavioral treatments for this type of disorder, and significantly more effective than absence of treatment (Riva, 2005; Scozzari & Gamberini, 2011). The use of VR environments has also been shown by several authors to have certain advantages over classic *in vivo* exposure, for example not having to wait until a certain event occurs in real life, greater control by the therapist of the stimuli and situations presented to the participant or the safety of this kind of environments, as nothing the person is afraid of really happens in the virtual world (Perpiñá et al, 2003).

It might be mentioned that to date, studies concentrating specifically on comparison of treatment by traditional exposure with exposure to 3D simulations have not been many compared the much more numerous studies evaluating the usefulness of 3D environments for triggering certain responses in persons exposed to these contexts. So focusing on the comparison of the two types of treatment, several questions could be pointed out.

In first place, several of the abovementioned studies have demonstrated that, in general, the effectiveness of the two types of treatment in their application to people with different types of mental disorders is very similar. Specifically, as discussed above, both procedures are equally effective in the various clinical applications studied (Scozzary & Gamberini, 2011). However, the choice of one or the other treatment (virtual reality exposure versus *in vivo* exposure) could be influenced by some of the characteristics that are derived from the use of 3D simulation environments instead of the classic exposure usually used. For example, the preference of some people with fear of spiders for one treatment or the other was evaluated, and significantly more motivation was found for participating in the VR exposure treatment than the traditional one, which could lead to more people unwilling to go through *in vivo* treatment accepting this type of treatment because of the greater acceptance and motivation generated by 3D simulation environments (García-Palacios et al., 2001). Furthermore, it has been observed that people who are subjected to this kind of 3D simulation environment prefer this type of procedures with VR to the classic *in vivo* exposure in the real world (Rothbaum et al., 2000, 2006). On the contrary, there is also evidence concerning possible advantages in using *in vivo* exposure instead of VR exposure, as shown by Wolitzky-Taylor et al. (2008), who found after a meta-analysis study in which the effectiveness of this treatment was compared to VR exposure for various specific phobias, that *in vivo* treatment is more effective than other types of interventions right after the application of the treatment, including VR exposure among these other interventions. Nevertheless, in the follow-up, that is, in the long-term, these differences were not maintained, and both VR and *in vivo* exposure treatments were equally effective. As similar results back both the usefulness and effectiveness of treatment with VR and traditional treatment usually used, the selection of one or the other would therefore be a matter of psychotherapist choice, depending on other variables, such as the inclination or preference of the patient for one or the other type of treatment, the time or cost of the treatment chosen, or the personal preference of the therapist, keeping in mind the empirical evidence backing the choice of one or the other.

In view of the results found in the various studies reviewed here, the use of 3D simulation environments is shown to be a promising tool in the area of evaluation, treatment and study of mental disorders, having demonstrated its usefulness and effectiveness in a wide variety of studies made to date.

Finally, it should be mentioned that future VR environment developments should make acquisition and use of 3D simulation systems in clinical practice less expensive. In this sense, several studies have shown that it is unnecessary to use costly 3D simulation systems (Krijn et al., 2004; Letosa-Porta et al., 2005; Carmona et al., in press). One of the great challenges for the future of VR environment development is therefore creation of effective 3D simulation programs which were more economical and easy to use, and thus more affordable to more therapists interested in the advantages of this type of technology for use in clinical practice and research.

5. Acknowledgements

Funding received from the Spanish Ministry of Science and Innovation (MICINN) (Project EDU2010-15186) is gratefully acknowledged. Álvaro I. Langer is been supported by FPU Research Program AP2007-02810.

6. References

Adams, R., Finn, P., Moes, E., Flannery, K., & Rizzo, A.S. (2009). Distractibility in Attention/Deficit/Hyperactivity Disorcer (ADHD): The Virtual Reality Classroom. *Child Neuropsychology*, Vol.15, No.2, (March 2009), pp. 120-135, ISSN 1744-4136

Anderson, P.L., Zimand, E., Hodges, L.F., & Rothbaum, B.O. (2005). Cognitive Behavioral Therapy for Public-Speaking Anxiety Using Virtual Reality for Exposure. *Depression and Anxiety*, Vol.22, No.4, (October 2005), pp. 156-158, ISSN 1520-6394

Banks, J., Ericksson, G., Burrage, K., Yellowlees, P., Ivermee, S., & Tichon, J. (2004). Constructing the Hallucinations of Psychosis in Virtual Reality. *Journal of Network and Computer Applications*, Vol.27, No.1, (January 2004), pp. 1-11, ISSN 1084-8045

Baumann, S.B., & Sayette, M.A. (2006). Smooking Cues in a Virtual World Provoke Craving in Cigarette Smokers. *Psychology of Addictive Behaviors*, Vol.20, No.4, (December 2006), pp. 484-489, ISSN 0893-164X

Bordnick, P.S., Graap, K.M., Copp, H., Brooks, J., Mirtha, F., & Logue, B. (2004). Utilizing virtual reality to standardize nicotine craving research: A pilot study. *Addictive Behaviors*, Vol.29, No.4, (December 2004), pp. 1889-1894, ISSN 0306-4603

Bordnick, P.S., Traylor, A.C., Graap, K.M., Copp, H.L., & Brooks, J. (2005). Virtual Reality Cue Reactivity Assessment: A Case Study in a Teen Smoker. *Applied Psychophysiology and Biofeedback*, Vol.30, No.3, (September 2005), pp. 187-193, ISSN 1090-0586

Bordnick, P.S., Traylor, A., Copp, H.L., Graap, K.M., Carter, B., Ferrer, M. et al. (2008). Assessing Reactivity to Virtual Reality Alcohol Based Cues. *Addictive Behaviors*, Vol.33, No.6, (June 2008), pp. 743-756, ISSN 0306-4603

Bordnick, P.S., Copp, H.L., Traylor, A., Graap, K.M., Carter, B.L., Walton, A. et al. (2009). Reactivity to Cannabis Cues in Virtual Reality Environments. *Journal of Psychoactive Drugs*, Vol.41, No.2, (June 2009), pp. 105-112, ISSN 0279-1072

Botella, C., Baños, R.M., Perpiñá, C., Villa, H., Alcañiz, M., & Rey, A. (1998). Virtual Reality Treatment of Claustrophobia: A Case Report. *Behaviour Research and Therapy*, Vol.36, No.2, (February 1998), pp. 239-246, ISSN 0005-7967

Botella, C., Baños, R.M., Villa, H., Perpiñá, C., & García-Palacios, A. (2000). Virtual Reality in the Treatment of Claustrophobic Fear: A Controlled, Multiple-Baseline Design. *Behavior Therapy*, Vol.31, No.3, (Summer 2000), pp. 583-595, ISSN 0005-7894

Botella, C., Osma, J., García-Palacios, A., Quero, S., & Baños, R.M. (2004). Treatment of flying phobia using virtual reality: data form a 1-year follow-up using a multiple baseline design. *Clinical Psychology and Psychotherapy*, Vol.11,No.5, (September/October 2004), pp. 311-323, ISSN 1099-0879

Botella, C., García-Palacios, A., Villa, H., Baños, R.M., Quero, S., Alcañiz, M. et al. (2007). Virtual Reality Exposure in the Treatment of Panic Disorder and Agoraphobia: A Controlled Study. *Clinical Psychology and Psychotherapy*, Vol.14, No.3, (May/June 2007), pp. 164-175, ISSN 1099-0879

Carlin, A.S., Hoffman, H.G., & Weghorst, S. (1997). Virtual Reality and Tactile Augmentation in the Treatment of Spider Phobia: A Case Report. *Behaviour Research and Therapy*, Vol.35, No.2, (February 1997), pp. 153-158, ISSN 0005-7967

Carmona, J.A., Espínola, M., Cangas, A.J., & Iribarne, L. (2010a). Mii School: New 3D Technologies Applied in Education to Detect Drug Abuses and Bullying in Adolescents. In: *Technology Enhanced Learning*, M. Lytras, P. Ordoñez, D. Avison, J. Sipior, Q. Jin, W. Leal, L. Uden, M. Thomas, S. Cervai, & D. Horner (Eds.). Springer, 65-72, ISBN 0805836659, Heidelberg, Germany

Carmona, J.A., Espínola, M., Cangas, A.J., & Iribarne, L. (2010b). Detecting drug use in adolescents using a 3D simulation program. *Psychology, Society & Education*, Vol.2, No.2, (November 2010), pp. 143-153, ISSN 1989-709X

Carmona, J.A., Cangas, A.J., García, G.R., Lánger, A.I., & Zárate, R. (in press). Early detection of drug use and bullying in Secondary School children using a 3-D simulation program. *CyberPsychology, Behavior, and Social Networking*, ISSN 2152-2723

Carter, B.L., Bordnick, P., Traylor, A., Day, S.X., & Paris, M. (2008). Location and longing: The nicotine craving experience in virtual reality. *Drug and Alcohol Dependence*, Vol.95, No.1-2, (November 2007), pp. 73-80, ISSN 0376-8716

Culbertson, C., Nicolas, S., Zaharovits, I., London, E.D., De La Garza, R., Brody, A.L. et al. (2010). Methamphetamine Craving Induced in an Online Virtual Reality Environment. *Pharmacology, Biochemistry and Behavior*, Vol.96, No.4, (October 2010), pp. 454-460, ISSN 0091-3057

Difede, J., & Hoffman, H. (2002). Virtual Reality Exposure Therapy for World Trade Center Post-Traumatic Stress Disorder: A Case Report. *CyberPsychology & Behavior*, Vol.5, No.6, (December 2002), pp. 529-535, ISSN 2152-2715

Emmelkamp, P.M.G., Krijn, M., Hulsbosch, A.M., de Vries, S., Schuemie, M.J., & van der Mast, C.A.P.G. (2002). Virtual Reality Treatment Versus Exposure In Vivo: A Comparative Evaluation in Acrophobia. *Behaviour Research and Therapy*, Vol.40, No.5, (May 2002), pp. 509-516, ISSN 0005-7967

Ferrer-García, M., & Gutiérrer-Maldonado, J. (2008). Body Image Assessment Software: Psychometric Data. *Behavior Research Methods*, Vol.40, No.2, (May 2008), pp. 394-407, ISSN 1554-3528

Ferrer-García, M., Gutiérrez-Maldonado, J., Caqueo-Urízar, A., & Moreno, E. (2009). The Validity of Vitual Environments for Eliciting Emotional Responses in Patients With Eating Disorders and in Controls. *Behavior Modification*, Vol.33, No.6, (November 2009), pp. 830-854, ISSN 1552-4167

Fornells-Ambrojo, M., Barker, C., Swapp, D., Slater, M., Antley, A., & Freeman, D. (2008). Virtual Reality and Persecutory Delusions: Safety and Feasibility. *Schizophrenia Research*, Vol.104, No.1-3, (September 2008), pp. 228-236, ISSN 0920-9964

Freeman, D., Slater, M., Bebbington, P.E., Garety, P.A., Kuipers, E., Fowler, D. et al. (2003). Can Virtual Reality be Used to Investigate Persecutory Ideation? *Journal of Nervous and Mental Disease*, Vol.191, No.8, (August 2003), pp. 509–514, ISSN 0022-3018

Freeman, D., Gittins, M., Pugh, K., Antley, A., Slater, M., & Dunn, G. (2008). What Makes One Person Paranoid and Another Person Anxious? The Differential Prediction of Social Anxiety and Persecutory Ideation in an Experimental Situation. *Psychological Medicine*, Vol.38, No.8, (August 2008), pp. 1121-1132, ISSN 0033-2917

Gamito, P., Oliveira, J., Rosa, P., Morais, D., Duarte, N., Oliveira, S. et al. (2010). PTSD Elderly War Veterans: A Clinical Controlled Pilot Study. *Cyberpsychology, Behavior, and Social Networking*, Vol.13, No.1, (February 2010), pp. 43-48, ISSN 2152-2723

García-Palacios, A., Hoffman, H., See, S.K., Tsai, A., & Botella, C. (2001). Redefining Therapeutic Success with Virtual Reality Exposure Therapy. *CyberPsychology & Behavior*, Vol.4, No.3, (June 2001), pp. 341-348, ISSN 2152-2723

García-Palacios, A., Hoffman, H., Carlin, A., Furness III, T.A., & Botella, C. (2002). Virtual Reality in the Treatment of Spider Phobia: A Controlled Study. *Behaviour Research and Therapy*, Vol.40, No.9, (September 2002), pp. 983-993, ISSN 0005-7967

Gutiérrez Maldonado, J. (2002). Aplicaciones de la Realidad Virtual en Psicología Clínica. *Aula Médica Psiquiátrica*, Vol.4, No.2, (April 2002), pp. 92-126, ISSN 1577-2950

Gutiérrez-Maldonado, J., Ferrer-García, M., Caqueo-Urízar, A., & Letosa-Porta, A. (2006). Assessment of Emotional Reactivity Produced by Exposure to Virtual Environments in Patients with Eating Disorders. *Cyberpsychology & Behavior*, Vol.9, No.5, (October 2006), pp. 507-513, ISSN 1094-9313

Jiménez-Murcia, S., Fernández-Aranda, F., Kalapanidas, E., Konstantas, D., Ganchev, T., Kocsis, O. et al. (2009). Playmancer Project: A Serious Videogame as an Additional Therapy Tool for Eating and Impulse Control Disorders. In: *Annual Review of Cybertherapy and Telemedicine 2009: Advanced Technologies in the Behavioral, Social and Neurosciences*, B. Wiederhold & G. Riva (Eds.), 163-166, IOS Press, ISBN 978-1-60750-017-9, Amsterdam, Holland

Josman, N., Schenirderman, A.E., Klinger, E., & Shevil, E. (2009). Using Virtual Reality to Evaluate Executive Functioning Among Persons with Schizophrenia: A Validity Study. *Schizophrenia Research*, Vol.115, No.2-3, (December 2009), pp. 270-277, ISSN 0920-9964

Krijn, M., Emmelkamp, P.M.G., Biemond, R., de Wilde de Ligny, C., Schuemie, M.J., & van der Mast, C.A.P.G. (2004). Treatment of Acrophobia in Virtual Reality: The Role of Immersion and Presence. *Behaviour Research and Therapy*, Vol.42, No.2, (February 2004), pp. 229-239, ISSN 0005-7967

Kuntze, M.F., Stoermer, R., Mager, R., Soessler, A., Mueller-Spahn, F., & Bullinger, A.H. (2001). Immersive Virtual Environments in Cue Exposure. *CyberPsychology & Behavior*, Vol.4, No.4, (August 2001), pp. 497-501, ISSN 1094-9313

Kurtz, M.M., Baker, E., Pearlson, G.D., & Astur, R.S. (2007). A Virtual Reality Apartment as a Measure of Medication Management Skills in Patients With Schizophrenia: A Pilot Study. *Schizhophrenia Bulleting*, Vol.33, No.5, (September 2007), pp. 1162-1170, ISSN 1745-1701

Lee, J., Kwon, H., Choi, J., & Yang, B. (2007). Cue-Exposure Therapy to Decrease Alcohol Craving in Virtual Environment. *CyberPsychology & Behavior*, Vol.10, No.5, (October 2007), pp. 617-123, ISSN 1094-9313

Letosa-Porta, A., Ferrer-García, M., & Gutiérrez-Maldonado, J. (2005). A Program for Assessing Body Image Disturbance Using Adjustable Partial Image Distortion.

Behavior Research Methods, Vol.37, No.4, (November 2005), pp. 638-643, ISSN 1554-3528

MacLay, R.N., Wood, D.P., Webb-Murphy, J.A., Spira, J.L., Wiederhold, M.D., Pyne, J.M. et al. (2011). A Randomized, Controlled Trial of Virtual Reality-Graded Exposure Therapy for Post-Traumatic Stress Disorder in Active Duty Service Members with Combat-Related Post-Traumatic Stress Disorder. *CyberPsychology, Behavior, and Social Networking,* Vol.14, No.4, (April 2011), pp. 223-229, ISSN 2152-2723

Maltby, N., Kirsch, I., Mayers, M., & Allen, G.J. (2002). Virtual Reality Exposure Therapy for the Treatment of Fear of Flying: A Controlled Investigation. *Journal of Consulting and Clinical Psychology,* Vol.70, No.5, (October 2002), pp. 1112-1118, ISSN 0022-006X

Mitchell, P., Parsons, S., & Leonard, A. (2007). Using Virtual Environments for Teaching Social Understanding to 6 Adolescents with Autistic Spectrum Disorders. *Journal of Autism and Developmental Disorders,* Vol.37, No.3, (March 2007), pp. 589-600, ISSN 0162-3257

Moussa, M.B., & Magnenat-Thalmann, N. (2009). Applying Affect Recognition in Serious Games: The Playmancer Project. In: *Motion in Games. Second International Workshop,* A. Egges, R. Geraerts & M. Overmars, (Eds.), 53-62, Springer-Verlag, ISBN 978-3-642-10346-9, Berlin-Heidelberg, Germany

Mühlberger, A., Wiedemann, G., & Pauli, P. (2003). Efficacy of a One-Session Virtual Reality Exposure Treatment for Fear of Flying. *Psychotherapy Research,* Vol.13, No.3, (June 2003), pp. 323-336, ISSN 1468-4381

North, M.M., North A.M., & Coble, J.R. (1997). Virtual Reality Therapy for Fear of Flying. *The American Journal of Psychiatry,* Vol.154, No.1, (January 1997), p. 130, ISSN 0002-953X.

Park, K., Ku, J., Park, I., Park, J., Kim, S.I., & Kim, J. (2009). Improvement in Social Competence in Patients with Schizophrenia: A Pilot Study Using a Performance-Based Measure Using Virtual Reality. *Human Psychopharmacology: Clinical and Experimental,* Vol.24, No.8, (December 2009), pp. 619-627, ISSN 1099-1077

Park, K., Ku, J., Choi, S., Jang, H., Park, J., Kim, S.I. et al. (in press). A Virtual Reality Application in Role-Plays of Social Skills Training for Schizophrenia: A Randomized, Controlled Trial. *Psychiatry Research,* ISSN 0165-1781

Parsons, S., Mitchell, P., & Leonard, A. (2004). The Use and Understanding of Virtual Environments by Adolescents with Autistic Spectrum Disorders, Vol.34, No.4, (August 2004), pp. 449-466, ISSN 0162-3257

Parsons, S., Mitchell, P., & Leonard, A. (2005). Do Adolescents with Autistic Spectrum Disorders Adhere to Social Conventions in Virtual Environments? *Autism,* Vol.9, No.1, (February 2005), pp. 95-117, ISSN 1461-7005

Perpiñá, C., Botella, C., Baños, R.M., Marco, J.H., Alcañiz, M., & Quero, S. (1999). Body Image and Virtual Reality in Eating Disorders: Exposure by Virtual Reality is More Effective that the Classical Body Image Treatment? *Cyberpsychology & Behavior,* Vol.2, No.2, (April 1999), pp. 149-159, ISSN 2152-2723

Perpiñá, C., Botella, C., & Baños, R.M. (Eds.) (2002). *Body image in eating disorders: Virtual reality assessment and treatment.* Promolibro, ISBN 84-7986-474-5, Valencia, Spain.

Perpiñá, C., Botella, C., & Baños, R.M. (2003). Virtual Reality in Eating Disorders. *European Eating Disorders Review,* Vol.11, No.3, (May/June 2003), pp. 261-278, ISSN 1099-0968

Perpiñá, C., Marco, J.H., Botella, C., & Baños, R. (2004). Tratamiento de la Imagen Corporal en los Trastornos Alimentarios Mediante Tratamiento Cognitivo-Comportamental Apoyado con Realidad Virtual: Resultados al Año de Seguimiento. *Psicología Conductual*, Vol.12, No.3, (September 2004), pp. 519-537, ISSN 1132-9483

Riva, G. (1998). Virtual Environment for Body Image Modification: Virtual Reality System for the Treatment of Body Image Disturbances. *Computers in Human Behavior*, Vol.14, No.3, (September 1998), pp. 477-490, ISSN 0747-5632

Riva, G., Bacchetta, M., Baruffi, M., Rinaldi, S., & Molinari, E. (1999). Virtual Reality Based Experiential Cognitive Treatment of Anorexia Nervosa. *Journal of Behavior Therapy and Experimental Psychiatry*, Vol.30, No.3, (September 1999), pp. 221-230, ISSN 0005-7916

Riva, G., Bacchetta, M., Baruffi, M., Rinaldi, S., Vincelli, F., & Molinari, E. (2000). Virtual Reality-Based Experiential Cognitive Treatment of Obesity and Binge-Eating Disorders. *Clinical Psychology and Psychotherapy*, Vol.7, No.3, (July 2000), pp. 209-219, ISSN 1099-0879

Riva, G., Bacchetta, M., Baruffi, M., & Molinari, E. (2002). Virtual-Reality-Based Multidimensional Therapy for the Treatment of Body Image Disturbances in Binge Eating Disorders: A Preliminary Controlled Study. *IEEE Transactions on Information Thechnology in Biomedicine*, Vol.6, No.3, (September 2002), pp. 224-234, ISSN 1089-7771

Riva, G, Bacchetta, M., Cesa, G., Conti, S., & Molinari, E. (2003). Six-month follow-up of in-patient experiential cognitive therapy for binge eating disorders. *CyberPsychology & Behavior*, Vol.6, No.3, (June 2003), pp. 251-258, ISSN 2152-2723

Rizzo, A.S., Buckwalter, G.J., Bowerly, T., Humphrey, L.A., Neumann, U., van Rooyen, A., et al. (2001). The Virtual Classroom: A Virtual Environment for the Assessment and Rehabilitation of Attention Deficits. *Revista Española de Neuropsicología*, Vol.3, No.3, (July 2001), pp. 11-37, ISSN 1139-9872

Rizzo, A.S., Difede, J., Rothbaum, B.O., Reger, G., Spitalnick, J., Cukor, J. et al. (2010). Development and Early Evaluation on the Virtual Iraq/Afghanistan Exposure Therapy System for Combat-Related PTSD. *Annals of the New York Academy of Sciences*, Vol.1208, No.35, October 2010, pp. 114-125, ISSN 0077-8923

Rothbaum, B.O., Hodges, L.F., Kooper, R., Opdyke, D., Williford, J.S., & North, M. (1995). Effectiveness of Computer-Generated (Virtual Reality) Graded Exposure in the Treatment of Acrophobia. *The American Journal of Psychiatry*, Vol.152, No.4, (April 1995), pp. 626-628, ISSN 0002-953X

Rothbaum, B.O., Hodges, L., Watson, B.A., Kessler, G.D., & Opdyke, D. (1996). Virtual Reality Exposure Therapy in the Treatment of Fear of Flying: A Case Report. *Behaviour Research and Therapy*, Vol.34, No.5-6, (May/June 1996), pp. 477-481, ISSN 0005-7967

Rothbaum, B.O., Hodges, L., Alarcon, R., Ready, D., Shahar, F., Graap, K. et al. (1999). Virtual Reality Exposure Therapy for PTSD Vietnam Veterans: A Case Study. *Journal of Traumatic Stress*, Vol.12, No.2, (April 1999), pp. 263-271, ISSN 0894-9867

Rothbaum, B.O., Hodges, L., Smith, S., Lee, J.H., & Price, L. (2000). A Controlled Study of Virtual Reality Exposure Therapy for the Fear of Flying. *Journal of Consulting and Clinical Psychology*, Vol.68, No.6, (December 2000), pp. 1020-1026, ISSN 0022-006X

Rothbaum, B.O., Hodges, L.F., Ready, D., Graap, K., & Alarcon, R. (2001). Virtual Reality Exposure Therapy for Vietnam Veterans with Posttraumatic Stress Disorder. *Journal of Clinical Psychiatry*, Vo. 62, No. 8 (August 2001), pp. 617-622, ISSN 0160-6689

Rothbaum, B.O., Hodges, L., Anderson, P.L., Price, L., & Smith, S. (2002). Twelve-Month Follow-Up of Virtual Reality and Standard Exposure Therapies for the Fear of Flying. *Journal of Consulting and Clinical Psychology*, Vol.70, No.2, (April 2002), pp. 428-432, ISSN 0022-006X

Rothbaum, B.O., Anderson, P., Zimand, E., Hodges, L., Lang, D., & Wilson, J. (2006). Virtual Reality Exposure Therapy and Standard (In Vivo) Exposure Therapy in the Treatment of Fear of Flying. *Behavior Therapy*, Vol.37, No.1, (March 2006), pp. 80-90, ISSN 0005-7894

Ryan, J.J., Kreiner, D.S., Chapman, M.D., & Stark-Wroblewski, K. (2010). Virtual Reality Cues for Binge Drinking in College Students. *CyberPsychology, Behavior, and Social Networking*, Vol.13, No.2, (April 2010), pp. 159-162, ISSN 2152-2715

Saladin, E.M., Brady, K.T., Graap, K., & Rothbaum, B.O. (2006). A Preliminary Report on the use of Virtual Reality Technology to Elicit Craving and Cue Reactivity in Cocaine Dependent Individuals. *Addictive Behaviors*, Vol.31, No.10, (October 2006), pp. 1881-1894, ISSN 0306-4603

Schneider, J.W. (1982). Lens-Assisted *In Vivo* Desensitization to Heights. *Journal of Behavior Therapy and Experimental Psychiatry*, Vol.13, No.4, (December 1998), pp. 333-336, ISSN 0005-7916

Scozzari, S., & Gamberini, L. (2011). Virtual Reality as a tool for Cognitive Behavioral Therapy. In: *Advanced Computational Intelligence Paradigms in Healthcare 6. Virtual Reality in Psychotherapy, Rehabilitation, and Assessment*, S. Brahnam & L.C. Jain (Eds.), 63-108, Springer-Verlag, ISBN 978-3-642-17824-5, Berlin-Heidelberg, Germany

Strickland, D., Marcus, L.M., Mesibov, G.B., & Kerry, H. (1996). Brief Report: Two Case Studies Using Virtual Reality as a Learning Tool for Autistic Children. *Journal of Autism and Developmental Disorders*, Vol.26, No.6, (December 1996), pp. 651-659, ISSN 0162-3257

Traylor, A.C., Bordnick, P.S., & Carter, B.L. (2008). Assessing Craving in Young Adults Smokers Using Virtual Reality. *The American Journal on Addictions*, Vol.17, No.5, (September-October 2008), pp. 436-440, ISSN 1521-0391

Vincelli, F., Anolli, L., Bouchard, S., Kiederhold, B.K., Zurloni, V., & Riva, G. (2003). Experimental Cognitive Therapy in the Treatment of Panic Disorders with Agoraphobia. *CyberPsychology & Behavior*, Vol.6, No.3., (June 2003), pp. 321-328, ISSN 2152-2715

Wald, J., & Taylor, S. (2000). Efficacy of Virtual Reality Exposure therapy to Treat Driving Phobia: A Case Report. *Journal of Behaviour Therapy and Experimental Psychiatry*, Vol.31, No.3-4, (September 2000), pp. 249-257, ISSN 0005-7916

Wald, J., & Taylor, S. (2003). Preliminary Research on the Efficacy of Virtual Reality Exposure Therapy to Treat Driving Phobia. *CyberPsychology & Behavior*, Vol.6, No.5, (October 2003), pp. 459-465, ISSN 2152-2715

Wallach, H.S., Safir, M.P., & Bar-Zvi, M. (2009). Virtual Reality Cognitive Behavior Therapy for Public Speaking Anxiety. *Behavior Modification*, Vol.33, No.3, (May 2009), pp. 314-338, ISSN 1552-4167

Wiederhold, B.K., & Wiederhold, M.D. (2010). Virtual Reality Treatment of Posttraumatic Stress Disorder Due to Motor Vehicle Accident. *CyberPsychology, Behavior, and Social Networking*, Vol.13, No.1, (February 2010), pp. 21-27, ISSN 2152-2715

Wolitzky-Taylor, K.B., Horowitz, J.D., Powers, M.B., & Telch, M.J. (2008). Psychological Approaches in the Treatment of Specific Phobias: A Meta-Analysis. *Clinical Psychology Review*, Vol.28, No.6, (July 2008), pp. 1021-1037, ISSN 0272-7358

Woodruff, S.I., Conway, T.L., Edwards, C.C., Elliott, S.P., & Crittenden, J. (2007). Evaluation of an Internet Virtual World Chat Room for Adolescent Smoking Cessation. *Addictive Behaviors*, Vol.32, No.9, (September 2007), pp. 1769-1789, ISSN 0306-4603

Yellowlees, P.M., & Cook, J.N. (2006). Education about Hallucinations Using an Internet Virtual Reality System: A Qualitative Survey. *Academic Psychiatry*, Vol.30, No.6, (November/December 2006), pp. 534-539, ISSN 1042-9670

6

The "ROC" Model: Psychiatric Evaluation, Stabilization and Restoration of Competency in a Jail Setting

Jerry L. Jennings[1] and James D. Bell[2]
[1]*Liberty Healthcare Corporation, Bala Cynwyd, PA*
[2]*Central State Hospital, Petersburg, VA*
USA

1. Introduction

Despite its well-meaning intentions, the movement toward deinstitutionalization has shifted more and more people with serious mental illness and co-occurring disorders from state hospitals to jails and prisons (Lamb and Weinberger, 2005; Human Rights Watch, 2003). There are now more than three times more seriously mentally ill persons in jails and prisons than in hospitals (Torrey, Kennard, Eslinger, Lamb and Pavle, 2010). The trend has intensified in recent years as public mental health resources, both at the state hospital level and at the local community level, continue to shrink. Even before the national recession of 2010 hit government agencies and forced them into profound and drastic cost-saving measures, reductions in public mental health services were already causing high numbers of people with severe and persistent mental illness to land in the criminal justice system. As early as 2007, Wortzel, Binswanger, Martinez, Filley & Anderson (2007) asserted that the systemic decline of public mental health resources had created a national crisis for persons judged Incompetent To Proceed (ITP) who are "log-jammed" in jails and prisons across the country. Calling it "the ITP crisis," the Wortzel group decried the practice of jailing persons with psychotic disorders, often for long periods of time, without adequate psychiatric treatment because there are not enough forensic beds available in state hospital systems.
"Hundreds of patients with severe mental illness deemed incompetent to proceed are languishing in jails around the nation, unable to access meaningful psychiatric care and not moving forward in the legal process as they await admission to grossly undersized and understaffed state hospitals... The combination of inadequate psychiatric care, the stress of incarceration and the long waits involved have yielded nightmarish results..." (Wortzel, et al., 2007, p. 357).

2. Alternative approaches

Budget cuts to state hospital systems and deficient community-based mental health resources will continue to shift the cost and services burden to local emergency rooms, county jails and law enforcement agencies. Efforts to address the problems of the ITP crisis have been varied and shown mixed results. Assertive Community Treatment has been shown to be effective for releasing high risk forensic patients (Jennings, 2009; Smith, Jennings & Cimino, 2010), but it is expensive and rarely available for most community mental health systems. "Outpatient commitment" and "court-to-community programs," used in combination with intensive case management, have been tried with some success to remove mentally ill defendants charged with less serious crimes (Gilbert, Moser, Van Dorn, Swanson, Wilder, Robbins, Keator, Steadman & Swartz, 2010; Loveland & Boyle, 2007; Swartz, Swanson, Kim & Petrila, 2006), but they cannot be used for those charged with violent and dangerous crimes. Housing programs and long-term residential services can help prevent recurrent relapses and reoffending, especially for homeless persons with mental illness (Miller, 2003; Trudel and Lesage, 2006), but these strategies cannot be exercised immediately to avert hospitalizations or detention.

In particular, "mental health courts" have multiplied across the country as a way to divert mentally ill defendants and substance abusers away from incarceration and toward appropriate treatment (Redlich, Steadman, Clark & Swanson, 2006; Grudzinskas & Clayfield, 2005). Mental health courts entail a variety of interventions, including non-adversarial process, training judges in mental health and collaborative inter-agency teams (Wortzel, et al., 2007), but there is no clear model that can be applied across jurisdictions and states.

As jails and prisons have been forced to take responsibility for greater numbers of persons with mental illness, they have had to increase and expand whatever mental health services they can offer. In fact, the largest facilities that house psychiatric patients in the United States are not hospitals, but jails and prisons (Rich, Wakeman & Dickman, 2011; Torrey, et al., 2010). Adding more psychiatry time or mental health clinic hours is not enough when the jail environment itself is highly stressful and can exacerbate symptoms of mental illness. Large state correctional systems may have more resources than local jails to offer emergency psychiatry, intensive stabilization, addictions treatment and even hospital-level inpatient mental health units, but these increased behavioral health services are proportionate to the ever-growing numbers of inmates with serious and persistent mental illness entering corrections. More importantly, this does not address the need to identify, evaluate, treat and stabilize persons with severe mental illness when they are first arrested and detained – well before they are convicted and incarcerated in long-term state and federal prisons.

The Restoration Of Competency ("ROC") model is a new approach to the ITP crisis that can intervene at the earliest point of arrest and detention by delivering forensic psychiatric evaluations and treatment, intensive stabilization and restoration of competency in a local jail setting. The ROC model evolved from a pilot project in Virginia in the late 1990's and has been further developed into a viable alternative to the ITP crisis. It can significantly accelerate needed treatment for mentally ill defendants, cut the demand for costly State Hospital forensic beds, and directly assist local jails and law enforcement in better managing this specialized high-risk population – yielding major cost savings and improved services for all.

3. Advantages of the ROC model

By diverting state hospital referrals to an alternative short-term restoration program in a local jail, the ROC model can help eliminate waiting lists for state hospital forensic beds, decrease the length of time to restore someone to competency, and relieve local jails from the responsibility of holding mentally ill defendants without adequate mental health resources. It can cost significantly more for a jail to hold an inmate with serious mental illness than a non-mentally ill inmate. This does not include the added liability, cost and personnel strain of managing individuals whose disabilities render them vulnerable to suicide, violence, medical emergencies and trauma in the non-therapeutic setting of a jail and therefore require much more intensive supervision and intervention.

The amount of time waiting in jail for a competency evaluation and/or a state hospital bed can be significant. There is the time from initial arrest to the defense counsel's recognition of competence as an issue; time from recognition until the competence evaluation can be done; time to complete the evaluation; and time from the receipt of the evaluation report until the court adjudicates the issue (Christy, Otto, Finch, Ringhoff & Kimonis, 2010). These critical delays in gaining needed psychiatric treatment can exacerbate clinical symptoms and problem behaviors. By accelerating access to skilled forensic psychiatric evaluation and treatment in the jail, the ROC model can make clinical interventions at the earliest onset of illness, which reduces risk and makes it easier to stabilize the individual and restore and maintain competency. Moreover, prompt forensic examinations can differentiate the cases that can be resolved more quickly and will not require full hospitalization (Zapf & Roesch, 2011).

In addition, the ROC model has the major advantage of facilitating access to local attorneys and the courts and family support. Individuals with mental illness can be evaluated, stabilized and restored to competency in their home community, eliminating the high cost of transporting patients to and from state hospitals and the courts. In a large and/or rural state, the distances can be enormous and expensive.

Finally, there are major cost advantages of performing competency evaluation and restoration in a local jail setting. The cost of a forensic hospital bed is far higher than a jail bed, even a jail bed designated for mental health. For example, currently in Virginia, where this ROC model was developed, the average cost for a patient bed in the state's maximum security forensic hospital is $776 per day; whereas, the average cost to house an inmate in the local Regional Jail is $70 per day (Commonwealth of Virginia, 2010). The challenge, of course, is how to be able to provide an equivalent level of humane and effective psychiatric treatment in a jail or prison space that is not designed, equipped or staffed to provide a therapeutic environment.

The following Table 1 summarizes the multiple advantages of the ROC model for state hospital systems, local jails, law enforcement and the persons served.

4. Transforming a jail pod into a restoration of competency "ROC" unit

Overcoming the jail environment: The main disadvantage of the ROC jail-based restoration model, and it is a major one, is that jails and prisons are simply not designed as mental health units. They are built for security, surveillance and control, not therapeutic calm and comfort. Jail buildings and units are typically austere, grim, noisy, crowded and uncomfortable. Even the few classrooms and program areas that are designated for more positive activities of education, recreation, leisure, visitation, or even treatment, are understandably limited in a jail – in number, size, appearance and amenities.

Given the harsh physical plant realities of correctional facilities, the success of the jail-based ROC treatment model therefore depends on how well the available program space can be modified into a therapeutic environment. This entails a creative combination of (1) physical renovations to create a more pleasant and practical space for behavioral health treatment, create a positive environment; (3) specialized behavioral health training and supervision for correctional officers and unit staff; and (4) consistent, well-coordinated interventions by an integrated interdisciplinary team in delivering therapeutic services within the secure setting. while mitigating the environmental risks that mentally ill offenders may use in attempts to inflict injury upon themselves or others; (2) application of behavioral engineering principles to

Challenges	Benefits
For State Hospital Systems	
• Increasing proportion of admissions to state hospitals are forensic patients. • State hospital systems have insufficient beds to meet demand. • Large and lengthy "waiting lists" for admission to state hospitals delay needed treatment. • The need to transport and escort forensic patients over long distances causes costly logistical problems. • Increased court pressure and administrative costs due to complications and delays in processing, treating and restoring patients. • Litigation from Advocacy agencies.	• Reduces number of individuals waiting for competency evaluation and restoration services. • Reduces length of stay for restoration through early intervention and targeted treatment. • Eliminates incentive for inmates to malinger by seeking "vacation" from jail or prison. • More convenient access for local courts, defense attorneys, prosecutors and law enforcement, which saves time and money and improves outcomes. • Seamless transition from ROC program helps maintain competence to stand trial.
For Local Jails, Emergency Rooms and Law Enforcement	
• High numbers of mentally ill patients must wait in the non-treatment jail setting. • Jail setting is not designed for treatment and jail personnel are not trained to manage mental illness. • It costs much more to house mentally ill inmates than regular inmates. • Symptoms and severity of mental illness can exacerbate without prompt psychiatric intervention and can further complicate and extend the time needed to restore competency. • Higher risk of suicide, aggression, injury, trauma and litigation in non-therapeutic jail setting. • High costs of escort staff and long-distance transportation to and from state hospitals, courts and jails. • Increased use of costly hospital emergency room visits to manage mental health crises in the community. • Negative cycle of competency restoration, relapse in jail while awaiting trial and re-hospitalization.	• Local county saves money by reducing the time spent in jail by mentally ill inmates. • County jail can gain new revenue to cover the expenses already incurred by holding mentally ill inmates. • Eliminates the time and cost of transporting patients to and from state hospitals and jails. • Reduces disruptions to jail operations caused by psychotic and disordered behavior. • Reduces risk of suicide, violence, injury and litigation. • Reduces costly Emergency Room visits. • More convenient access for local courts, defense attorneys, prosecutors, law enforcement and family support. • On-site clinical support can potentially be extended to support mental health crises for other inmates.

Table 1. Advantages of the ROC Model

Some of the key ingredients for setting up a ROC program in a local jail include the following:
Choice of facility: The ideal site for the ROC model is a jail that has many Incompetent to Stand Trial (IST) or Incompetent to Proceed (ITP) defendants, who are either waiting for admission to the state hospital for evaluation and restoration and/or defendants who have been restored and returned from the state hospital to await court proceedings. Based on the available space in the jail, the ROC program requires about 20 beds to be cost effective, but it can be flexed to accommodate a larger capacity of up to 40 or more.

Program space requirements: The ROC provider must work collaboratively with the local Sheriff or jail authorities to assess and configure the pod, unit or area within the jail that can separately house the mentally ill inmates (forensic patients) and provide the primary program space for delivering the restoration of competency services. The main need is to separate the mentally ill inmates from the general population and establish an area that is sufficiently quiet, clean, orderly and safe to serve as the therapeutic environment. As illustrated in the case study below, many activities can be held in the common area of the jail pod, but other cells or multi-purpose rooms in the unit or jail can be adapted, if available, into clinician offices, exam rooms and group rooms. For recreation, the ROC patients should have scheduled access to a gym, recreation room or exercise yard separate from the general inmate population.

Specially trained security staff: The ROC unit should have its own dedicated staff of specially trained security officers, who are separate from the traditional correctional officers working in the rest of the jail. The ROC provider must work closely with the jail leadership to select, train and coordinate the work of security officers who will be assigned to the ROC mental health unit. Candidates should be carefully interviewed and evaluated to determine if they are suited to using a very different approach to managing and interacting with inmates. They should demonstrate values, attitudes and behavior that will be congruent with the program's therapeutic orientation. They will be trained in the recovery model and the use of positive behavioral techniques and will continually interact with the inmate/patients and clinical staff alike. They are expected to play an active and meaningful role in maintaining the therapeutic milieu. A designated ROC Deputy is also recommended to supervise the other security officers on the ROC unit, serve as an intermediary with jail leadership, and directly participate as a member of the interdisciplinary treatment team.

Interdisciplinary treatment team: The ROC treatment team would be interdisciplinary like that of a traditional forensic psychiatric unit, typically including a forensic psychiatrist, forensic psychologist, psychiatric nurse, social worker, rehabilitation therapist and clerk to coordinate scheduling, court dates, transports and forensic reports. A larger ROC program would have a larger team of professionals. The direct care staff would be security officers (see above), who are dually trained in security and treatment functions.

Approach to competency restoration: The ROC program uses a recovery model that focuses on individual strengths and targets abilities that are related to competency, including remediation of deficits and alleviation of acute symptoms. The primary goal for most IST patients is to resolve the psychosis, when present, to enable the patient to regain general thinking abilities. The second goal is to educate the patient in court process such that he is able to cooperate with his counsel in mounting a defense. If there is a failure to achieve either of the these goals, the third goal is to compile documentation to credibly opine that the patient is unrestorable to competency. The ROC team combines the proactive use of psychiatric medications, motivation to participate in rehabilitative activities, and multi-modal cognitive, social and physical activities that address competency in a holistic fashion. This includes the essential component of providing individual tutorials in competency issues by a psychologist. Some treatment modules/groups can be offered at two cognitive levels to better match higher and lower levels of functioning and understanding. The ROC model also avoids the problem of involuntary psychiatric medication by establishing and delivering incentives that result in voluntary agreement to medication.

Motivation using a milieu management system: One of the strongest ways to motivate treatment and medication compliance is the use of a milieu management system that rewards meaningful participation in treatment and positive behaviors with points or privileges, such as points to "buy" various canteen items. It is better to deliver such rewards frequently and at the time of the positive behavior rather than accumulating points over a full day. By breaking the day into short half-hour periods during which one or two points can be gained, patients are better able to comprehend expectations, consequences and progress toward desired goals. For example, if the patient is expected to attend a restoration group at 10 am, he gets one point if he attends and none if he doesn't. But he can earn two points if he exerts earnest efforts to learn the material.

Admission/assessment and treatment planning: Treatment begins with the intake assessment. The clinical team evaluates the person's psychological functioning, suicide and behavioral risk, current level of trial competency, and likelihood of malingering. A standard battery of psychological tests is used to evaluate cognitive abilities, social and psychological functioning, psychiatric symptoms and potential malingering. As needed, the ROC psychologist has other tests/screenings available for specific targeted areas of deficit. Assessment continues through the course of the admission to measure response to treatment and identify new problems to target for restoration of competency. A measure such as the self-developed Competence-related Abilities Rating Scale (CARS) can be used to monitor the individual's progress (Hazelwood & Rice, 2011). Based on the assessments, the treatment plan is individualized and geared toward one of two curriculums for lower and higher functioning patients. But treatment planning continues to be flexible and vigorous. It is common for the treatment team to discuss the treatment plan informally on a daily basis and to formally discuss treatment issues at least once a week.

Rehabilitative services and coordination of medical care: Individuals in the program typically meet with a treatment professional one-on-one about issues related to regaining their mental health, or competency issues, at least twice daily, and are engaged in 3.5 to 5.5 hours of group-based psychosocial rehabilitative activities each day depending on the individual's current capacities. (Experience showed that the lower functioning patients could not tolerate more than 3 to 4 hours of focused work per day.) For the most part, the clinical professionals can largely work during traditional weekday business hours, but evening and weekend programming is important for maintaining the therapeutic milieu. The clinical team can maintain on-call support during afterhours, and if necessary, come into the jail to evaluate and assist with a psychiatric crisis.

Treatment activities are structured and delivered across four domains: restoration of competency, mental illness and medication management, mental/social stimulation, and physical/social stimulation. Basic residential and health care, including all medical care and medications, can be provided on-site through a service agreement with the Sheriff/jail to utilize its existing pharmacy, medical records and medical service delivery system.

Discharge planning: Discharge planning begins at the time of admission. The ROC establishes a link with the designated mental health professional at the referring jail to discuss the case and provide aftercare information that will assist the jail in managing the inmate/patient upon return. Information may include continuation of medications based on those available in the jail's formulary; use of resources at the jail to help with behavior management (e.g., available mental health cells, paraprofessional assistance, etc.); and recommended protocols for managing the individual, particularly someone who might use malingering for secondary gain (e.g., restrictions on personal property, defined triggers for acting out behaviors, etc.).

Performance measures: The ROC model is organized to track multiple measures of efficiency, effectiveness, access to care, reduction in risk, and consumer satisfaction. Key performance measures can include the timeliness and results of evaluations, length of stay to achieve restoration, diagnostic and demographic data, hours of service by type and clinician, interventions, timeliness of court reports, customer satisfaction (including jail personnel, local law enforcement, courts, defense and prosecuting attorneys, state hospitals, patients and patient families, advocates and other stakeholders), recidivism and more.

5. ROC Case Study: The Liberty Forensic Unit at Riverside Jail

The pilot program: In 1997, Central State Hospital in Petersburg, Virginia needed to renovate its aging forensic units to accommodate a growing state-wide demand for forensic beds. The Department of Mental Health, Mental Retardation and Substance Abuse Services devised a bold plan to temporarily create a licensed forensic psychiatric hospital unit within the newly constructed Riverside Regional Jail in nearby Prince George County. A private company called Liberty Healthcare Corporation was selected to implement the pilot project. In just four weeks, the jail pod was transformed into an inpatient psychiatric unit with a complete staff of forensic clinicians, medical personnel, security and direct care staff and received initial state licensure as an inpatient behavioral health care facility and subsequent JCAHO certification as an inpatient psychiatric hospital unit. The unit then functioned as the acute, male admission unit for the state's maximum security forensic hospital.

Minimal renovation required: The first challenge was to modify the two-level jail pod into an acute inpatient psychiatric unit without impacting its correctional functionality. This was achieved with very minimal renovation. Of the 48 single-occupancy cells within the pod, 35 were simply converted into individual patient bedrooms using the original bed, toilet, sink and dresser/desk. Beds were removed from cells in one quadrant of the pod to create ten staff offices, one treatment team room and two behavior stabilization rooms (i.e., quiet/seclusion rooms). Brighter colored paint replaced the original institutional gray. A non-secure page-fence was added to the mezzanine walkway to prevent anyone from falling or jumping.

The creative use of behavioral engineering averted the need for other renovations. As part of the behavior management system, the mezzanine level bedrooms were designated for patients who had earned higher levels of responsibility and privilege in the treatment program. Also, patient movement from the floor to the mezzanine level was restricted to the central ramp, while the stairs on either side were restricted for staff use only. Otherwise patients were free to move about the unit. Boundary lines were marked on the floor using colored tape to delineate the few specific areas where patients were not allowed to travel without permission, such as the medical records room and the staff offices.

Use of space for treatment and activities: The pod included one small conference room that could be used for treatment groups, competency groups and other therapeutic activities. Certain subareas of the common area could also be used for community meetings and socialization and group activities at designated hours of the day, such as a "Current Events" discussion group or to watch a psychoeducational videotape or TV program. For recreational activities, the patients could use an enclosed patio/basketball court and enjoyed exclusive use of the prison's gymnasium at scheduled hours every day, separate from the general inmate population.

Restoration to competency: Efforts to restore a defendant to competency to stand trial primarily consist of medications to remediate active symptoms of mental illness, when present, and group and individual education about court and criminal justice processes with correlative documentation of response to these efforts at education. Group-based education included mock court run-throughs in which every patient took a turn at playing the various roles in court. Individual tutorials in court procedure were provided by the unit psychologists to move the patient more quickly toward competency and a defensible opinion for the court (when possible), but also helped document the thorough efforts made by ROC for cases that concluded in an opinion of unrestorability.

Individual forensic evaluations, psychological testing, clinical interviews and counseling could be conducted in one of the single rooms or the small group room. One-to-one sessions were frequent because the psychologist conducted individual competency tutorials with most patients and each patient would meet regularly with his designated primary therapist.

The host jail provided housekeeping, food services, and laundry. The ROC unit provided its own primary medical care and pharmacy and would refer serious and emergent medical issues to the state hospital infirmary or local civil medical hospitals.

Team-based interventions and milieu management: The ROC program was highly proactive and preventative. Great emphasis was placed on maintaining a therapeutic environment characterized by calm, quiet, safety, predictability and interpersonal respect. A vigorous schedule of therapeutic activities helped to prevent boredom and provided opportunities for positive interactions. The key, however, was use of intensive team-based staff supervision. The security officers/direct care personnel were trained to be mobile, engaged observers, who could promptly identify and respond to precursors of disruptive behavior on the unit. The goal was to intervene gently as a team at the earliest point of concern – well before the patient might escalate into a full-blown episode of disruption and/or violence that could quickly undermine the vital climate of calm and safety for the rest of the unit.

When disturbances occurred, as expected with an inmate population that was acutely ill and volatile, the ROC staff were trained to quickly, but quietly migrate to the scene as a team. This was accomplished with subtle cues and nonverbal communication between staff and performed without the need for rushing movements, loud verbal commands or calls for emergency assistance. Effective prevention and early intervention had the tremendous advantages of reducing the need for seclusion/restraint as well as lowering the risk of trauma and injury to patients and staff alike (see outcomes below).

As a team, the staff were continually reviewing the therapeutic environment and monitoring patient behavior. This teamwork extended across working shifts. Problematic patient behaviors occurring on one shift were not allowed to carry over onto the next shift. When new risk factors were identified for patients, the team developed strategies to address individual needs. For example, patients themselves were taught and encouraged to use "time out" sessions on a voluntary basis. They understood they could go to a special area with close staff support if they were beginning to feel agitated or losing personal control.

For all these reasons, the use of seclusion and restraint was minimal. When necessary, the team used the same calm efficiency in employing physical intervention techniques that were designed to preclude trauma to patients. In fact, the Local Human Rights Commission commended the unit for creating and implementing a Protocol for Recurrently Aggressive Patients because it introduced a lesser restrictive measure than seclusion and restraint, while enhancing the general safety of the unit.

6. Patient data and ROC program outcomes

In five years of operation, the Liberty Forensic Unit at Riverside Jail (LFU) evaluated and treated over 1,400 inmate-patients and completed 572 formal forensic evaluation reports for the courts. The following patient and outcome data summarizes the work and achievements of the ROC model at the LFU.

Diagnostic profile: The patients served by the LFU were extremely disordered, suffering from acute psychotic symptoms, extreme behavioral disturbances, substance abuse disorders, impaired cognitive functioning, or combinations of these problems. In fact, half (49%) suffered from a major mental illness, including schizophrenia, schizoaffective, bipolar, Psychosis NOS, dementia, and major depressive disorders. Nearly one quarter (23%) also suffered from substance abuse or substance abuse-induced disorders as the primary Axis I diagnosis. When Substance Abuse was identified as a concomitant diagnosis, the number of patients with substance abuse/dependence increased to 56%. It is notable that well over one third of the admissions to the LFU also had an Axis II Diagnosis (43%), including 34% with a diagnosed Personality Disorder. In particular, 10% of the patients had a diagnosis of Borderline Intelligence or Mental Retardation.

Criminal offense profile: The most common criminal offenses were Property Crimes (20%), Assault (18%), Sex Offenses (13%) and Assault on an Officer/Resisting Arrest (13%). Two thirds of the patients who were charged with violent crimes (67%). Of note, over half (54%) had committed violence against persons, including 6% charged with murder.

Primary Clinical Diagnoses		Primary Criminal Offenses	
Psychotic Disorders		**Violent crimes**	
Schizophrenia	15%	Assault	18%
Schizoaffective	10%	Assault on police/Resist arrest	13%
Bipolar disorder	6%	Sex Offenses	13%
Psychotic Disorder NOS	8%	Robbery	8%
Major Depressive Disorder	8%	Murder	6%
Subtotal	47%	Arson	5%
Substance Abuse		Abduction	2%
Substance Abuse Induced		Domestic violence	2%
Mood or Psychosis	12%	Subtotal	67%
Substance Abuse	11%		
Subtotal	23%	**Nonviolent crimes**	
Other Disorders		Property Crimes	21%
Adjustment Disorder	16%	CDS Offenses	6%
Dementia	2%	Weapons (no injury)	3%
Malingering	2%	Parole/Prob. violation	3%
All other diagnoses	8%	Subtotal	33%
Subtotal	28%		

Table 2. Diagnostic and Criminal Profile

Forensic categories served: The Liberty Forensic Unit at Riverside Regional Jail provided three basic categories of forensic psychiatric service:

- The "Evaluation" category was comprised of patients referred specifically for forensic evaluations, including pre-sentence evaluations, Competency to Stand Trial evaluations (CST), Mental Status at time of Offense evaluations (MSO) and combined CST/MSO evaluations.
- The "Incompetent to Stand Trial" (IST) category was comprised of patients admitted for the purpose of restoring them to competency to proceed with the judicial process.
- The "Temporary Detention Order" (TDO) category was comprised of pre-sentence and pre-trial jail transfers in need of acute inpatient psychiatric treatment to stabilize them and enable them to be returned and maintained in the jail setting. Note: The unit received acute referrals from dozens of jails across the Commonwealth.

Volume of forensic services provided by type: The following chart summarizes the volume of patients served by forensic category over the history of the program operation. It also shows the proportion of patients requiring IST, TDO and Evaluation services shifted from year to year. In particular, the primary focus of the program shifted from the provision of acute psychiatric stabilization (TDO) in the first two years to the restoration of competency in the last two years.

Number of Patients Served by Forensic Category

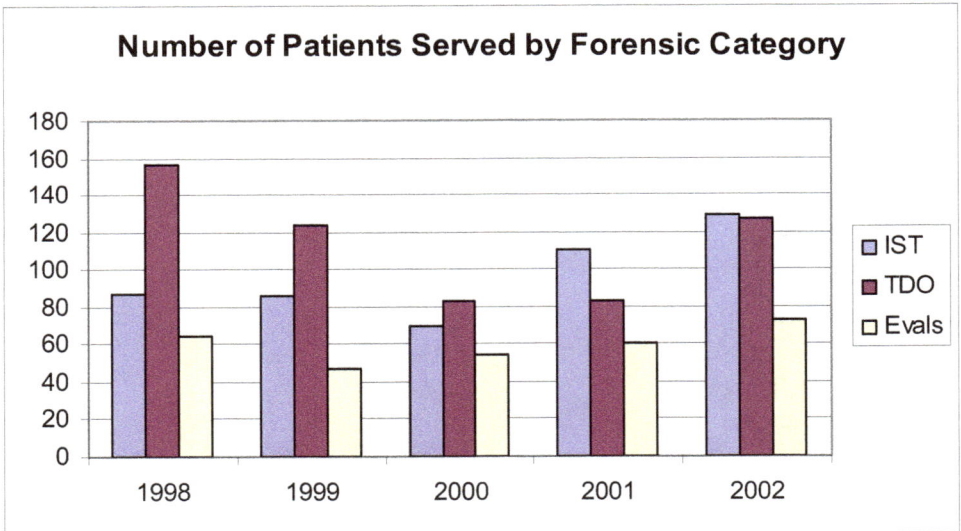

Length of stay by forensic category: Over a five year period, the LFU discharged forensic evaluation cases in an average of 21 days and provided psychiatric stabilization to return inmate patients to their referring jails in an average of 32 days. The ROC program achieved an overall competency restoration average of 83% while restoring full competency in an average of 77 days. Notably, in its final year and a half of operation, the ROC program was restoring competency in an average of just 69 days.

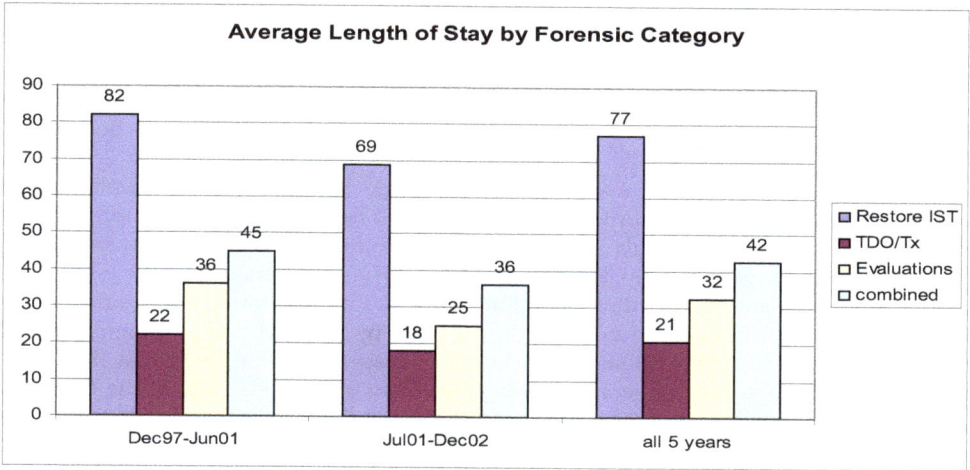

Average Length of Stay by Forensic Category

Seclusion and restraint rates: The LFU maintained very low rates of seclusion and restraint throughout its five years of operation. Seclusion was almost never used on the unit and was not employed at all in the final year of operation. Using data from the NASMHPD Research Institute for comparison, one study compared the number of restraint hours used in the LFU against the national average for forensic psychiatric units for the same period. Despite the high volatility and acuity of the forensic patients served, use of restraint on the LFU was typically less than half of the national average in the same year.

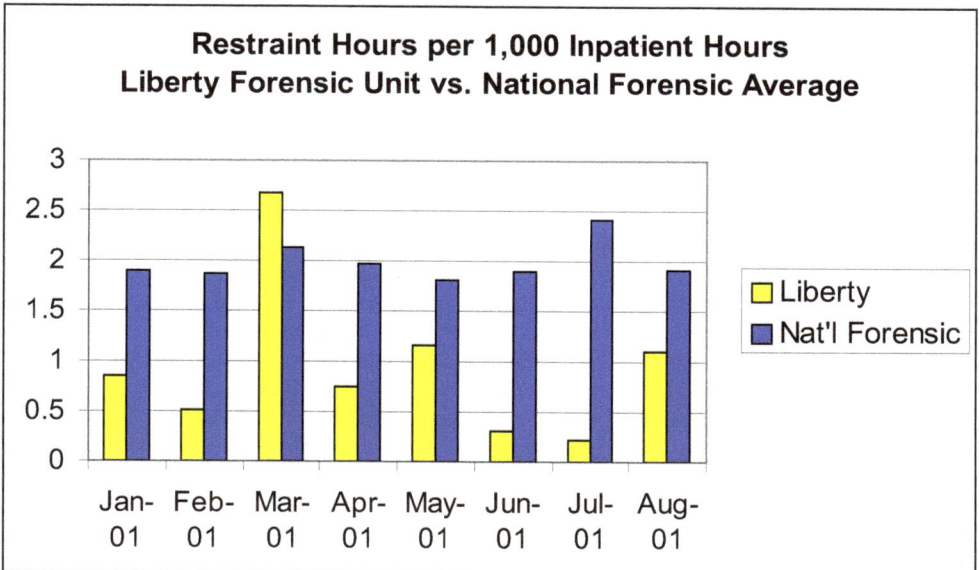

Restraint Hours per 1,000 Inpatient Hours
Liberty Forensic Unit vs. National Forensic Average

Customer satisfaction: The Liberty Forensic Unit at Riverside (LFU) was widely respected for the consistent delivery of excellent psychiatric and forensic services. It received formal commendations by the state chapter of the National Alliance of the Mentally Ill and the Local Human Rights Committee and frequent unsolicited praise from patients, patient families, Judges, State and Defense Attorneys, local jails, Community Service Boards and human rights advocates.

Customer satisfaction surveys were given to referring jails, community mental health centers (called CSBs), courts, attorneys and other entities being served. Results reflected the exceptional forensic services, high quality treatment and the collaborative responsiveness of the treatment team. 96% of the CSBs affirmed that LFU staff contacted them within one week of admission and provided regular clinical updates on the status of the patients. The clinical and treatment follow-up information provided by the LFU was also highly valued by both local jail staff and CSB staff. 90% and 87% respectively indicated that they were better able to manage their patients following treatment at the LFU. 96% of the CSB staff were better able to perform service linkages based on the information provided from the LFU. 87% of the referring jails affirmed that they were able to participate in both treatment and discharge planning for their patients and 93% acknowledged that the LFU treatment had been helpful. 92% of the referring entities received the discharge plan in a timely fashion, 97% acknowledged that aftercare recommendations were helpful, and 97% received some kind of follow-up support from the LFU team. 92% also affirmed that the recommended medication regimens at discharge remained unchanged for the inmate/patients served.

Commonwealth attorneys and defense attorneys were also satisfied with the quality of services received from the LFU unit. Whether on the side of the defense or the prosecution, the attorneys were nearly unanimous in their satisfaction with the clarity, utility and timeliness of the forensic reports received. Likewise, all but one attorney were satisfied that they could readily communicate with the ROC unit about their patients and that their patients had benefited from treatment at the LFU.

7. Conclusion

At a time when state hospital and community mental health resources are increasingly limited by critical financial realities, more and more people with severe and persistent mental illness and co-occurring disorders are becoming involved in the criminal justice system. In turn, the responsibility of caring for the mentally ill has shifted to the jails and prisons of America. One of the major areas is the ITP crisis in which inmates with mental illness are subjected to extended stays in jails awaiting competency evaluation and restoration. The ROC model is a cost-effective, clinically-effective and more humane model for this common problem. It calls for the provision of intensive psychiatric stabilization, forensic evaluation and restoration and maintenance of competency in the local jail

Despite the apparently aversive physical constraints of most jails and prisons, the ROC model shows that mental health providers can transform a jail pod into a true mental health facility with a remarkably therapeutic milieu. By combining an effective behavior management system, a lively treatment schedule, and some simple environmental modifications, such as marking "boundary lines" on the floor, a well-trained team of clinicians and direct care/security personnel can maintained a climate of safety, predictability and respect. The ROC model can accelerate needed treatment and restoration for mentally ill defendants, cut the demand for costly State Hospital forensic beds, deliver competency services at significantly lower cost per bed and directly assist local jails and law enforcement in better managing this specialized high-risk population – yielding major cost savings and improved services for all.

8. References

Bell, J. (2003). A proven model for placing an inpatient psychiatric unit within a jail. Presentation to the National Conference on Correctional Health Care, Austin, TX, October 2003.

Christy, A., Otto, R., Finch, J., Ringhoff, D., & Kimonis, E. (2010). Factors affecting jail detention of defendants adjudicated incompetent to proceed. *Behavioral Sciences and the Law, 28,* 707-716.

Commonwealth of Virginia. (2010). FY 2009 Jail Cost Report: Annual Jail Revenues and Expenditures Report. Report from the Compensation Board to the General Assembly, November 1, 2010.

Gilbert, A., Moser, L., Van Dorn, R., Swanson, J., Wilder, C., Robbins, P., Keator, K., Steadman, H., and Swartz, M. (2010). Reductions in arrest under assisted outpatient treatment in New York. *Psychiatric Services, 61,* 996–999.

Hazelwood, L. and Rice, K. (2010). Competency-related Assessment Rating Scale (CARS). Unpublished forensic assessment tool developed by Liberty Healthcare Corporation, Bala Cynwyd, PA.

Human Rights Watch. (2003). *Ill-equipped: U.S. Prisons and Offenders with Mental Illness.* New York: Human Rights Watch.

Jennings, J. (2009). Does Assertive Community Treatment work with forensic populations? Review and recommendations. *The Open Psychiatry Journal, 3,* 13-19.

Lamb, H. and Weinberger, L. (2005). The shift of psychiatric inpatient care from hospitals to jails and prison. *Journal of American Academy of Psychiatry and Law, 33,* 529-534.

Loveland, D. and Boyle, M. (2007). Intensive case management as a jail diversion program for people with a serious mental illness: A review of the literature. *International Journal of Offender Therapy and Comparative Criminology, 51,* 30-150.

Miller, R. (2003). Hospitalization of criminal defendants for evaluation of competence to stand trial or for restoration of competence. Clinical and legal issues. *Behavioral Sciences and Law, 21,* 369-391.

Smith, R., Jennings, J. and Cimino, A. (2010). Forensic continuum of care with ACT for persons recovering from co-occurring disabilities: Long term outcomes. *Psychiatric Rehabilitation Journal, 33,* 207-218.

Swartz, M., Swanson, J., Kim, M. and J. Petrila, J. (2006). Use of outpatient commitment or related civil court treatment orders in five U.S. communities. *Psychiatric Services, 57,* 343-349.

Torrey, E., Kennard, A., Eslinger, D., Lamb, R. and Pavle, J. (2010). *More mentally ill persons are in jails and prisons than hospitals: A survey of the states.* Arlington, Va.: Treatment Advocacy Center.

Trudel, J. and Lesage, A. (2006). Care of patients with the most severe and persistent mental illness in an area without a psychiatric hospital. *Psychiatric Services, 57,* 1765-1770.

Redlich, A., Steadman, H., Clark-Robbins, P. and Swanson, J. (2006) Use of the criminal justice system to leverage mental health treatment: Effects on treatment adherence and satisfaction. *Journal of American Academy of Psychiatry and Law*, *34*, 292-299.

Rich, J, Wakeman, S. and Dickman, S. (2011). Medicine and the epidemic of incarceration in the United States. *The New England Journal of Medicine*, *364*, 2081-2083.

Wortzel, H., Binswanger, I., Martinez, R., Filley, C. and Anderson, A. (2007). Crisis in the treatment of incompetence to proceed to trial: Harbinger of a systematic illness. *Journal of American Academy of Psychiatry and Law*, *35*, 357-363.

Zapf, P. and Roesch, R. (2011). Future directions in the restoration of competency to stand trial. *Current Directions in Psychological Science*, *20*, 43-47.

Part 3

Treatments

7

The Vitality of Fragmentation: Desublimation and the Symbolic Order

Geoffrey Thompson
Saybrook University, San Francisco, CA
USA

1. Introduction

This chapter will focus on theoretical, clinical and personal challenges surrounding my work as an art therapist in an adult outpatient service of a psychiatric hospital. The evolution of my thinking pervades my clinical work with the client discussed in the vignette, as I sought to integrate desublimation from art theory and philosophy with psychoanalytic theory. (Thompson, 2007). When I first met Evelyn, who is diagnosed with Schizoaffective Disorder, she was hospitalized, constantly agitated and psychotic with auditory hallucinations, severe labile mood, disorganization in cognition and behavior and paranoid delusions, linked to her experience of the polarizing states of grandiosity and inferiority. She constantly sought to expel the experience of being belittled and hurt by projections and hostile attacks on other patients and clinicians. As a result, she was frequently expelled from verbal group psychotherapy after vicious angry attacks on peers and therapists. She could frequently be seen pacing the hospital corridors while engaged in an angry verbal monologue of diatribes. Evelyn's physical appearance was also notable for her reliance on trailing scarves, jewelry, and numerous bags and necklaces, strung impossibly around her body. Staff and fellow patients at the center would consciously avoid her when she approached, anticipating the inevitable hostile barrage of affect, fueled by paranoid ideation.

In this chapter I will describe the process, challenges and outcome in our work together over a four-year period. I hoped that the seemingly impossible task of developing a meaningful relationship with Evelyn, one, that might support therapeutic growth through the intermediary container of art, could be accomplished. Ironically, some of the later breakthroughs of our time together were the direct result of a Derridean deconstructive approach to initial models of art therapy. (Derrida, 1997). Evelyn had become part of the complex narrative of the institution, the psychiatric hospital, which co-creates shared meanings. In the case of Evelyn the hopelessness surrounding her pervaded the milieu and was mirrored leading to a shared sense of marginalization and failure. This was a familiar narrative when I met her and it extended to her tentative and abortive relationship with art and art therapy. (Fig. 1) Traditional models of art therapy that are quintessentially modernist employ some basic assumptions regarding pivotal aspects of art and creativity. These will be explored in the chapter and include the Symbolic Order, sublimation, desublimation, and embedded in these areas are the roles of regression, repression, self-identity, rationality and the irrational.

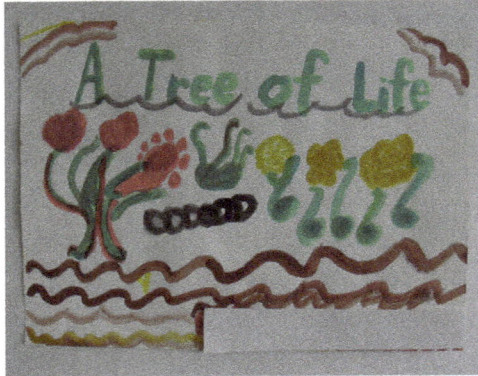

Fig. 1. A Tree of Life. Watercolor on paper. 12X18.

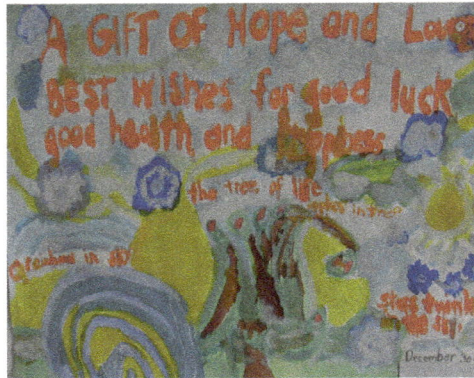

Fig. 2. A Gift of Hope and Love. Tempera on paper. 12x18.

2. The Symbolic Order

The Symbolic Order pertains to the conception of art and language within cultural parameters and is relevant in this case because it can either assist or hinder an understanding of what constitutes art. Art therapy has historically adopted the symbolic order of modernism without questioning its validity, and especially its relevance or efficacy with challenging populations such those individuals seen within the psychotic spectrum disorders. This approach has contributed to the sense of impasse and failure of art, thus joining the psychoanalytic understanding that psychotic patients are unable to participate in the shared discourse of symbolic meanings prominent in language. (Wrye, 1993).

During the course of modernism art has developed along a continuum of new, avant-garde movements each progressing in a temporal rhythm. Art history has tended towards reading ontological development of a system codifying visual form. This type of codification is the substance of the modernist epoch that stressed logical and organic growth so that, at least officially, it appeared the multiple "isms" flow naturally from one to another. The end game of modern art became entrenched in what the art historian Greenberg (1965, 2003) described as formalism. Formalism, briefly, postulated that modern art was driven to advance only those characteristics deemed integral to a specific medium. The metaphor of art originating and developing as an organism bears similarities to developmental theories and especially psychoanalytic drive theory that stresses mastery and maturation of biologically derived stages of growth and development.

Both fields harnessed movement towards rationalism and integration but there are exceptions. The site and the specifics of these exceptions are important because they point towards alternative means of generating meaning. Exceptions can be seen as ruptures that provide opportunities to reconfigure the generation of meaning and in this particular case offer a reparative window through which Evelyn could find beauty and success. As if anticipating these difficulties and minimizing potential ruptures and impurities, cubism's radical departure was interpreted smoothly within this continuum. Differences are swept aside in the overarching historical reading that stresses the continuum of visual form.

One of these sites is the historical period of Impressionism, where modernism supported the development in both art and early psychoanalysis of the symbolic order. The graphic supremacy of the line disappeared in the impressionist's small individual dabs of color as the form is designed to appear magically in our own eyes as a direct result of optically mixing the separate colors. Nineteenth century color theories were influential in lending a measure of scientific respectability to the avant-garde. The final reading and cognitive grasp of the painting in the (optical) unconscious took place through the cohering of all the separate interacting colors. Voila! The haystack, bridge or landscape is there to behold in Technicolor, magically solidified as the visual proof of the artist's authentic vision. Clark (1999) reiterates the connection between the optical mix integral to the impressionists and both Helmholtz and Freud. Freud (as cited in Clark, 1999) states,

"The intention of this project is to furnish us with a psychology which shall be a natural science: its aim, is to represent psychical processes as quantitatively determined states of specifiable material particles and so to make them plain and void of contradictions." (p. 139) Clark (1999) explains more on this connection that a young Freud (writing in 1895) is "still struggling to think the unconscious in a language borrowed from Helmholtz and Fechner." (p. 142). The coherence of visual images configured as an aspect of unconscious processing informed Freud's psychology of the unconscious and these in turn would then be reapplied throughout modernism by providing the ready model that Ehrenzweig (1971) used to advocate a *hidden order*. Sense can always be made of seemingly irrational images or forms because all will conform to this biological drive to cohere incoming perceptions. Even analytic cubism and the drip paintings of Jackson Pollack could then be made conform to the cultural expectation of the symbolic order, as the significance of the seeming irrational and sheer incomprehensibility of this radical form of painting suddenly conforms after all.

The connections between "high art" and psychological theory colluded spawning alliances such as Winnicott's (1971) squiggle technique and the use of such spontaneous images in art therapy. (Cane,1989; Naumburg, 1987). This model has repercussions in contemporary art and in art therapy practices, where non-conforming art is marginalized, unless it can be retrieved within the dubious frame of "Outsider" art. In Evelyn's case her fragmented paintings (see Fig. 1) embody the frustration that taps the parallel process of her own psyche and the apparent failure to enter true symbolic communication.

3. Sublimation and art therapy

Evelyn's sense of failure emanates partly from the therapeutic frame that can pathologize intrapsychic fragmentation and from the pivotal model of art therapy that relies heavily on the psychoanalytic concept of sublimation. Freud (1989) on sublimation explains, "the transformation of object-libido into narcissistic libido which thus takes place obviously implies an abandonment of the sexual aims, a desexualization-a kind of sublimation, therefore. Indeed the question arises, and deserves careful consideration, whether this is not the universal road to sublimation, whether all sublimation does not take place through the mediation of the ego, which begins changing sexual object-libido into narcissistic libido and then, perhaps, goes on to give it another aim." (pp. 24-25)

An early pioneer of art therapy, Edith Kramer (2001) echoes this, "whereby primitive urges, emanating from the id, are transformed by the ego into complex acts that do not serve direct instinctual gratification." (p. 28). Sublimation completes a temporal sequence that takes place from the innate and primitive drives culminating in a final form, transformed by the dynamic mechanism of psychic process that can then communicate within the accepted norms of cultural speech, the symbolic order. This takes the shape of interpersonal communication in language or in art the product and its imagery, may be referred to as Naumburg (1987) did as *symbolic speech*. Green (1999) charts the original course of sublimation from Freud's early work where it was conceived in direct relationship to the drives acting as a kind of bridge between sexual energy and aims, becoming diverted or displaced within the matrix of society (p. 217). As regression loosens the ego's control on primary process some of the newly tapped energy must escape repression; "sublimation has indeed to be considered in relation to repression: namely, as the outcome of a certain drive quota which has *partially* escaped its action." (p. 218). Green explains that the duality of repression and sublimation is a continual process, with repression occurring, "each time there is a return of the repressed liable to 'let through' repressed material." (p. 218).

Sublimation, according to Green (1999) is a "vicissitude of the drive but also as a deviation of this same vicissitude." (p. 218). This deviation particularly interests Green because it focuses on the *negative* or anti-sexual aspect of sublimation. Green describes this negative as reinforcing the narcissistic self from "a retreat into the ego, corresponding to a desexualisation, [that] results in a unification, a kind of total unity [and] the ego, thus invested (through identification) with the finery of the object, has desexualized its relations with the latter and, ceasing to love it, sets itself up as its rival." (p. 226).

Kramer (1971) proposed five distinct ways of using art materials, precursory activities, chaotic discharge, art in the service of defense, pictographs and finally formed expression (p. 54) The five stages echo developmental theory and constitute a hierarchy with formed expression as the most advanced and desirable. As such it is also where sublimation has been most successful; it attains "the production of symbolic configurations that successfully serve both self-expression and communication." (p. 55). With all systems of hierarchies inferiority lurks and so it is with these stages that privilege a certain pedigree of aesthetic form. The form that is favored by Kramer is usually representational and aspects from the earlier stages are described using the focus on what is lacking or deficient, for example "scribbling, smearing; exploration of physical properties that does not lead to creation of symbolic configurations, [or] banal conventional production... pictographs are, as a rule, crudely executed" (p. 54). Kramer linked the five stages to the relationship between the sublimated images to how successful the therapeutic encounter as a measure. When difficulties arise with sublimated art, Kramer sometimes used the term pseudo-art, a term that resembles Green's (1986) characterization of pseudo-sublimation.

Henley (1992) weighs in on Kramer's linkage of sublimation of *formed expression* with how successful a given therapeutic intervention is, coming down with some reservations, in support. Henley believes that "a model of aesthetics and even art criticism can be constructed that is commensurate with the aims of therapy without diluting the intent of either discipline." (p. 153). Henley questions Kramer's criticism of the primitivism associated with Art Brut that "an intelligible communication is either obscured or so alien that it invites speculation regarding the problems of its maker." (p. 154). Primitive art is irreconcilable in Kramer's paradigm because it fails to meet certain judgments regarding its ability to communicate inviting Kramer to speculate about the health of the artist/client.

Severe psychopathology characteristic of extreme regression of psychosis can compromise artistic integrity and at such times "aesthetic expectation should be all but suspended." (Henley 1992. p. 161). Knafo (2002) describes the way that regression in the service of creativity can produce mental states that have similarities to psychosis, stating:

"These processes resemble childlike states or characteristics generally associated with madness…[except]…they are under the artist's control in the sense that he or she has the capacity to make the transition from these states to others requiring observation, discipline, and criticism." (p. 46)

The ability to step back and forth in this regressed state is the hallmark of creativity and the specialization of the artist. This phenomenon relates to the function of the observing ego and the way the art object occupies transitional space (Winnicott, 1971) providing psychic distance between self and other. Through the use of art the ability to navigate between these different realms of the psyche could be accomplished.

Given this particular scenario does it really make sense to abandon aesthetic criteria since this is the substance of the regressive/creative state of mind? This is the intertwined relation between madness and art and the aesthetic imperative perhaps is to focus on their meeting rather than abandoning the task. Foucault's (1973) observation that madness is incompatible with art persistently shadows this discussion; Foucault stated, "Artaud's madness does not slip through the fissures of the work of art; his madness is precisely the absence of the work of art, the reiterated presence of that absence, its central void experienced and measured in all its endless dimensions." (p. 287). Nietzsche's demise, Foucault explains comes at the point when the philosopher's art disappears from the "very annihilation of the work of art, the point where it becomes impossible and where it becomes silent …[and]… Van Gogh, who did not want to ask 'permission from his doctors to paint pictures,' knew quite well that his work and his madness were incompatible." (p. 287).

4. Fragmentation, regression and creativity

A psychoanalytic concept developed by Kris (1952) called *regression in the service of the ego* illustrates how creativity is intertwined with regression. Kris was interested in delineating the role of regression in both pathological and non-pathological states, acknowledging that with important differences this phenomenon taken to its logical conclusion on the one hand can lead to the type of psychosis found in schizophrenia and on the other the highest cultural products in art. Kris (1975) explains the difference between a creative individual and a "psychotic artist" is the concrete nature of the depictions, "…words are not signs but acts, pictures tend to become verdicts, and creation may mean 'making' in a literal and magical sense." (p. 488). The ability of the ego to loosen control as a result what Freud (1989) called a *flexibility of repression* while not becoming engulfed was seen by Kris (1975) to be an essential element of the creative process. This permits primary process to be used in the service of the ego, which retains control of the psychic processes, and art is communicative rather than in psychotic experience, concrete and magical.

The healthier characterization of creativity that Kris (1975) formulated were taken up by the psychoanalytic theorists that comprise of the group referred to as ego psychology; this movement was oriented towards an understanding of the adaptive functions and structure of the ego and its relative defenses. More recently, Knafo (2002) summarized Kris' theories regarding creativity and his assertion of two main phases, "During the first inspirational phase, the artist is passively receptive to id impulses [that are] otherwise hidden and unavailable, emerge to communicate with the ego." (p. 26). The second phase of elaboration "calls for the artist's active use of such ego functions as reality testing, formulation, and communication." (p. 27). This resembles Freud's (1966) concept of *secondary revision*, and Ehrenzweig's (1971) application of secondary process to locate rationality in art. The artist displays a flexibility regarding relative control in the dynamic relationship between the ego and the id and the ability to move back and forth in these levels of consciousness. Freud (1989) describes the substance of primary process relating to instinctual drives that seek satisfaction through discharge and, that an instinct deriving from one particular erotogenic source can make over its intensity to reinforce another component instinct originating from another source, that the satisfaction of one instinct can take the place of the satisfaction of another. (p. 43)

The source of energies emanates from the vast store of id characterized by sexual, aggressive and narcissistic instincts or drives and Freud (1989) theorized that as these energies are cathected to objects, the satisfaction of instinctual impulses can be displaced. Freud explained, "it was in dream-work that we first came upon this kind of looseness in the displacements brought about by primary process." (p. 44). Freud continues, if this displaceable energy is desexualized libido, it may also be described as sublimated energy; for it would still retain the main purpose of Eros-that of uniting and binding-in so far as it helps towards establishing the unity, or tendency toward unity, which is particularly a characteristic of the ego." (p. 44)

Freud (1989) writes concerning obsessional neurosis that "through a regression to a pregenital organization, for the love impulses to transform themselves into impulses of aggression against the object." (p. 55). When the tendency towards unity fails due to severe pathological states fragmentation can result. The aggression unleashed upon objects can fragment and potentially destroy the object. While Knafo (2002) and Kris (1952) before her sought to depathologize regression, the dual processes that lead to either art or psychosis are linked and share the same foundational psychological processes. Therefore, "if regression predominates the symbols used in the artwork are egocentric and take on private meaning" (Knafo, 2002, p. 27) which pushes the work towards the continuum of psychosis. Egocentric might mean personal and inscrutable because in psychosis the images are often characterized as private, falling short of partaking in the community of either visual or verbal forms of symbolic speech.

The psychology of the self and the generation of meaning that is dependent on growth within the symbolic order could perceive this as precipitating a crisis of faith. This is the prevalent frame that Wrye (1993) discusses, when "very disturbed patients often begin treatment unable to enter into the therapist's verbal-symbolic framework. Without the capacity to communicate with and understand symbolic language, experience remains concrete. Such individuals cannot enter into the world of consensual meaning." (p. 115). The incomprehensible images, words and behavior reinforce Evelyn's and the institution's sense of the symbolic void. Desublimation will illustrate an alternative means of generating meaning where comprehension reigns. The regression to magical procedure might contribute to confusion with reality but the navigable path out of this could be the same creative process.

The fragmentation involved in the creative process can find itself at odds within the frame of art therapy when the broken, fragment, piece, or unintegrated meshes with psychological conception of splits, schizoid, schizophrenic and psychotic process. An integral part of creativity is then linked to pathology and may be seen as interesting but unformed and essentially lacking the integration that is necessary for wholeness.

5. Desublimation in art and art therapy

The transcendent function of art that has been the hallowed ground of the modern era has been challenged by the philosophy of structuralism and post-structuralism. Krauss (1987) explains the depth of these ramifications:
"On the one hand, structuralism rejected the historicist model as the means to understand the generation of meaning. On the other, within the work of poststructuralism, those timeless, transhistorical forms, which had been seen as indestructible categories wherein aesthetic development took place, were themselves opened to historical analysis and placement." (p. 2)
Thinking about a work of art as a structure challenges the dominant ontological model and permitted radically new discussions of how meaning in art can be generated. One gap or rupture in the symbolic order is the conception of a revitalized gestalt operating in analytical cubism (roughly the period between 1908–1912). The desperate attempt to rationalize the fragmentary and split planes of cubism was required to maintain the historical evolution of progressive modern art. Form can be reconfigured, as it was in cubism, so that it will not cohere into a logical and hence progressive order that makes sense. As the cubist forms lurch, fragment and unravel there may in fact be the flavor of irrationality, but of a qualitatively different character to the primary process more characteristic of regression.

Desublimation in my text is not the reverse of sublimation, not pseudo-sublimation or un-sublimation, or the type of overt sexual images that Jones (2003) describes as desublimation occurring in surrealism. (p. 122). Rather, it originates from the insight that gestalt could be seen as resembling a state of flux as it offers a multiplicity of possible configurations rather than a correct one that compels the order of the good gestalt. Einstein (2004) wrote "...by means of art, one attempts to contest deadly generalizations and the rationalistic impoverishment of the world, to sever the chains of causality, to unravel the web of significations." (p. 174).

The separate planes that Einstein refers to in cubism are deliberately fragmentary to subvert the nature of vision by preventing and interrupting the tendency to order form. Desublimation works in cubism by undermining the concept of the mnemonic in art, radically altering the cognitive sense of seeing a work of art as a totality with a fixed structure. The fragments of planes do not make sense in the usual way of building an image in the mind from scanning the temporal sequences and utilizing memory and causality to connect this piece with the next. Zeidler (2004) describes the challenge that was evoked in the critical texts of Einstein who began to question the idea of a work of art that exists as "a sublimated version of everyday experience." (p. 5). The idea of the art object in modernism representing an epistemological regime was one of the main challenges of the work of Einstein. He identified the work produced during Analytic cubism as a testament to a rupture in the episteme.

Perhaps Ehrenzweig (1971) was right after all when he envisioned cubism as an attack on conscious sensibilities. However the source of this affront was not the characteristic of schizoid fragmentation awash in primary process resulting from the alienating destruction of humanism, that he feared, but rather the optical challenge to the notion of form as a fixed and hence predictable and logical organism. The desublimated form challenges the idea of the connection to the work of art transformed into "a reconfiguration of the world into a 'world seen.'" (Zeidler, 2004. p. 30). In this methodology of embodied vision the artist presents for the viewer, the potential to construct a subjective identity construction: "…a world made over into a set of stimuli to be synthesized by a subject's vision: a world in which appearance takes precedence over object and where pictorial means no longer served to clarify the objective order of things." (p. 30).

The preceding discussion helps to illustrate that art history, theory and even criticism brings an urgency as well as agency to the pivotal role of art in art therapy. The opening that desublimation affords changes the context for meaning making and challenges the prevailing theories outlined. The foundational theory involving sublimation, regression and repression bends the art to conform to this paradigm, This has resulted in pathologizing work that reflects incompleteness. Kramer (1971) wrote, "we know in particular that disturbances in feelings of identity and personal intactness invariably reveal themselves by distortions and fragmentations of the visual images" (p. 29). The relationship of the un-sublimated and fragmented work of art to satisfying the demands of the pleasure principle will be at best an incomplete wish fulfillment "limited by his pathology, the state of his ego, his manual skill, his 'talent,' and many other factors." (p. 29). Green (1986) also examined pseudo-sublimation that might also be named a *defensive sublimation* or a *failed sublimation* and states "undeniably, there do exist sublimations which are the offspring of certain pathological forms. These can be viewed as emergency exits from conflict" (p. 132).

Green (1986) links pseudo-sublimation to personality types who demonstrate a *moral narcissism* and the partial pleasure afforded by incomplete sublimation to the potential of "the essential part of this observation of the ego is the completion of the constitution of what Winnicott calls a *false* self." (p. 133). The identification with the false self blocks the connection to the generative inner core where true creativity resides. The false self "also functions to limit and to block the symbol-making capacities of mental life, because of the important role that unconscious processes play in the image-making processes of the mind."(Dragstedt, 1998. p. 498). This state of "living is superficial, and it often contributes to states of claustrophobia, preoccupation with self-image, and acting-out archaic relationships with the body." (p. 498).

Deconstructing the relationship between sublimation, regression, and art helps to reveal how subjective identification emerges within culture to circumscribe belief systems. Dualism informs this or that, high/low, true/false logic whereas desublimation leads to another kind of mental space free of these stifling parameters. Embedded in these structures are power relations in which Foucault (1984) sought to understand the "…modes of

objectification which transform human beings into subjects." (p. 417). This is primarily achieved through *dividing practices*,
"The subject is either divided inside himself or divided from others. This process objectivizes him. Examples are the mad and the sane, the sick and the healthy, the criminals and the 'good boys.'" (p. 417)
Fragmentation in the art in art therapy is enormously difficult to separate from this kind of dividing practice, where it easily can be linked or interpreted as evidence of pathology or a kind of "not good-enough" sublimation. The undoing of form, honoring fragmentation as a gestalt ever changing, permits a dialogue with these archaic relationships to the body, accessing the regenerative healthy core, giving it form and substance as it pulls apart conventions.

6. Vignette

Evelyn is a sixty eight year old woman who currently attends a Community Mental Health partial hospitalization service for severely mentally ill adults. She was first diagnosed with mental illness at age twenty-four after an aborted suicide attempt. She earned a college degree and worked as a Kindergarten teacher for twenty-seven years before retiring on a medical disability related to her current psychiatric diagnosis of Schizoaffective Disorder Bipolar type. She participates in psychotherapy and other therapeutic regimes including art therapy producing many paintings like the example in Figure 1 and Figure 2 that lend clarity to the stages described by Kramer (1971). These paintings are crudely executed and seem to accentuate the fragmented split between Evelyn and the reality of the world around her. They fit with the following description and as such they seem to fall short of Kramer's coveted status of formed expression, (p. 54) belonging instead to the level characterized as pictographs and "art in the service of defence" (p. 121) reflecting, "bland stereotypes that are dull, repetitious, and conventional; work that is rigid and stereotyped but presents unusual or bizarre configurations; work that is filled with false sentiment, such as saccharine sweetness, hollow heroism, or false piety." (p. 122)
Evelyn had produced many of these bland paintings with daubed text describing sentimental messages and depictions of flowers incongruent with her frequent paranoid raging attacks. Empathic support and various interventions all appeared inconsequential to this repetitive cycle that provided the artistic equivalent of acute fragmentation with the resulting negativity and frustration. With traditional materials such as paint and pencils Evelyn stubbornly derailed any attempts to continue in an engaged, prolonged manner with the images. Green's (1999) conception of the negative relates to Evelyn's wall of incomprehension. Green cites Bion's work on the positive (+K) and the negative (-K) attributes of knowledge when "-K is not content with qualifying the negative in terms of an insufficiency or deficit; it gives it status. Not-understanding is brought into play by the patient's psyche when it is in his interest to stop understanding. This is a widely encountered phenomenon. It is with psychotic patients, or in Bion's terminology, with the psychotic part of the personality, that the specific nature of this mechanism can be pinpointed." (p. 8-9)
The concept of *attack on linking* (Bion, 1967) meshes with the process by which Evelyn at times appears incapable of knowing or understanding. The splitting of parts of the self and others into *bizarre objects* that are then perceived "out there" as inhabiting the dangerous and destructive world infects the milieu. The theories outlined earlier now appear to make sense with this dynamic, when the art experience follows a format that would require linking, integration and sublimation, working images towards a sense of completion and wholeness

the psychic level of fragmentation intrusively impinges upon the process. The smoothness of paint and the insubstantiality of pencils were quickly sabotaged and aborted as a result of the fragmented nature of Evelyn's cognitive and affective chaos, leading to further disconnection and fragmentation.

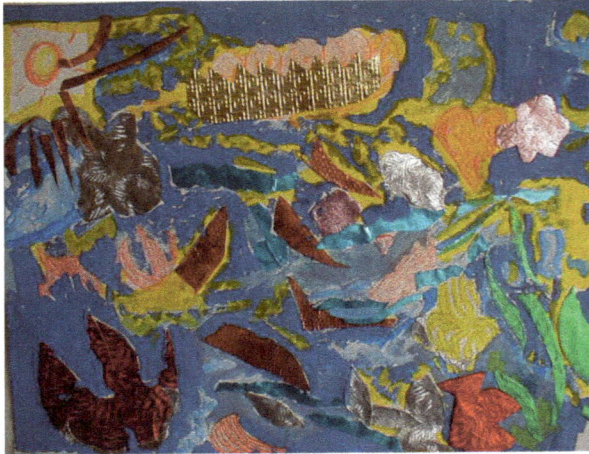

Fig. 3. Collage. Tempera & Paper on Paper.

I wanted to introduce what Derrida (1997) calls the *absolute break* by introducing a radical newness without discarding the existing framework, instead finding a phenomenological openness to art, materials and intersubjective space. Part of this orientation involves a slow temporal discovery of the sense of self as an artist, initially through a sustained focus on the constituents of artistic sensibility. (Thompson, 2009). After introducing collage to Evelyn many significant changes took place. Collage confronts fragmentation directly with the potential to hold disparate ideas and affects while honoring fragmentation and differences. (Figure 3) I thought of the desire of Close (2004) to use multiple fragments in his paintings to subvert and prevent the image from cohering into a whole. What would happen if Evelyn began making images that do not cohere from an aesthetic perspective as opposed to the incomplete sublimation resulting from regression?

The sculpture that Evelyn titled appropriately "A Portrait of Beauty" (Figures 4 & 5) resulted from her increased investment, *going-on-being* (Winnicott, 1986) over the period of one year, realizing her vision of beauty, standing as a testament to the strong therapeutic alliance that developed between us. The apparent contradictions in the work are a mark of its complexity and result in part from the slow temporal unfolding. In this way the individual history that informs the way the materials are joined has now become a palpable presence. The sculpture has the embodied affect contained in the visible fragments that are tied together and the invisibility of the negative three-dimensional space that almost magically supports the structure.

The sculpture reiterates Lyotard's (1984) description, "What is important in a text is not what it means, but what it does and incites to do. What it does: the charge of affect it contains and transmits." (pp, 9-10) The desublimated form can harness this affective charge in a powerful way. Since this sculpture was so large (eight feet tall) the phenomenon of

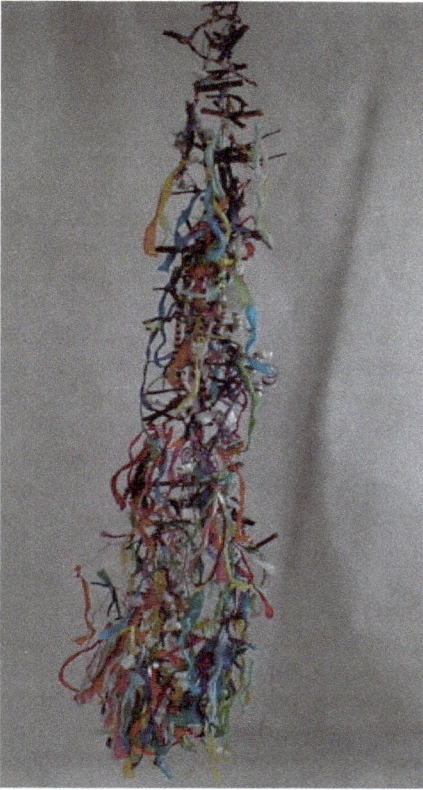

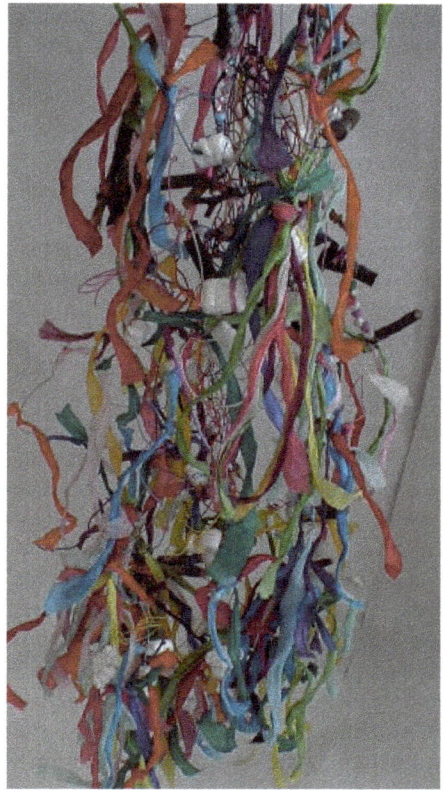

Tissue, wood, beads and wire. Height 8'

Fig. 4. A Portrait of Beauty. Syrofoam,   Fig. 5. A Portrait of Beauty. Detail.

being inside heightened the sense of play that Winnicott (1986) describes as transitional space, the intermediate zone between what is *me* and *not me* (p. 45). Stepping in and out and back and forth was necessary to complete this work and required careful negotiation and increased self- and body-awareness heightening the physical presence that in turn strengthened Evelyn's spatial-kinesthetic sense – previously she had a history of falls (not explained medically) that now had stopped.

The slow incremental use of the disparate fragments of wood, paper, tissue, wire, beads, and styrofoam derailed the derailing from the internal attacks on linking. *Aesthetic action* (Thompson, 2010) guided Evelyn as she found herself freed from the confines of the symbolic order. Evelyn discovered that desublimation leads to a new and exciting configuration where a lack is not a hindrance; the negative becomes knowledge since it is operating beyond the reach of the dualistic parameters of whole/broken or integration/disintegration. Thus, it relates to the stage of being or becoming that is related to *unintegration;* a value-neutral process of being that Winnicott (1986) describes as necessary for the development of ego integration. Abandoning convention does not mean spiraling through a regression where primary process abounds; rather it permits possibility by embracing all the separate pieces, fragments, thoughts, affects embodied and worked on through the safe, meditative action of tying and binding. The abstraction of form also released the cultural and self-imposed constraints that influence how representational art should appear as the sculpture now reads as a self-portrait. Evelyn revealed during the course of this work that she had been estranged from her twin sister for many years, a disclosure that throws new light on the twin roles that The Portrait of Beauty may hold for her. Her jealousy of her healthy, successful sister with a loving family had been intolerable for Evelyn, since she is acutely self conscious of failure, the stigma of severe mental illness and the debilitating physical effects of Hailey-Hailey's disease (hereditary skin eczema).

This sculpture had been made during an art therapy group with non-English speaking patients, an unusual paradoxical example of the positive attributes of the language barrier – Evelyn felt safe enabling her paranoid ideation to subside and the group-as-a-whole were blissfully unaware of her anger and sadistic attacks which also rapidly discontinued. The tilt of the final piece captures Evelyn's gait and posture and strikingly she shed her bizarre manner of dress with multiple scarves, necklaces and handbags, as the symbolic equivalents were bound together in aesthetic form. A Portrait of Beauty exceeds the stage of *formed expression* achieved with the fragmentary now sublimated in the desublimated form that permits this new conception; the fragments remain distinct. The sculpture surprises and overpowers clinicians and peers alike as testament to the generative power of creativity allowed to develop and unfold on Evelyn's own terms. This phenomenon desublimates the viewer's sensory experience forcing a radical new appreciation of the artist and her oeuvre. (Marcuse, 1978). Seasoned clinicians marveled at her work leading to a positive reappraisal of Evelyn, unimaginable prior to this undertaking! It was selected from over several hundred submissions to an Outsider art Exhibition in New York City and later exhibited and subsequently sold, in the gallery at the hospital she attends, completing the cycle from studio to gallery within the institution that is confronted with Evelyn, now visible as a unique, skilled and beautiful person, rather than a patient with severe mental illness (Thompson, 2009).

Desublimated art can alter form, freeing it from the stifling repressive symbolic order, to permit coherence within an alternative paradigm while remaining fragmentary. Desublimation is the aesthetic dismantling of form, supporting the multiplicity of self. The sculpture shows the process of Evelyn's attempt to construct recognizable and knowable patterns and arrangements that contain new patterns. Amidst these new patterns the poetic containment of trauma, ruptures, attacks and nihilistic yearnings can be empathetically perceived, as perhaps the sculptural form of desublimation accesses both the return of the repressed and the dissociated experiences caused by trauma. (Van der Kolk and Van der Hart, 1995). The holistic totality of this experience had several parallel effects on the therapist, the client, and the institution itself leading to openings based in the real and tangible feeling and experience of success and hope. Evelyn now at times co-leads groups with therapist and has returned to more conventional painting that is now invested with tremendous care, love and she has progressed closer to the goal she shares with the notable artist Agnes Martin, (1992) to find inspiration and beauty in oneself and in the world. Evelyn has after all integrated self, accepting imperfections while tolerating many stressful situations that previously may have triggered severe decompensation and possible hospitalization.

7. References

Bion, W. (1967). *Second thoughts; Selected papers on psychoanalysis.* Northvale NJ: Aronson.

Cane, F. (1989). *The artist within us.* Craftsbury Common, VT: Art Therapy.

Clark, T. J. (1999). *Farewell to an idea: Episodes from a history of modernism.* New Haven, CT: Yale University Press.

Close, C. (2004). April 29, 1987. Studio, SoHo. In J. O. Richards (Ed.), *Inside the studio: Two decades of talks with artists in New York,* (pp. 35-37). New York, NY: Independent Curators International.

Derrida, J. (1997). *Deconstruction in a nutshell: A conversation with Jacques Derrida.* (Ed. J. Caputo). New York, NY: Fordham University Press.

Dragstedt, N. R. (1998). Creative illusions: The theoretical and clinical work of Marion Milner. *Journal of Melanie Klein & Object Relations,16,* (3), 425-536.

Ehrenzweig. A. (1971). *The hidden order of art.* Berkeley, CA: University of California Press.

Einstein, C. (2004). Gestalt and concept. In *October, Carl Einstein.* A special issue, pp. 169-176. Cambridge, MA: The MIT Press.

Foucault, M. (1973). *Madness and civilization. A history of insanity in the age of reason.* New York, NY: Vintage Books.

Foucault, M. (1984). The subject and power. In B. Wallis (Ed), *Art after modernism. Rethinking representation.* (pp. 416-434). New York, NY: The New Museum of Contemporary Art.

Freud, S. (1966). *The interpretation of dreams.* New York, NY: Avon Books.

Freud, S. (1989). *The ego and the id.* New York, NY: W. W. Norton.

Green, A. (1999). *The work of the negative.* London, England: Free Association Books.

Green, A. (1986). *On private madness.* Connecticut: International Universities Press, Inc.

Greenberg, C. (1965). *Art and culture.* Boston, MA: Beacon Press.

Greenberg, C. (2003). *Clement Greenberg. Late writings.* Ed. R. Morgan. Minneapolis, MN: University of Minnesota Press.

Henley, D. (1992). *Exceptional children: Exceptional art.* Worcester, MA: Davis.

Jones, A. (2003) *Irrational modernism. A neurasthenic history of New York Dada.* Cambridge, MA: The MIT Press.

Knafo, D. (2002). Revisiting Ernst Kris's concept of *regression in the service of the ego in art. Psychoanaytic Psychology,19*(1), 24-29.

Kramer. E. (1971). *Art as therapy with children.* New York, NY: Schocken Books.

Kramer, E. (2001). Sublimation and art therapy. In J. Rubin (Ed.), *Approaches to art therapy theory and technique,* (pp. 28-39). Philadelphia, PA: Brunner-Routledge.

Krauss, R. E. (1987). *The originality of the avant-garde and other modernist myths.* Cambridge, MA: The MIT Press.

Kris, E. (1952). *Psychoanalytic explorations in art.* New York, NY: International Universities Press.

Kris, E. (1975). *The selected papers of Ernst Kris.* (Foreword by Anna Freud). New Haven, CT: Yale University Press.

Lyotard, J. F. (1984). *Driftworks.* New York, NY: Semiotext(e).

Marcuse, H. (1978). *The aesthetic dimension: Toward a critique of Marxist aesthetics.* Boston, MA: Beacon Press.

Martin, A. (1992). *Writings.* (H. von Dieter Schwartz, Ed.). Winterthur, Germany: Hatje Cantz.

Naumburg, M. (1987). *Dynamically oriented art therapy; its principles and practice.* Chicago, IL: Magnolia Street Publishers.

Thompson, G. (2010). *The contextual aesthetic: Artist identity within the psychotherapeutic matrix.* Grand Rounds Lecture at Maimonides Medical Center, Brooklyn, NY.

Thompson, G. (2009). Artistic sensibility in the studio and gallery model: Revisiting process and product. *Art Therapy: Journal of the American Art Therapy Association, 26*(4), 159-166.

Thompson, G. (2007). *The vitality of fragmentation: Desublimation and the symbolic order.* Paper presented at the 38th Annual Conference of the American Art Therapy Association, Albuquerque, NM.

Van der Kolk, B. A., & Van der Hart. O. (1995). The intrusive past. (C. Caruth Ed) *Trauma. Explorations in memory,* pp. 158-182. Baltimore, MD: John Hopkins University Press.

Wrye, H. K. (1993). Hello, the hollow: Deadspace or playspace. *Psychoanalytic Review, 80*(1), 101-121.

Winnicott, D.W. (1986). *The maturational processes and the facilitating environment: Studies in the theory of emotional development.* New York, NY: International Universities Press.

Winnicott, D. W. (1971). *Playing and reality.* Middlesex, England: Pelican.

Zeidler, S. (2004). Introduction. In S. Zeidler (Ed) October 107. *Carl Einstein a special issue,* pp. 3-13. Cambridge, MA: The MIT Press.

8

Homelessness as an Incurable Condition? The Medicalization of the Homeless in the Swedish Special Housing Provision

Cecilia Hansen Löfstrand
Department of Sociology, University of Gothenburg
Sweden

1. Introduction

In Sweden, the prevailing model for combating homelessness has been, and to a large extent still is, the disciplining staircase model, which stresses absolute sobriety as a criterion for eligibility for municipally organized special housing. The model builds on a view of the homeless as individuals incapable of independent living, albeit ones who are (potentially) *able to become* capable of independent living and (at least theoretically) of securing an ordinary apartment for themselves on the regular housing market, with the help of discipline and self-regulation (by adhering to the principle of absolute sobriety and complying with a number of other rules). In the staircase model, self-regulation is characteristically seen as a necessary precondition for this gradual improvement in the help receivers' housing standard, their increasing independence (living without rules, regulations, and surveillance), and the stability of their living situation more in general (Sahlin, 2005).

Of the country's population of nine million, approximately 17,800 are homeless, in the latest estimate of the National Board of Health and Welfare (National Board of Health and Welfare [NBHW], 2006). According to the same statistics, 62 percent of the homeless have problems with addiction and 40 percent suffer from a variety of mental disorders. The Board's figures, however, likely fail to accurately capture the size and nature of the homeless problem in the country. Due to respondent selection issues in its survey, there was, for example, no way to adequately assess the number of homeless individuals *not* suffering from addiction or mental health problems; nor could the number of homeless families be ascertained. Nonetheless, if the results are to be trusted, in 2005 there were 2,620 homeless persons in Gothenburg, Sweden's second largest city, with the municipality becoming singled out as having proportionally speaking the highest number of homeless in the country (54 homeless per 10,000 inhabitants).

In subsequent years, new measures to combat homelessness have been introduced in a number of municipalities in the country. In 2007, for example, the city of Gothenburg officially abandoned the staircase model it had been using until then (see Hansen Löfstrand, 2010), adopting in its stead the so-called Housing First model, as it was named when originally launched in the United States (see Tsemberis et al., 2004). In Gothenburg, the new approach has thus far been limited to a few housing units assigned for the experimentation with it. However, even though is the fundamental principle behind the Housing First model is to provide homeless with first-hand apartment contracts, this has thus far not been done in the Gothenburg case; instead, the city has settled into providing what amounts to permanent special housing for the homeless. In effect, what this has meant, as I will argue below, is that instead of marking a genuine shift in the city's homeless policy, the new model has simply been adapted for old purposes: the purpose of finding a way to deal with the problem of "the truly homeless." Who those "truly homeless" are, how they are identified and diagnosed, and what the prognosis is claimed to be is what I will elaborate on in what follows.

More broadly, in this chapter I investigate two concurrent trends in Swedish homelessness policy: the increasing medicalization of the homeless and a shift towards the Housing First approach, with its attendant emphasis on what among the local practitioners is called "symptom tolerance." How should these trends be understood in the particular country context in question, both in isolation and in relation to one another? At first glance, they might seem even contradictory, but, as my analysis will show, they are in fact all mutually related. Indeed, the medicalization of the homeless provided a prerequisite for the consideration of the Housing First model as a possible solution in the first place. However, in the Gothenburg context, the policy recommendations regarding normal housing arrangements based on first-hand apartment contracts that the model implied were taken to simply mean *permanent* housing arrangements with no expectation of sobriety, sometimes referred to as symptom-tolerance housing, which were based on second-hand rentals. Symptom-tolerance housing or, as it is also called, low-threshold housing has subsequently become a popular solution in the homeless policy of many of the country's larger cities, building on the basic idea that it is necessary to "relinquishing previous demands on people to be drug-free before they are offered housing" (Olsson & Nordfeldt, 2008, p. 165).

The local adaptations of the Housing First approach in contexts generally prescribing disciplinary measures have thus led to two different models coexisting in parallel. The first of these I call "homelessness as an incurable condition," and it used mostly for homeless deemed incurably ill, or to be suffering from an incurable condition. The goal is to provide permanent special housing and palliative care, which is regarded as a last-resort solution adopted only on account of the perceived failure of medical institutions to accept their responsibility for this group among the homeless: the best solution for it, in this view, would be hospitalization. The second model could be called "homelessness as a curable condition." This model is used for those homeless who are assumed to still be able to develop into capable and independent individuals with the help of regulation and self-regulation applied through the housing staircase model. The goal is for the homeless individuals to ultimately be able to obtain and manage an ordinary apartment of their own, although few actually reach this stage. The reasoning behind the two models goes, respectively, as follows: If suffering from an incurable condition, the homeless individual should be entitled to permanent housing (special housing units for the homeless) even when he or she acts in contravention of the relevant rules (continues to use alcohol, acts violently, threatens others, etc.), for which reason "housing first" is prescribed. If *not* incurably ill (i.e., still "curable"), the individual has to earn his or her way to housing, by demonstrating ability to comply with the demands of the disciplining staircase system. In other words, when the homelessness of the individual is considered an incurable condition, housing is to be facilitated and "the coercive social control strategies" of the staircase model should be bypassed (Willse, 2010, p. 156). Following Willse, what I will be arguing in what follows is that an important precondition for this new initiative was the "invention of chronic homelessness" (Willse, 2010, p. 157).

The research on which this chapter is based was carried out within a broader project entitled "Homelessness as Business: The Marketization of Social Housing in Gothenburg" and funded by the Swedish Council for Working Life and Social Research. The empirical material collected for it thus far consists of transcripts of 36 interviews (with politicians, civil servants, NGO and company representatives, homeless individuals), tenders submitted in the latest two procurement processes for special housing for the homeless, internal documents related to the try-out phase of the municipality's Housing First project, and the returns of a telephone questionnaire distributed to social service offices in the municipality of Gothenburg. For this chapter, I analyzed in depth the interviews with politicians and civil servants responsible for managing the problem on homelessness in the city, along with the interviews with nonprofit and for-profit providers of special housing for the homeless. A central analytical question guiding this analysis was: How is the problem of homelessness – and homeless persons – understood and how is the category of "the homeless" constructed and defined among the city's decision-makers and administrators? In addition, recent policy shifts and the planning and implementation of the local Housing First project in the city of Gothenburg were examined investigated. In the sections that follow, I will first review the main arguments put forward by Willse concerning the policy shifts that implementing a Housing First model implies and the possible motives behind it, before presenting my main theoretical framework. The presentation of the research findings then proceeds as follows: I start out by analyzing the views of key politicians and civil servants regarding the issue of homelessness in the city of Gothenburg. After that, I discuss the recently launched Housing First project in Gothenburg (its target group, main features and principles). Finally, I examine the way in which nonprofit and for-profit service providers interpreted and adapted their activities in response to the ongoing changes in the city. The chapter ends with a few concluding remarks on what the policy shift in question has really meant and what likely motivated it.

2. The Housing First model: The end of medicalization?

In the US American – just as in the Swedish – context the invention of (chronic) homelessness as a medical problem is connected to the basic idea behind the modern social service agencies, that it is necessary to "work on oneself" in order to gain access to and keep an apartment of one's own:

> Medicalization treats housing deprivation as a symptom of personal pathologies that must be cured by experts.... Thus, the medicalization of housing insecurity or deprivation opens a ground for the intervention of disciplinary techniques. (Willse, 2010, p. 165)

The dominant model in combating homelessness has for long consisted of a social worker who "assumes responsibility for guiding the client, or case, through a process of self-evaluation to determinate the individual causes at the root of their problem" (Willse, 2010, p. 165). This process has often involved drug and/or alcohol addiction treatment or comparable. Very frequently, absolute sobriety has thus been made a precondition for eligibility for special housing units for the homeless, in both Sweden (Hansen Löfstrand,

2010) and in the United States (Willse, 2010). This is described by Willse (2010) as an instance of the medicalization of homelessness. The Housing First approach, Willse (2010, p. 166) suggests, "represents a potential break" from such medicalized models since it involves a "separation of shelter provision from health and social services." Precisely because of this, the model was initially viewed with suspicion by social workers working within a system built on the assumption that health and social services are necessary "for making people 'housing-ready'" (Willse, 2010, p. 166). In a like fashion, the model, upon its introduction, met with skepticism by the local authorities in both Gothenburg and elsewhere in the country. Only recently have there been signs of interest among the country's municipalities in giving the approach a green light.

As Willse (2010, p. 168) has pointed out, to understand the developments in the United States that lead to the shift in focus and the subsequent introduction of the Housing First model, one has to understand "the economic dimension of the invention of chronic homelessness." Some American researchers (Culhane and his colleagues) have successfully argued that, apart from its other positive contributions, the Housing First model is also a more economical way to manage homelessness. At the municipal level where fiscal constraints and budget cuts must frequently be accommodated, the model has indeed come to be viewed as an economically more viable and efficient solution. It is thus the limited economic resources of the municipalities rather than the needs and wants of the individual help-seeking citizens that has to a large extent motivated the policy change (Willse, 2010, pp. 169–172). For many cities and municipalities, the Housing First model has become "*the most economically efficient means of managing* [the homeless] *population*" (Willse, 2010, p. 172; emphasis in the original). In this fashion, notes Willse, researchers have been able to "mobilize a neo-liberal discourse on costs and efficiency to advocate successfully what humanist and ethical discourses have failed to do – that people in need of shelter should be housed as quickly as possible," thus by "recasting housing insecurity in terms of financial costs their research provides an economic justification for permanent, long-term housing" (Willse, 2010, p. 171).

In the Swedish context, too, the neoliberal discourse on cost and efficiency has doubtless played a part in influencing the willingness of municipal authorities to try out the model. While a great majority of the Swedish municipalities still adhere to the old model based on disciplining techniques, sobriety, and personal development as prerequisites for eligibility to housing and keeping one's apartment or room, several of them today show a positive attitude towards experimenting with the new Housing First-based model. The main argument used in favor of this policy adjustment has been that the established way of managing homelessness has become too expensive without still bringing the desired results, with the rhetoric remaining silent about the (previously express) goal of reestablishing homeless individuals in the regular housing market or the (hitherto implied) desire to transform deviant individuals into disciplined citizens complying with societal norms, rules, and regulations. Yet, at least in Gothenburg, the willingness to try out the Housing First model has been premised on a more pervasive medicalization of homelessness, rather than bringing about the kind of de-medicalization often associated with Housing First initiatives in the research literature.

3. Theoretical framework

3.1 Medicalization
Medicalization is "a process by which nonmedical problems become defined and treated as medical problems, usually in terms of illnesses and disorders" (Conrad, 1992, p. 209). At the

same time, the medicalization of a problem does *not* automatically mean that it has been assigned to the jurisdiction of the medical profession (Conrad, 1992, p. 210). This is made clear in Conrad's own definition of the phenomenon:

> Medicalization consists of defining a problem in medical terms, using medical language to describe a problem, adopting a medical framework to understand a problem, or using a medical intervention to "treat" it. This is a sociocultural process that may or may not involve the medical profession, lead to medical social control or medical treatment, or be the result of intentional expansion by the medical profession. (Conrad, 1992, p. 211)

It is important to bear in mind that medicalization of – a medical gaze at – the problem at hand usually does not "fully supplement earlier modes of social control": the medicalization might remain incomplete, competing definitions might exist, or "remnants of previous definition [may] cloud the picture" (Conrad, 1992, p. 218). The coexistence of previous and/or competing definitions will then naturally affect the degree of medicalization itself (Conrad, 1992. p. 220). Furthermore, drawing attention to the process of medicalization, or disclosing instances of medicalization, is not the same as saying that the problem should *not* be looked at as a medical problem (Conrad, 1992, p. 212). Nevertheless, medicalization may, at least potentially, result in a problem's (such as homelessness) becoming decontextualized and individualized (Conrad, 1992, pp. 223–224), leaving any structural causes overlooked with the result that the responsibility for solving the problem becomes more easily rejected by politicians and civil servants. For this reason, the process whereby deviant behaviors are given medical meanings is always a profoundly political one, one, moreover, that has "real political consequences" (Conrad & Schneider, 1992, p. 1). In the concluding part of this chapter, I will return to some of such consequences that the process of the medicalization of the homeless brings. It is, however, even at this stage important to bear in mind that what we are discussing here is a very specific version of medicalization: while to some extent the problem of homelessness is defined in medical terms – the "truly" homeless as mentally ill substance abusers suffering from severe functional impairments – what is nonetheless prescribed is care and (in some cases) medication rather than comprehensive treatment. While the "truly" homeless are certainly viewed as needing the kind of treatment that medical professionals working in mental hospitals provide, these institutions are criticized for rejecting what is claimed to be their caring responsibility. Thus, what is actually provided is not a kind of medical intervention that "treats" the problem, that is, one which makes the "truly" homeless housing-ready and capable of independent living in an ordinary apartment, but instead palliative care – easing of the symptoms of an incurable condition – and access to a permanent special housing unit meant for the homeless clients of the social services.

3.2 Diagnosis and prognosis

As Conrad and Schneider (1992, p. 8) have argued, "the authority to define certain behaviors, persons and things" is the "greatest social control power." This authority belongs to institutions and the people who represent them. In this section, I discuss how the people with this authority, in the Swedish city of Gothenburg, define the problem of homelessness and diagnose homelessness in persons. In this same connection, I will also bring up what the politicians and civil servants interviewed for this study stated about what they thought should be done to successfully combat homelessness.

My analysis is inspired by the theoretical concept of framing as first put forth in the work of Erving Goffman and subsequently developed by others. The framing processes can be of many different kinds. In their study of homeless social movement organizations, Cress and Snow (2000), for instance, have made a useful distinction between *diagnostic* and *prognostic* frames. Diagnostic frames "shape how the issue is perceived, and identify who or what is culpable," while a prognostic frame "stipulates specific remedies or goals" (Cress & Snow, 2000, p. 1071). In my analysis in this article, I focus on "accounts of the problem and who or what is to blame (diagnostic framing), and what needs to be done in order to remedy it (prognostic framing)" (Cress & Snow, 2000, p. 1072). The two types of frames are generally "mutually facilitative," but "prognostic frames might sometimes develop in the absence of articulate diagnostic frames" (Cress & Snow, 2000, pp. 1099–1100).

The focus on diagnostic and prognostic frames as expressed in accounts means that I look mostly at the way in which claim-makers such as politicians and civil servants construct a condition, in this case homelessness. Loseke (2003, p. 59) has defined diagnostic framing as the activities by which claim-makers "construct a condition as a particular type of condition [while] this, in turn, constructs blame and responsibility." The first step in the analysis of actors' accounts of the problem (who or what is to blame) and what is to be done about it was thus to find out if the diagnostic frame constructed the causes as social – that is, as something having to do with the social structure (the housing market or the welfare system) – or as individual (the behavior, personality, or condition of the unique individual or individuals of this type). According to Loseke (2003, p. 61), successful claim-making strategies ignore the complexity of the issue, relying instead on the construction of simple diagnostic frames.

Social problems are, by definition, "conditions we believe can and *should* be changed" (Loseke, 2000, p. 97). A central analytical question is therefore: According to claim-makers in the field of homelessness, what should be done in order to combat the problem and who is, explicitly or implicitly, made responsible? Prognostic framing concerns precisely this question:

> *Prognostic frames* [answer] audience members' questions about what should be done. This frame constructs a general line of action (what should be done) and it constructs the responsibility for that action (who should do it). These claims are important because they legitimize some solutions (and not others), they construct some indicators of success (and not others), they assign some people (and not others) the responsibility for changing the condition. (Loseke 2000, p. 98)

4. Homelessness as an incurable condition

What made it possible for Swedish politicians and civil servants to at once medicalize the issue of homelessness *and* introduce (aspects of) the Housing First model into the context of local homelessness work? While, in light of the discussion thus far, it may seem like a contradiction from a more theoretical point of view, for local politicians and civil servants the intensified medicalization of homelessness in fact served as a precondition for the introduction of the Housing First model, or, as we shall see, a certain key aspect of it: permanent (but not regular) housing.

4.1 Politicians' position: Homelessness as a psychiatric care problem forced on the municipal special-housing provision

The driving force behind the medicalization – and I would say, more accurately, the *intensified* medicalization – of homelessness in the city of Gothenburg was a local politician responsible for the homeless questions in the city government. His own long professional career in psychiatric nursing might have contributed to the new problem construction. In his interview for this study, he stated that for patients experiencing psychoses, it is detrimental to change their daily environment by moving them to another room or apartment:

> What I've seen also in my own work [as a psychiatric nurse] is that it may take three, four, five years for a person suffering from a psychosis to adapt to his or her new environment, and then, if you have to move [to another place], the process starts all over again and so on.

The politician's previous knowledge about mental health patients was transmitted onto a from his perspective new group of clients: the homeless. What he held to be true about mental health patients was thereby thought to be true also of the homeless. Taking his previous professional experience as his starting point, and using it as his main frame of reference, the politician therefore decided to recommend the dismantling of the existing housing staircase model, which was built upon the idea of stepwise progression until the achievement of the end goal, an apartment of one's own in the regular housing market. To replace the idea of housing staircase, the politician introduced the metaphor of an elevator: instead of moving through all the steps of the staircase to gradually come closer and closer to the final destination of gaining an apartment of one's own, an individual should take the elevator directly to the correct floor, get off there, and permanently stay there. The long-term strategy he outlined to make all this possible was to turn the city's stock of short-term housing for the homeless into permanent housing units, so as to change the policy of providing temporary accommodation for the homeless.

Another decision the politician made was to initiate collaboration between, on the one hand, the city's social authorities having the responsibility for the local homelessness work and, on the other hand, the local university hospital. This he thought was needed for the necessary outreach programs. During his interview, he stated that "if there is a person who lives in a tent in the woods and does not want any help from us," the first thing to do was "to check that this person does not have any psychiatric problems," something which in his opinion was ideally done through a joint outreach intervention by staff from the local social services and the university hospital. A third decision he took was then to make it the responsibility of the municipality to offer housing to those who were excluded from, or refused by, the city's current special-housing system. The city's stock of special housing units for the homeless had been expanding, but even though a lot of new units were built, "the most difficult cases," or the categories of homeless individuals declared as the official target group of the city's special-housing organization, were still excluded from them (Hansen Löfstrand, 2010; Löfstrand, 2005):

> So we were complaining about that, and then we said, "No; everything we build from now on should be for the most difficult cases." And then we got [two new housing

complexes], you know. And they're specifically for the double-diagnosis cases, the really tough ones, with lots of staff there and so forth.... And then we also hired three nurses to work there to help them with their medication and so on. Because – well, I come from psychiatry, so I know that when a person ends up at a psychiatric ward, after a month or so they feel better, they get their medication and so on, and then they are discharged and sent to the outpatient clinic, then they go there, get a bag of medicines which they will not take, and after two or three months they are just as aggressive again and that's when they are discharged from there and left on their own. So now we employ nurses to deal with this problem.

The strategy that the municipality came to employ – of defining the problem in medical terms, dismantling the housing staircase model, and offering long-term and even permanent special housing to the homeless – did, however, not agree with the requests coming from the municipality's social service offices for access to regular housing for their clients. While the interviewed politician stated that he was "aware of" such requests, he had nevertheless opted not to act on them, continuing instead with the process of further medicalization of the homeless as incurably ill, with the intent of securing more special housing units for the municipality where this category of homeless individuals could live permanently while receiving medical care. While indeed he did much to contribute to the continued medicalization of homelessness, it is true that also his predecessor had focused on those in the wider category of the homeless who are often referred to as double-diagnosis cases, arguing them to be ill but not ill enough to be admitted to the hospitals' psychiatric wards. In the interview excerpt below this politician expresses his frustration with "psychiatry" which, according to him, rejects its responsibility for the "mentally ill people" among the homeless population:

> *Politician*: They are too ill to be managed in ordinary housing, but they are not ill enough for us to have them forcibly hospitalized in a psychiatric ward. The municipality doesn't have any means of coercing them, apart from the cases where somebody is about to die from drug use.... If you are mentally ill and do a little drugs, it's not possible to force anyone.... So here's a group, then, that's not doing well but nobody takes the responsibility for.
> *Interviewer*: But a group nonetheless that has been regarded as a target group for the municipality's own special-housing system?
> *Politician*: Yes, exactly, but they are usually refused or excluded on work environment grounds as they create problems for the staff working there.

To be able to handle this group of homeless individuals more effectively, it was decided to employ staff with previous experience of working within mental health care at some of the special housing units for the city's homeless.

When analyzing the two politicians' accounts about the problem of homelessness, it becomes clear that the diagnostic framing operating in them constructs homelessness as something caused by mental illness that is self-medicated through use of alcohol and drugs, with the diagnostic term used for the condition being "double diagnosis." Nothing is mentioned about other possible causes, such as factors related to the housing market.

Although the first interviewed politician knew of the local social service offices' express need for something completely different for their clients, their requests for access to ordinary housing in no way featured in his ways of acting on, talking about, or redefining the problem. His case, then, provides an example of the more general tendency to ignore the complexity of the issue in order to construct simple and thus more convincing diagnostic frames (Loseke, 2003, p. 61).

In their accounts about the problem, both of the politicians individualized the problem and presented it as something having to do with illness. One consequence of this way of constructing the homeless as individuals who are ill and suffer from an incurable condition is that they cannot be then held responsible for their homelessness in the manner that other homeless persons are. This, in turn, has enabled the municipality to effect a partial change in its policy: in contrast to the previous situation where the double-diagnosed "most difficult cases" – often referred to as "the truly homeless" – became constantly evicted from different special housing units due to rule breaches, the new policy is to put a stop to the recurrent evictions and offer these individuals permanent special housing. Housing offered by the municipality's special-housing organization is thus regarded as a *permanent solution* for them (as far as the municipality is concerned). A by-product of the solution is the fact that the homeless individuals benefiting from these new permanent housing arrangements are no longer subject to the kind of disciplining rules and regulations that characterized the housing staircase model. A central concept of the new policy – and something that is required from nonprofit and for-profit providers of social housing for the homeless – is "symptom tolerance": as a provider of special housing for the homeless, one has to tolerate the symptoms of the illness, especially since the illness is regarded as an incurable condition. Furthermore, as evident from the interviews with the above two politicians, public medical services were seen as having the primary responsibility for this category of homeless citizens. Both of the two – and, as we shall see, also the civil servant responsible for the municipality's own special-housing organization – nonetheless claimed that the city's medical services had failed to accept this responsibility by refusing or otherwise excluding these "incurably ill" patients as "not ill enough." This fact, in turn, was then construed as *causing* the homelessness problem as the two interviewees had come to know it. The problem was thus not construed as a housing problem, but was instead described as a medical care problem. Both the politicians and the high-ranking civil servants interviewed for this research thus effectively claimed the city's medical services to be responsible for both causing and solving the problem, but, since they refused to recognize this responsibility, the municipal special-housing organization was forced to deal with it in practice.

How did it become possible, then, that some version of the Housing First model could be introduced locally? From a purely theoretical point of view, constructing homelessness as an incurable medical condition while simultaneously presenting it as a housing problem seems like a contradiction of terms. As shown by Cress and Snow (2000, pp. 1099–1100), the diagnostic and prognostic frames need not always be "mutually facilitative." From a perspective in which homelessness is regarded as a housing problem, the emergent prognostic frame (access to permanent housing first) does not follow from the diagnostic frame (homelessness as incurable illness), but seems to have evolved rather independently of the latter. One possible interpretation for this is that the "modern" solution provided by

Housing First, which was vocally advocated in Sweden by (some parts of) the research community, and the criticism that the municipal special-housing organizations were not functioning very well and were costing too much, made it possible to introduce the solution even though it really did not marry well with the prevailing diagnostic frame. As evidenced by the two Gothenburg politicians above, the city's preferred solution was in fact medical treatment and medication, but since the medical services system, according to the perception of the decision-makers, in effect denied its responsibility for those "incurably ill" in the wider homeless population, the next best solution, which was permanent special housing for this category of the homeless, was resorted to instead. This was also presented as the rationale for the new policy of employing mental health care workers as staff at the city's special housing units, and for hiring nurses to pay regular visits and provide medical (somatic) care to the clients at some of the special housing units for the homeless (Sennemark, 2009). In the below quote, an interviewed civil servant in charge of Gothenburg's municipal special-housing organization discusses this new initiative:

> The idea is that, since these people rarely come for treatment at our healthcare facilities or in some other way get to receive medical care, we now have a two-year project where we hire three nurses who will work at some of our special housing units, and then we'll follow up on it to see if it makes any difference in these people's lives that they get access to medical care, get their wounds looked after, get to talk to a nurse who might get them to go to a psychiatrist if they need that, or whatever their problem might be…. Then we will review all this and see…if their lives indeed became any better, if their quality of life improved at all.

The first special housing unit in Sweden offering medical care to its homeless clients opened in Stockholm in 2005 (Ingermarson & Holmdahl, 2010). A few years later, in 2007, medical care to homeless persons staying at special housing units was put on the political agenda also in Gothenburg (Sennemark, 2009). Also the establishment of healthcare centers catering for homeless persons only, in Stockholm in 2001 and in Gothenburg in 2005, provides an example of the medicalization of homelessness, reflecting the tendency to regard homelessness not as a housing issue but as a medical/healthcare problem. The homeless were seen as excluded from the scope of the ordinary healthcare and medical treatment system, which nevertheless was supposed to be equally serving all citizens, or as not really fitting within it well. They were, moreover, considered as needing three different types of medical care: psychiatric care, addiction treatment, and somatic care. The choice to then create separate solutions for the homeless – special housing and special medical care institutions – has, however, only exacerbated their exclusion, as they thereby de facto become treated as almost non-citizens.

What is important to bear in mind is that, in reality, the term "homeless" is a very heterogeneous category. In considering the kind of instances of medicalization of homelessness as described above (homelessness framed as a result of mental illness and self-medication with alcohol and/or drugs), it needs to be noted that, for instance, those presenting the diagnoses in the above quotes are laymen and not part of the medical establishment. Furthermore, these interviewees had no experience of direct contacts with homeless clients. The street-level bureaucrats at local social welfare offices often propose and act on definitions of their homeless clients as either double diagnosis cases or not, at least implicitly in their decisions about where to refer them for placement (to which kind of special housing unit). Like politicians and high-ranking civil servants in general, they lack the medical education ordinarily considered as necessary for performing such diagnoses. It is, moreover, also important to bear in mind that it was primarily politicians and civil servants who contributed to the intensified medicalization of homelessness, in the Gothenburg context at least. As powerful claim-makers, their diagnosis of homelessness as an incurable condition, accompanied by their prescription of special housing where homeless clients can receive palliative care and medication, had a great impact in the policy process. Even though (some of) the street-level bureaucrats claimed that there was a great need for ordinary housing for the homeless clients of the city's social services (and for homeless help-seeking individuals and families refused by the social services as not suffering from any "medical" or "social" problems), the solution put forward was nevertheless *permanent special housing for the "truly" homeless*, or those suffering from an incurable and irreversible condition and deemed never to be able to live in an apartment of their own in the regular housing market.

4.2 Civil servants' position: The "truly" homeless as individuals with brain damage, functional disabilities, and a need for permanent special housing

In her interview, the civil servant responsible for the municipal special-housing organization in Gothenburg connected the problem of homelessness with a contested major reform in psychiatric care that was initiated in Sweden in 1995. The reform, aimed at reducing the number of mentally ill living in large institutions and integrating them more in society, has been widely criticized for leaving mentally ill persons isolated and without proper care. While indeed the proportion of homeless persons regarded as mentally ill has increased since the introduction of the new care policy, no direct correlation has nevertheless been found between the two (Halldin, 2000; NBHW, 1998). All the same, the interviewed civil servant claimed that many of those in the city's homeless population today in the past "used to live in mental institutions." According to her, the psychiatric reform "changed the whole concept of homelessness," because with it, the target group changed so that it now included many more mentally ill homeless. She described the mentally ill as individuals with "functional impairments." Also those in the wider category of the homeless who abuse alcohol were described by her as suffering from such "functional impairments," caused by damage to the brain from prolonged alcohol abuse. These two subcategories were then seen as together constituting the category "the truly homeless" that formed the most important target group for the municipality's special-housing organization. As the interviewee herself described it:

> Before, one wasn't even really aware of what long-term alcohol or substance abuse does to the human brain and one's abilities.... Of course, the hard part is the human beings with functional impairments...who also suffer from brain damage. Many of them do.

The interviewee further explained that even though integration into society might serve as a fine ideal, one nevertheless had to face "the reality" – a reality in which the public medical services cannot cope with the homeless addicts, as can neither the psychiatric care services nor the wards for somatic care or hospice care. Accordingly, it was the local social services that had to deal with homelessness as a medical care problem:

> The fact that they are here [being cared for by the municipal special-housing organization] is because the medical care system cannot manage the integration [of the homeless].... Have you ever seen a double-diagnosed homeless person at a local healthcare center?

Just like the politician responsible for homelessness in the Gothenburg municipality, the interviewed civil servant in charge of the municipality's special-housing organization pointed to the recent changes in the local policy that brought an emphasis on permanent placement at special housing units. Initially, she interpreted this political will as a will to offer the homeless more or less ordinary apartments, albeit within the framework of the municipal special-housing organization (without first-hand contracts and normal lease terms). In her understanding, the need for "ordinary housing" had meant "ordinary apartments," at least when it came to their material standard:

> When I started out here [in the municipal special-housing organization], I thought: "We have to refashion [one of the special Gothenburg housing units] into fully adequate apartments and then people may stay on." For precisely this group of people with early disturbances – those who are violent, those who look for conflicts, who brawl and fight at the social service offices and are refused admission.... And then, instead, we'd be like: "Here you've got your key, now you have your apartment, you can do whatever you want, here you may live, you can take care of yourself here…you never need to move" – things like that, you know.

The interviewee then went on to describe a process of gradual realization and increasing comprehension, a process leading her to understand that there nonetheless were some people – those in the homeless population who can be categorized as suffering from an incurable illness – who should *not* be placed in regular-type housing. She could not view an apartment in the regular housing market through a first-hand contract as a good solution or even an appropriate end goal for the process of integration into society, because "integration will never be possible." On the other hand, according to the interviewee, this category of the homeless should not be placed in housing units either where, due to predictable rule breaches, they were liable to be moved to another special housing unit "every other night." Accordingly, permanent special housing for the homeless, instead of permanent regular housing first, became the preferred political model to combat long-term homelessness in the municipality. The interviewed civil servant claimed this kind of homeless to be unable to live in ordinary apartments:

> We cannot heal people just because we're the municipal special-housing organization.... Sometimes people in general don't realize what kind of functional impairments there actually are out there…because they have never in their entire lives made a cup of coffee or boiled an egg or even a kettle of water. You don't think that there are that types of functional impairments…. But they can stay there in any case, we

say, as long as they want. We don't think that...the pathway out of homelessness is an apartment of one's own.

In consequence, some of the city's housing units that had previously functioned as short-term shelters were converted into long-term special housing units. Today, these units are to offer a permanent solution for those homeless diagnosed as suffering from an incurable condition. This policy shift was described by the interviewed civil servant as a result of a learning process in which she, too, initially thought that everyone should have their own apartment "with a kitchen and all that." However, her new colleagues with a long experience in homelessness work had made her revise her initial thinking that subsequently appeared almost naïve:

> Then they started telling me, "But have you thought about this, that it might not be – that they might not be able to enjoy it; on the contrary, it might prove an obstacle to their coping." So we gave up on the idea of providing them with regular, fully functioning apartments. We could be wrong, too, of course – I don't know. But that's the way we do it, anyhow.

Another interviewed civil servant, who at the time of the interviews was responsible for coordinating the outreach work carried out by the municipality in collaboration with certain nongovernmental church-based organizations, explained that many of the homeless individuals encountered by the outreach staff had been refused admittance to the special housing units "because they threaten the staff or other people staying there, which is actually very common." In fact, a list of barred persons had been created at the unit where the interviewee worked, which was maintained by the municipality and offered shelter-like temporary accommodation. Contrasting with these individuals, there was "a group of people who land in [name of the housing unit] and don't have social problems" and thus did not end up on the list of barred persons. The interviewee differentiated this latter category of "the houseless" from "the homeless," who were "barred" not only from the regular housing market but also from most units within the city's special-housing sphere (Löfstrand, 2005). She described "the homeless" as individuals with mental disabilities who proved a challenge for the organization to handle: they were often "people who come in here with guns.... It's not all that easy [to deal with them as] the staff are human beings, too." Just as the politicians and the civil servant quoted above, also this civil servant depicted "the truly homeless" as mentally ill. The interviewee further claimed the general public to think that "nobody cares" about this group of homeless persons; this was an illusion, however, since:

> these are persons we have worked with for many years already, basically trying to lure them into the van [used in the outreach work] just so that they would come with us and not be harmed, and drive them to hospital.

"The truly homeless" thus suffered from an illness, and homelessness was portrayed as an incurable condition, impossible for the local social services authorities to manage. The "truly homeless" were, moreover, in need of medical treatment and healthcare, not ordinary housing. The city's longstanding special-housing organization, based on a disciplinary model where access to housing required both regulation by others and self-regulation, had thus not been replaced by a Housing First model based on the idea that regular housing (including first-hand apartment contracts) provided a necessary precondition for the ability to handle all other possible problems (economical, medical, mental, or addiction problems). What thus happened when the new trend – the Housing First model – was interpreted within this specific local professional culture, becoming used for its own particular ends, was that only *some* of its aspects were incorporated into the framework of the local special-housing organization. A catchword used in the debates around the new model was *permanent housing* for the homeless. This suited the municipal politicians and civil servants who wanted to put an end to the endless movement of the homeless between shelter-like special housing and sleeping in the rough. Correspondingly, it became possible for the municipality to introduce special housing as a permanent solution for the homeless (as well as for the municipality). In this way, the in reality rather old solution (special housing for the homeless with "symptom tolerance," which had been the norm for long until the period of the preceding staircase model commenced in the 1980s) could thus be made to appear as something modern, simply by refashioning it in terms of the latest trend – the Housing First model. This way of on the surface adapting to the latest trend while in reality still following the old model has been described as path dependence, in which previous choices affect which decisions will be taken in the future, with the path already taken rendering some choices and decisions seemingly unthinkable while leaving others appear only natural (Pierson, 2000). The local interpretation of the Housing First approach deviated from the original model in at least one important aspect: while a first-hand apartment contract with normal terms of occupancy formed the most important aspect of the new model, the same starting point did not inform the local interpretation and adaptation of it. Since, as it was perceived, the medical service and healthcare system rejected its responsibility for "the truly homeless" (the homeless who are mentally ill or addicts or have brain damage) suffering from an incurable condition marked by functional impairments, permanent special housing was introduced as a solution to serve both these individuals and the municipality itself. It remains to be seen if, with the new hybrid model in place, the endless evictions for rule breaches will cease and, to the extent that happens, what kind of sanctions might remain for the city's special-housing agency to use for its purposes, since the principle is now that the homeless individual is to be allowed to stay on permanently even when he or she "misbehaves" by acting in contravention to the agency's rules.

4.3 The Housing First model translated

In fall 2010, the local social service authorities in Gothenburg started planning for a new project openly influenced by the Housing First model as originally developed in United States. The model had been advocated by Swedish researchers working on homelessness issues, especially at Lund University where the Housing First model was heavily promoted as the best choice for Swedish municipalities. According to some of the key figures working at the university (Heule et al., 2010), the basic principles relied on by the model are the following: (1) Homelessness should first and foremost be considered as a housing problem; (2) homeless persons should be reestablished in the regular housing market as quickly as possible; (3) access to housing of one's own forms an important precondition for subsequently solving other problems; (4) permanent and safe housing is to be considered a basic human right that belongs to everyone. The authors recommend that these basic features be incorporated into local homelessness work in general, with the long-term goal of integrating them into the municipal special-housing organizations and their overall operation as their constitutive principles. As important preconditions for its successful implementation, it is generally considered that the model depends on access to ordinary housing through first-hand rental contracts, that the support offered through it should always be optional, and that the homeless should be allowed to stay in their apartments permanently. In addition, any social and geographical segregation is to be avoided by incorporating the apartments offered to homeless persons into the city's ordinary rental housing stock (and not confined to separate apartment buildings for the homeless clients of the social services). To facilitate the achievement of these goals, Lund University offers the municipalities willing to try out the model a range of education and evaluation services, along with access to research on the topic (see http://www.soch.lu.se/o.o.i.s/21367). Some of the Swedish municipalities have, as a result, expressed interest in giving the model a try. The factors behind their reasoning often relate to the high cost of their current programs to combat homelessness and the persistence of the problem of homeless individuals sleeping in the rough. While the city of Gothenburg is among the municipalities not receiving guidance from the researchers at Lund University, its approach is nevertheless very much inspired by the Housing First model as promoted at Lund University and by US American researchers such as Tsemberis and his colleagues.

In a manner much like in the municipalities acting in direct collaboration with Lund University, in 2010 politicians and civil servants from Gothenburg's municipal special-housing organization issued a statement to the effect that the city was going to try out the Housing First model, by launching a small-scale project in which a few apartments were to be acquired for the purpose of offering direct access to independent housing to homeless individuals thus far excluded from the city's special-housing services as too "difficult" to manage within their framework. There was one major difference, however: the homeless clients were not to be offered first-hand apartment contracts, not in Gothenburg nor in any other municipality trying out the model. In Gothenburg, the civil servants responsible for homelessness were well aware that this meant significant deviation from the original model. The method was, consequently, interpreted as being all about housing as the first intervention and a foundation:

> In its original and orthodox form [the model] means first-hand apartment contracts, issued directly and without any intermediaries or conditions other than those stipulated in the Rental Act. Most of those who adopt the approach are not very "orthodox" in every respect, however. [In many municipalities] the possibility offered to the homeless comes with additional terms and limiting conditions or initially issued second-hand rental contracts. (City of Gothenburg, 2011, p. 1)

The Housing First project in Gothenburg was named "Housing as a Foundation," and it was launched when an opportunity for it arose with one of the city's a special-housing units scheduled for closing towards the end of 2010. The facilities involved, consisting of sixteen individual apartments in one building and an additional nine apartments spread out in the area, were then adopted for use in the Housing First project. The apartments were rented by the local social authorities and then sublet to these authorities' homeless clients; in other words, the local social services signed the first-hand contracts, with their clients then entering into second-hand contracts with the social services. No additional terms and conditions for occupancy were included other than those enumerated in the country's Rental Act that apply to all tenants in the regular rental market. The formerly homeless clients occupying the apartments were considered to need support in their everyday life (to make sure they paid rent, did not disturb their neighbors, took care of their apartments), and the involvement of medical care and addiction care institutions was considered necessary (City of Gothenburg, 2011).

The local adaption of the Housing First model to combat homelessness in the form of the this project was presented as a way to solve an urgent and long-standing problem: the exclusion of certain categories of homeless individuals not only from the regular housing market, but also from the city's special-housing sphere consisting of all the beds, rooms, and apartments offered to the homeless clients of the city's social services and run by different actors (municipal, nonprofit, and for-profit) (see Löfstrand, 2005). The task at hand was to provide housing for a small group of homeless persons who were regarded as exceptionally hard to handle for all the practitioners and authorities involved (Holm, n.d.). The size of the target group in the municipality is described as "fairly limited," estimated at 15 to 30 persons. These are described as individuals whose behavior (as either violent or otherwise excessively unpleasant) has made them unsuited for living together with others in ordinary conditions. They are, furthermore, described as mostly men who are well known to the city's social service offices, nongovernmental organizations, and medical care institutions. The support to these individuals was to be organized in line with the "case management model," in that all authorities in contact with homeless individuals were to gather together in working groups so as to coordinate their efforts in a more efficient manner and that way help facilitate and enhance the support work and possible interventions. The groups meet regularly and share the responsibility for the clients in question (Holm, n.d.). The approach adopted by the municipality thus clearly mixes elements of the Housing First model with disciplinary interventions associated with the hitherto dominant housing staircase model.

4.4 The adaptation of nonprofit and for-profit housing providers to the "new" politics of "symptom tolerance"

In keeping with the prevailing policy as practiced until now, the municipality, nonprofit organizations, and (to a lesser extent) private companies had been evicting special-housing residents on the grounds that they had appeared at their housing units under the influence of alcohol or consumed alcohol on premises. The new policy, however, clearly stated that the actors involved – whether municipal, nonprofit, or for profit – were to provide long-term special housing without the ability to consider relapses as grounds for eviction. The housing providers are to explicitly describe how they "work with symptom tolerance." As noted above, among the municipal authorities the "truly homeless" are regarded as suffering from an incurable condition. The new catchword of "symptom tolerance" then fit very well with the manner homelessness was defined in medical terms: the symptoms of an incurable condition (such as incapacity to abstain from alcohol and/or drugs) had to be tolerated. In consequence, the non-municipal providers of special housing (both nonprofit and for-profit ones) therefore had to adapt their practices to the new policy, introduced to put an end to the endless circulation of "the truly homeless" between shelter-like housing units and sleeping in the rough. In response to the question of what sort of providers (among the nonprofit and for-profit ones) the municipality should contract for its initiative, the interviewed civil servant responsible for the city's special-housing organization explained that, contrasting with the earlier situation, the effect of the new policy was that:

> [The providers of special housing for the homeless] can no longer come in here and just offer housing where everybody's required to stay sober; we also need housing where...[the principle of] symptom tolerance is observed. But even then you can still say that boozing is not allowed here. They can't do that at [the municipality's own special-housing units], either. You can come home when you are drunk, but you can't have a drinking party in your apartment or on premises, to put it that way. You can't do that at our own units, either. But then [the providers] have to explain to us how they work with symptom tolerance, how they deal with relapse cases.

In a focus group interview with nonprofit providers of special housing for the homeless, these providers linked what they termed "the new municipal strategy" to "symptom tolerance," which was described as "the dominant term everywhere right now" and as "a key phrase." To more effectively pursue its goal of minimizing the constant drift between temporary accommodation and sleeping in the rough among the city's more problematic homeless population, the municipality made a decision to give precedence in the official procurement process to providers who offered special housing where the principle of symptom tolerance would be followed. Organizations that for one reason or another are unable to provide "symptom tolerance housing" have in consequence had hard time surviving. Indeed, the nonprofit providers often understood the new policy to imply that the clients could "have relapses a hundred times over and still be able to stay on [in their apartments]," which made the new policy unpopular and difficult to implement in their eyes, as, over the years, they had slowly but steadily just managed to adapt to the previous policy of drug-free units and absolute sobriety as preconditions for housing. According to the interviewed nonprofit providers, the central message from the politicians to the civil servants and actors involved in the provision of special housing for the homeless was: "As little people as possible on the city streets." The interviewees criticized what they saw as the new official view of the municipality: that there are "hopeless cases" unable to "escape their situation" (which for them meant "unable to overcome their addiction"). This was regarded as something that only contributed to cementing the marginalized situation of certain categories of the homeless, leaving them permanently outside of the regular housing market and society. According to the nonprofit providers, the municipality construed "the truly homeless" as ill individuals who were fundamentally "incurable" and thus represented what amounted to hopeless cases: "Addicts who have been taking heroin for five, six years are incurable.... They have this idea that these people, they have to live with their symptoms, this illness; it's more and more about that sort of thinking."

Although the new policy has resulted in fewer homeless people on the streets of the city center, it has at the same time become even more difficult for those among the homeless population who are categorized as "truly homeless" to reestablish themselves in the regular housing market or even gain access to self-contained "reference apartments" in the city's special housing units, which in the prevailing system provide a chance for them to prove their readiness for and practice independent living. As noted above, the politician in charge of the problem of homelessness issues in the Gothenburg city council had received signals from the municipality's local social service offices that what was really needed for their homeless clients was apartments integrated into the regular rental market. The interviewed nonprofit providers of special housing judged the need in the same way: "There are far too few [of such] apartments; they [the homeless residents of special housing units] cannot advance, they will only get stuck."

Regardless of what was requested from them, then, the politicians and civil servants in charge of homelessness in the municipality have continued to develop local homelessness policy in just the opposite direction. To be sure, this has happened, to some extent at least, as a result of a feeling that their hands are tied, given their basic inability to provide regular apartments due to a general housing shortage and the current housing market situation in the city, the reluctance of local landlords, and other similar factors curtailing their leverage. At the very minimum, however, the politicians in charge should, at least in theory, be able to influence the rental policy of the municipal housing companies. To a significant extent, the current shift in policy has thus come about a result of the more or less conscious construction of "the truly homeless" who are diagnosed as suffering from an incurable condition. The prognosis for them reads as follows: housed permanently in municipally provided special housing units or in units provided by other actors providing symptom-tolerant special housing, they will never gain access to an apartment of their own in the regular housing market.

5. Conclusion

The "new" politics of "symptom tolerance" and (more or less) permanent special housing for the homeless as a way of combating long-term homeless in the city of Gothenburg very much resembles an earlier model followed by the municipality up until the end of the 1980s: the hostel system. The one notable exception is that during the earlier period, the "symptoms" of the incurable condition could be, and also were, "tolerated" at hostels that provided no more than *temporary* accommodation for the homeless individuals targeted, whereas today they are offered permanent or semi-permanent but in principle fully functional small apartments. The apartments, to be sure, are not fully "standard," coming as they do for example without a proper kitchen and a first-hand rental contract. Both *before* the disciplining staircase model was introduced in the late 1980s, and *after* it was officially abandoned in 2007 (see Hansen Löfstrand, 2010), homeless persons were – and still are – portrayed as suffering from an incurable condition, with the solutions to the homelessness problem based on that premise. The current model for combating homelessness, the Housing First approach, is, however, even where officially adopted, at best embraced at arm's length (Åkerström, 2006). Where it has been put in place and made operative, it (or, rather, some selected aspects of the original model) has been harnessed for the municipality's own, locally defined and determined purposes. As a result, individuals who are long-term homeless continue to be denied any possibility for first-hand apartment contracts.

Willse (2010, p. 165) has connected the invention of (chronic or long-term) homelessness as a medical problem to the basic notion inspiring the work of modern social service agencies, namely, that it is necessary to "work on yourself" to gain access to and keep an apartment of your own. In this respect, the Housing First model, as already noted, promises to bring a break from the medicalized models by separating shelter provision from health and social services (Willse, 2010, p. 166). Much as a consequence, the reactions to it among social workers, still working on the old assumption that health and social services are necessary for preparing homeless clients for independent living, have been notably reserved. In the city of Gothenburg, too, where some of the model's features have been adopted for use, the approach has been modified to fit locally defined and largely inherited purposes. In line with the original model, the importance of immediate access to permanent housing is emphasized by the municipality, with the result that "the truly homeless" – the homeless regarded as incurably ill – are now being made eligible to it. The housing in question, however, is not regular housing obtained from the rental market that comes with a first-hand rental contract, but instead special housing that is adapted to the perceived special needs of the homeless and comes without standard facilities and standard terms of occupancy. In other words, certain aspects of the Housing First model have been strategically incorporated by adopting them for use for local purposes that, paradoxically enough, are still centered on the framing of long-term homelessness as a medical problem. At the same time, by adhering to the principle of the Housing First model that stresses the need for permanent housing solutions for the homeless while simultaneously defining the problem of homelessness in medical terms, the fact that the goal is no longer to reestablish the homeless in the regular housing market is legitimized. By linking policy shifts to a model perceived as "modern" and "legitimate," the morally questionable strategies of diagnosing homeless people as suffering first and foremost from an incurable condition and of prescribing them permanent special housing in combination with treatment and medical care are camouflaged and thus made less vulnerable to criticism. In effect, then, one might even conclude that the moral legitimacy of the Housing First model is being strategically used for (other) local purposes, to hide from sight what is going on in actual reality: an intensified medicalization of homelessness and a constant narrowing of the category of "the truly homeless." The politics of homelessness manifest in, and in turn propelling, such developments can then but render the pathway out of homelessness even more difficult to traverse. For as long as "the truly homeless" are depicted as suffering from an incurable illness, the problem of homelessness can be "solved" by permanently housing the homeless in special housing units falling short of ordinary standards, with the occupants lacking first-hand rental contracts. Meanwhile, the attention to the structural causes (such as the housing market, housing politics and welfare politics) producing homelessness may comfortably lapse (cf. Conrad, 1992; Lyon-Callo, 2000).

While not ultimately guiding the actions of the decision-makers and high-ranking civil servants in Gothenburg (or in Sweden more broadly), then, where it was used only strategically and selectively for local, pre-existing purposes, we might nevertheless note that the Housing First model with its key objective of promoting access to *regular housing* with first-hand rental contracts has been fully and successfully implemented elsewhere, for instance in the United States (see Padgett, Gulcur, & Tsemberis, 2006; Stefancic & Tsemberis, 2007; Tsemberis et al., 2004), providing a precedent to follow. Furthermore, besides prescribing palliative care and medication to homeless clients considered incurably ill (and placing them in long-term or semi-permanent special housing), as was done in Gothenburg, also other measures could have been resorted to that have been offered for consideration as potentially effective means for dealing with mental and physiological problems in this respect. For instance, approaches have been proposed that stress the benefits of extended social networks (the health benefits of good relations with friends, family, partners, and pets), activities for enjoyment and relaxation, nutritious food, and involvement in group-discussion programs (Harwood and L'Abate, 2010; L'Abate, 2007b). Through self-initiated and self-administrated self-help where good social relations, enjoyment of life, and general well-being are the goal, it might be possible to promote rehabilitation and self-reliance in this area as well. Such measures to promote good health seem, moreover, to be not just effective but also notably cost-efficient (Harwood & L'Abate, 2010; L'Abate, 2007a; L'Abate, 2007b). It is hard to see why they could not be considered in the context of the Swedish special-housing provision as well, as a measure to address the mental and physiological problems among the country's homeless population. At the same time, however, one might ask whether the image increasingly promoted of homelessness as an incurable condition – with the "truly homeless" depicted as the hopeless cases – might effectively prevent this from happening, at least in the foreseeable future.

6. References

Åkerström, M. (2006). Doing Ambivalence: Embracing Policy Innovation – at Arm's Length. *Social Problems*, Vol.53, No.1, pp. 57–74, ISSN 0037-7791

City of Gothenburg (2011). Bostad som grund [Housing as a foundation]. Internal working document, City of Gothenburg, Social Resources Department, dated 19.1.2011

Conrad, P. (1992). Medicalization and Social Control. *Annual Review of Sociology*, Vol.18, pp. 209–232, ISSN 03600572

Conrad, P. & Schneider, J.W. (1992). *Deviance and Medicalization: From Badness to Sickness*, Temple University Press, ISBN 13: 978-0-87722-999-5, Philadelphia, USA

Cress, D.M. & Snow, D.A. (2000). The Outcome of Homeless Mobilization: The Influence of Organization, Disruption, Political Mediation, and Framing. *American Journal of Sociology*, Vol.105, No.4, pp. 1063–1104, ISSN 0002-9602

Halldin, J. (2000). Avinstitutionaliseringens betydelse för hemlösheten – myter och fakta [The effect of deinstitutionalization on homelessness: Myths and facts], In: *Hemlöshet – en antologi om olika perspektiv och förklaringsmodeller* [Homelessness: Perspectives and Explanations], W. Runquist & H. Swärd, (Eds.), 135–148, Carlssons, ISSN 91-7203-977-9, Stockholm, Sweden

Hansen Löfstrand, C. (2010). Reforming the Work to Combat Long-Term Homelessness in Sweden. *Acta Sociologica*, Vol.53, No.1, pp. 19–34, ISSN 0001-6993

Harwood, M.T. & L'Abate, L. (2010). *Self-Help in Mental Health: A Critical Review*. Springer, ISBN 1441910980, New York, USA

Heule, C., Knutagård, M., & Swärd, H. (2010). Bostad först – ett innovativt försök [Housing First: An innovative approach]. *Alkohol & Narkotika*, No.1, pp. 9–12, ISSN 0345-0732

Holm, P. (n.d.). Uppdrag svårplacerade klienter med utagerande beteende [Assignment: Clients who are difficult to place and have impulsive behavior]. Social Resources Department, City of Gothenburg, Sweden

Ingemarson, M. & Holmdahl, J. (2010). *I lugn och oro. En brukarstudie över Erstabacken, ett medicinskt boende för svårt sjuka hemlösa* [In peace and quiet: A study of Erstabacken, a hospice for severely ill homeless persons]. Ersta Sköndal University College, ISSN 1402-277X, Ersta Sköndal, Sweden

Löfstrand, C. (2005). *Hemlöshetens politik – local policy och praktik* [The Politics of homelessness: Local policy and practice]. Égalité, ISBN 91-975231-4-3, Malmö, Sweden

L'Abate, L. (2007a). Low-Cost Approaches to Promote Physical and Mental Health, In: *Low-Cost Approaches to Promote Physical and Mental Health: Theory, Research, and Practice*, L. L'Abate (Ed.), 3–40, Springer, ISBN 0387368981, New York, USA

L'Abate, L. (2007b). *Low-Cost Approaches to Promote Physical and Mental Health: Theory, Research, and Practice*. Springer, ISBN 0387368981, New York, USA

Loseke, D.R. (2003). *Thinking about Social Problems: An Introduction to Constructionist Perspectives* (2nd ed.), Aldine de Guyter, ISBN 0-202-30684-4, New York, USA

Lyon-Callo, V. (2000). Medicalizing Homelessness: The Production of Self-Blame and Self-Governing within Homeless Shelters. *Medical Anthropology Quarterly*, Vol.14, No.3, pp. 328–345, ISSN 0745-5194

National Board of Health and Welfare (1998). *Psykiatrireformen: Årsrapport 1998. Reformens första tusen dagar* [Psychiatry reform: Annual report 1998: The first 1,000 days]. Norstedts Juridik, ISBN 91-7201-286-2, Stockholm, Sweden

National Board of Health and Welfare (2006). *Hemlöshet i Sverige 2005. Omfattning och karaktär* [Homelessness in Sweden, 2005: Scope and nature]. National Board of Health and Welfare, Stockholm, Sweden

Olsson, L.-E. & Nordfeldt, M. (2008). Homelessness and the Tertiary Welfare System in Sweden: The Role of the Welfare State and Non-profit Sector. *European Journal of Homelessness*, Vol.2, pp. 157–173, ISSN 2030-3106

Padgett, D.K., Gulcur, L., & Tsemberis, S. (2006) Housing First Services for People Who Are Homeless with Co-Occurring Serious Mental Illness and Substance Abuse. *Research on Social Work Practice*, Vol.16, No.1, pp. 74–83, ISSN 1049-7315

Pierson, P. (2000). Increasing Returns, Path Dependence, and the Study of Politics. *The American Political Science Review*, Vol.94, No.2, pp. 251–267, ISSN 0003-0554

Sahlin, I. (2005). The Staircase of Transition: Survival through Failure. *Innovation: The European Journal of Social Science Research*, Vol.18, No.2, pp. 115–136, ISSN 1351–1610

Sennemark, E. (2009). *Medicinsk kompetens på sociala boenden i Göteborg – behövs det?* [Medical competence at social housing units in Gothenburg: Is it needed?]. The Gothenburg Regional Association of Local Authorities (GR), Gothenburg, Sweden

Stefancic, A. & Tsemberis, S. (2007). Housing First for Long-Term Shelter Dwellers with Psychiatric Disabilities in a Suburban County: A Four-Year Study of Housing Access and Retention. *Journal of Primary Prevention*, Vol.28, Nos.3–4, pp. 265–279, ISSN 1573-6547

Tsemberis, S., Gulcur, L., & Nakae, M. (2004). Housing First, Consumer Choice, and Harm Reduction for Homeless Individuals with a Dual Diagnosis. *American Journal of Public Health*, Vol.94, No.4, pp. 651–656, ISSN 1541-0048

Willse, C. (2010). Neo-liberal Biopolitics and the Invention of Chronic Homelessness. *Economy and Society*, Vol.39, No.2, pp. 155–184, ISSN 0308-5147

9

Adolescents with Mental Disorders: The Efficacy of a Multiprofessional Approach

Michela Gatta[1], Lara Dal Zotto[1], Lara Del Col[1], Francesca Bosisio[2],
Giannino Melotti[2], Roberta Biolcati[2] and Pier Antonio Battistella[1]
*[1]Neuropsychiatric Unit for Children and Adolescents and Pediatrics Department,
ULSS 16 and University of Padua*
[2]Psychology Department, University of Bologna
Italy

1. Introduction

Approaches to mental health problems can historically be grouped into three theoretical-methodological systems, i.e. the psychological, the bio-pharmacological and the socio-environmental. Operators often tend ideologically to support one of these approaches, thereby emphasizing a distinction that originates from an old-fashioned separation between body and mind, and between individual and setting. The therapist with a biological education thus often brings the issue down to choosing the appropriate drug to eliminate the symptom; the therapist with a background in psychology is only interested in giving patients the most fitting interpretation of their symptoms to enable the latter to deal with them; and the educational therapist tends to search for social breakdowns (seen as the reason for the patient's pathological behavior) and suggest more adequate relational models. The different types of therapist remain locked in their own world and often mistrust the other possible approaches, running the risk of misunderstanding the patient's needs and providing only partial or ineffective intervention as a result.

Many studies have focused on and compared the benefits of different treatment settings for different mental disorders (psychoses, eating disorders, mood disorders, behavioral problems, ADHD, etc), and reviewed the various treatment methods that have proved helpful in managing young patients (Bachmann et al., 2008a, 2008b; Connor et al., 2006; MTA, 2004; Velligan et al., 2009). Although different settings and a multimodal treatment approach (including individual psychotherapy, pharmacology and family-based interventions) are described and recommended, evidence-based findings on the effects of the various treatment methods are still limited (Herpertz-Dahlmann & Salbach-Andrae, 2009; Masi et al., 2008; Nützel, Schmid, Goldbeck & Fegert, 2005; Steiner & Remsing, 2007).

2. Theoretical and clinical background

2.1 Clinical assessment and diagnosis in adolescence

Adolescence, more than any other stage in an individual's life cycle, poses the problem of normality and disease; it is a period of development characterized by discontinuity, rupture and existential uncertainty. Though it is difficult to trace a precise boundary between normality and disease in adolescence because of the complexity of this period of development, with its characteristic multiple behavioral deviations and often contradictory psychological functioning, it is of fundamental importance to arrive at a correct diagnosis in order to plan effective treatment strategies and establish a prognosis. What makes the psychopathological diagnosis of an adolescent's condition so particular is its prognostic aspect, i.e. the risk of a disorder interfering with the adolescent's global developmental process and consequently on their acquisition of a stable identity, which is the premise for an adequate social and relational adaptation (Pissacroia, 1998).

Adolescent disorders are strongly characterized by evolutionary elements and psychological traits specific to this time of life, so efforts to understand and diagnose the disorder cannot avoid considering the broader, more complex dynamics of the individual's development as a whole. The clinical evaluation of mental disorders in adolescents must consequently be intimately correlated with the specificity of the psychological development theory and models of psychic functioning in this age group (Ammaniti & Sergi, 2002). Every psychopathological symptom must be seen as part of the child's development process (Gatta et al., 2005a) and analyzed in relation to the various settings in which the child is involved, be it the family, or peer groups, or society at large; it is essential to consider this expanded relational context, or "enlarged psychic space" (Jeammet, 1980).

For this purpose, clinicians and researchers increasingly use empirical assessment tools that enable them to shed light on the risk factors, the processes and the etiological mechanisms of psychopathology in adolescence, including the fundamental role played by environmental variables, be they interpersonal or contextual, in relation to the specific dynamics of this period of life.

The understanding deriving from individual differences in adaptive and maladaptive functioning, both in normal development processes and in dysfunctional and psychopathological conditions, is useful in the prevention, diagnosis and care of patients in the adolescent age-group.

Given the intrinsic characteristics of adolescence (bodily changes and interest in the self, psychological separation from internalized parental figures and the search for objects outside the family, construction of an identity in its psychological, social and sexual expressions) that make value the boundaries between normality and disease vague, the problem of which criteria or theoretical references to adopt in assessing any pathological conditions - be they transient or at risk of persisting and evolving - becomes particularly difficult.

The psychodynamic approach emphasizes the *clinical assessment* of the case – rather than its psychiatric diagnosis – in which symptoms are placed in relation to desires and fears, defenses, cohesion and stability of the self, types of objective relationships, and quality of affective control. A psychiatric diagnosis restricted to considering these domains seems more like a formal procedure than a method capable of explaining the complex nature of mental suffering. On the other hand, the medical model on which most of current psychiatry relies is characterized by important, closely correlated elements: 1. a study of the etiology, 2. an analysis of the set of signs and symptoms that tend to be associated and significantly repetitive; 3. a diagnosis based on an analysis of the clinical course and the underlying causes; 4. a possible prognosis; 5. a differential diagnosis; 6. a study of the epidemiology; 7. a choice of therapy. Although the etiopathogenetic aspects are unsuited to psychopathologies because the causes of mental disorders are not known, the use of such model is justified by the strong logical link between diagnosis and therapy, which underscores the role of the diagnostic process *per se*; it is also fundamentally important to be able to use a universal diagnostic language to facilitate communication between specialists in the field. It is thus a matter of interweaving the data relating to the set of signs and symptoms, which phenomenologically identify a psychiatric disorder using descriptive criteria, with details on an individual's psychological functioning interpreted in the light of the developmental role of adolescence.

2.2 Adolescent patients and how they are taken into care

According to a recent study by Costello et al. (2005), as many as 12% of adolescents suffer from a psychiatric disorder severe enough to interfere with their functioning. From the various data available in the literature it also emerges that many disorders of developmental age (60% on average) continue into adult life (Bittner et al., 2007; Hofstra et al, 2001; Kessler et al., 2005; Kim-Cohen et al., 2003). Moving from this finding, many authors have wondered about the variables capable of better predicting the stability or susceptibility to change of developmental-age psychiatric disorders. For the time being, however, no general model has been developed to explain the mechanisms behind the continuity or discontinuity of a psychopathological condition (Rutter et al., 2006).

There are still no global epidemiological data on the long-term future of patients who had various problems in adolescence, nor any comparative studies on the nature of these difficulties and their treatment. Clinical experience and the various studies conducted on some such disorders would nonetheless converge in suggesting a strong correlation between disorders of adolescence and even severe problems in the long term (Fava Vizziello, 2003; Jeammet, 1980).

Most studies in the literature on these issues have focused on following up patients with various psychiatric diagnoses, and the persistence of a given disorder would depend primarily on its diagnostic category (Fonagy et al., 2003). Other studies indicate, however, that the degree to which the disorder interferes with the patient's functioning is equally important for prognostic purposes, even in the absence of a diagnosis of frank psychopathology (Angold et al., 1999; Gatta et al., 2009a, 2010a, 2010b). In the light of these considerations, and given the worrying epidemiological data pointing to a marked persistence of such problems, it is worth taking a look at the type of work done by the services for developmental age to treat and prevent psychopathologies in adolescents.

In this setting, a central role is occupied by services designed specifically for adolescents, for this age of transition from childhood to adulthood involving changing and personality structuring processes that lay the foundations for and shape the type of functioning of the future adult. Sadly, it is for this particular age group that we often find shortcomings in the health services and inadequacies in their specialization, in Italy at least - to such a degree that it is still true to say, as De Martis said many years ago (1997), that the organization of health care mirrors the problems of identity typical of these individuals, giving rise to a no man's land (neither children or adults) where we often see a destructive game in which competences and responsibilities are batted backwards and forwards between psychiatrists, hospitals, families, schools, social services and, in many cases, even the police and the law courts.

While the more recent literature reflects the uncertainty of the services, there is clearly still a paucity of documentation – even on an international level - on the efficacy of therapeutic-rehabilitation treatments offered by the services for developmental age, as regards the methods for taking them into care without resorting to hospitalization for cases with moderate-severe disorders (Gatta et al., 2009, 2010a, 2010b). Day centers would seem to be a good resource for the more severe cases, thanks to their flexibility and capacity to adapt to different circumstances, but unfortunately not enough research has been done to compare the efficacy of residential treatments as opposed to day centers or the patient's living environment for the various types of patient and severities of their conditions (Green, 2002). All too often, the available studies report generic outcome measures in relation to different psychiatric disorders without specifying the type of therapeutic intervention provided, while studies comparing groups of hospitalized patients with groups treated elsewhere are still entirely inadequate in providing practical indications on how to organize the services (Shepperd et al., 2009). Unlike the situation for other types of therapeutic intervention in the living environment (such as multisystem therapy and case management), we could find not one comparative study including intensive treatments at day centers or in semi-residential settings (Lamb, 2009).

Given the lack of information from controlled randomized studies, in a recent meta-analysis published in Cochrane, Shepperd et al. (2009) pointed to the need to conduct prospective studies at the various services, based on clear clinical and demographic parameters at the time of a patient's admission and using precise, standardized outcome measures at the time of their discharge.

As for the best approach to these patients, studies are focusing on the hypothesis that a multimodal and multidisciplinary approach is more effective than single, sectorial approaches (Dimigen et al., 1999; Gatta et al., 2010a; Pazaratz, 2001) and that this approach - with a coordinated action involving several operators sharing in the project- may be best for taking adolescents into care in many situations in which their psychopathology is severe.

The multi-professional therapeutic team shares the investment between people in different relational settings, while remaining united in its global view of the project, offering a response that facilitate the process of differentiation between dependence and development, so difficult to achieve without the aid of a "third party". Clearly, focusing on the numerous aspects of the relationship with the patient and working as a team can contribute to a better outcome and improve the clinical efficacy of the intervention (Palareti & Berti, 2010; Pazaratz, 1996). This therapeutic method is applicable to various mental disorders, both in developmental age and in adults, and its efficacy has been acknowledged internationally (Bartels et al., 2004; Bond et al., 2001). Within this network, it is also worth emphasizing the importance of the cooperation with the adolescents' families and the proper exploitation of a personal relationship with them so that they can share the experiences of suffering caused by their child's disorder, also with a view to reinforcing the working alliance with them (Gatta et al., 2009b, 2010b, 2010c; Hawley & Weisz, 2005; Marcelli, 2009; Woolfenden et al., 2009).

2.3 The Semi-residential Adolescent Psychopathology Service

The study involved patients attending the Daily Service for Adolescents at the Neuropsychiatric Unit for Children and Adolescents in Padua. The main purposes of this service are the care and rehabilitation of adolescents with severe psychopathological disorders (mood disorders, psychotic disorders, antisocial behavior and personality disorders), particularly optimizing their welfare and providing intervention for these young patients through an integrated clinical and pedagogical approach. Various professional figures cooperate on the therapeutic project and this multi-professional team includes a child and adolescent neuropsychiatrist, a psychologist and two educators and a social worker. Adolescents attending the center undergo an initial diagnostic process, leading to a psychiatric diagnosis formulated according to the ICD 10 (World Health Organization, 1992) and the therapeutic project involves attending a day center.

The centre receives adolescents (males and females from 12 to 18 years of age) with various types of psychiatric and behavioral disorder of moderate to severe degree: it has a capacity to treat approximately 25 patients in all and can simultaneously accommodate up to six adolescents, with the ratio of one operator to every two patients.

The adolescents attend from Monday to Friday from 09.00 to 17.00. Access to the structure is based on individual projects prepared by the team, which establishes the number of weekly visits and their duration. The educators can also implement tailored and/or home-based interventions in situations where an adolescent suffers from significant social isolation, and in acute cases requiring temporary hospital stays, acting as companions and providing support while the patient is in hospital. Patients can also be received in emergency situations (moments of acute crisis, or when a "buffer intervention" is needed while a patient is waiting to join a residential community). These latter interventions do not follow the normal enrolment protocol.

The general goals of the service are:

- to optimize the patient care and education measures for adolescents in situations of particular mental illness and at particularly crucial times;
- to support the families in their educational role;
- to construct an integrated clinical and pedagogical project with the various services on different levels and with different institutional roles;
- to improve the social involvement of adolescent in their living environment.

The multidisciplinary team consists of: a developmental neuropsychiatrist responsible for the service, a psychologist-psychotherapist, two educators, a social worker, a coordinator, and an administrative assistant.

There are also trainee psychologists, trainees on the degree course for professional educators at the Faculties of Education Sciences and Psychology, and physicians training in developmental neuropsychiatry.

The team holds the following meetings:

- a weekly meeting to coordinate their clinical-pedagogical work and program the educational activities;
- a weekly team meeting to discuss the cases;
- periodical meetings with social-sanitary operators and clinicians to report on the cases being treated in the semi-residential setting to discuss the clinical issues, assess the adolescent's progress, and recommend new patients for the treatment;
- a monthly supervisory team meeting with an outside psychiatrist-psychotherapist.

2.3.1 Protocol for enrolling new patients at the semi-residential center

The phase for assessing and enrolling an adolescent at the semi-residential center for adolescent psychopathologies is completed according to the following protocol.

1. The case is presented to the team operating at the semi-residential service for adolescent psychopathologies by the psychologist or neuropsychiatrist proposing their enrolment at the Neuropsychiatric Unit for Children and Adolescents and a file is prepared for the patient being recommended.

2. The case is discussed and, where applicable, a preliminary period of observation and assessment of the adolescent is decided.

3. A meeting is held with the patient and family to formalize the proposal to start with a preliminary period for the adolescent to get to know the semi-residential service. In addition to patients and their parents, this meeting is also attended by the clinician referring them and an educator.

4. The observation period starts, normally involving four meetings according to the following schedule:

    -   the first meeting is for introductions, observations and free activity (playing, computer, exploring spaces);
    -   the second meeting is when an observation file is completed (a semistructured interview) by a "third party" educator, i.e. an educator who has had the least to do with the adolescent so far, in order to guarantee the utmost neutrality in the administering the assessment tool. Then activities are proposed in small groups to see how the adolescent functions in group situations;
    -   at the third meeting activities are proposed on the basis of the adolescent's interests emerging from the previous interview;
    -   the fourth and last meeting is where, in addition to the activities already begun at the third meeting, there is also space for a conversation and exchange of ideas with the adolescent, to provide feedback relating to the previous meetings, the adolescent's mode of participation and greater or lesser willingness to enroll at the semi-residential center.

5. The reference educator completes an initial observation file on the trend of the four meetings.

6. The team assesses the observation period within two weeks after its completion and decides whether to recommend that the adolescent continue with the semi-residential experience or terminate it.

7. The patient and family are informed about the child's progress so far and there is an exchange of ideas relating to the adolescent's and the family's experiences and motivations. If all concerned agree to the semi-residential program, this decision is shared and signed jointly by the family and by the physician referring the case to the team, and these parties agree on a first integrated, tailored therapeutic and educational project, and an initial schedule for the adolescent's attendance at the center.

2.3.2 The path for taking the patient into care

1. *Formulation of the tailored educational project and schedule of attendance at the semi-residential center*

This phase is completed by the working team and the object is to prepare a first project in the light of the findings during the preliminary observation period. A record is made of patients' and their families' demographic details, the motives for enrolment on the program, the internal and external activities conducted, the established goals, the general and specific objectives of the course of therapy, a description of the integrated intervention designed for each adolescent of and the timing for assessing their progress and the project.

Access is always formulated on the basis of a tailored individual project and the adolescent's weekly attendance is constantly monitored. Punctuality and adherence to the agreed frequency of attendance is an important tool for assessing the adolescents' and their families' compliance with the agreed educational project, as well as being a necessary premise for implementing the semi-residential program. For each patient, a schedule is agreed with the family, the specialist and the adolescent concerned, starting from a minimum of two attendances a week (lasting four hours each).

2. Periodical clinical interviews and progress monitoring

For each patient, there are periodical clinical meetings with their own doctors to monitor their psycho-developmental trends and personal response to the therapy. The parental couple is also followed up with regular meetings with a clinician (neuropsychiatrist or psychologist), possibly with the support of an educator.

This action on the families needs to be supported and empowered to help parents establish a different image of their child from the one they knew before, and make sense of the changes taking place in the child during the period in semi-residential care, as well as providing input on how the parents themselves need to respond to the child on a daily basis. A course of psychotherapy proper for both the adolescents and their parents is often recommended and implemented.

3. Completion of a file for recording changes and reviewing the therapy

After the first six months of attendance at the semi-residential centre, the educational project is reviewed, and the goals and/or operating methods are expanded and/or diversified, based on a first structured assessment of the adolescent's progress that involves completing and checklist of specific indicators relating to the various areas of intervention (relational, social, autonomy).

4. Ongoing assessment

The ongoing assessment of the adolescent's progress is based on various methods:
- periodic team discussions,
- periodic meetings with reference clinicians
- periodic meetings with family
- periodic meetings with teachers
- periodic assessment of files completed by the reference educator
- observation/assessment charts recorded before and after laboratory activities
- the periodic administration of standardized tests (Youth Self Report 11-18) at the baseline, when the patient is taken into care and subsequently every six months
- the periodic completion by the team of the Global Assessment of Functioning test (GAF) (at the time of compiling the therapeutic and educational project and subsequently every six months).

This assessment and constant monitoring procedure enables the ongoing adjustment of the objectives of the integrated individual projects, which is normally done every 3-6 months. The tests can also be used as a tool for pre- and post-assessment of the effects of the intervention at the start and end of a specific laboratory activity to evaluate it efficacy.

5. Discharge

The end of the course of therapeutic intervention can be decided by various factors. In the most favorable of outcomes, the project may be concluded because the preset goals have been achieved and the adolescents have regained their social contacts and schooling experience, and the course of therapy undertaken can be consolidated.

Attendance at the centre may also be interrupted due to poor compliance on the part of the adolescent and/or the family (with repeated and unjustified failures to attend appointments at the semi-residential centre or meetings with clinicians, or inadequate cooperation). The program may also be stopped by the need to include the patient in a residential community. In each case, the conclusion of the project is confirmed during the course of a final meeting attended by all the parties involved (the adolescent, the family, the reference educator, the psychologist and the neuropsychiatrist).

2.3.3 Pedagogical activities

The object of the pedagogical activities is to support the adolescents in the course of their development by means of a relationship with the figure of the educator, who serves as an "auxiliary ego" and consequently as a supportive companion. This is achieved by providing a space, which takes practical shape in the rooms at the semi-residential centre, and by designing a project that involves customized objectives and timings.

In experiences of research applied to different educational settings, various functions have been identified on which the educator's action is concentrated. The educator thus has several functions (Marcelli & Braconnier, 1989; Pani et al., 2009):

- as a mediator between the adolescent and the adult world;
- to provide protection in relation to the adolescent's interior conflicts;
- to accompany the patient on a path towards a normalizing educational context;
- as containment, providing stability and helping the adolescent to manage the dynamics of his/her daily life.

The *general educational goals* of the educational process providing the starting point of an individual educational project tailored to each patient include:

- helping the adolescents to gain awareness of their own sentiments, impulses and behavior;
- helping them to test their abilities in a protected setting and to raise their self-esteem;
- helping them to realistically assess their living environment.

The *activities* in which the psycho-educational process takes shape are designed to achieve the individual objectives of each adolescent's project and rely on fundamental tools, such as providing a setting as a framework in which to enable to the experience of meeting, using the operator's capacity for empathy to create a relationship that can help the adolescent to let their emotional experiences resound inside themselves and thereby increasingly gain control over them, promoting organized behavior patterns, abilities and motivations that can pave the way to satisfactory social relations and an adequate performance in the completion of tasks and the achievement of goals. During their attendance at the center, the adolescents conduct activities designed to develop their personal interests, acquire skills and reinforce their self-esteem. Outings, the preparation of a newspaper, painting, watching films, playing, writing, and dramatizations are activities conducted at the center, individually and in small groups, in the constant presence of the educators. There are also structured laboratories involving pet therapy, horse therapy, art therapy and naturalistic experiences at teaching farms organized in cooperation with other associations, as well as participation in therapeutic winter and summer holiday camps. For many young people, these activities are the only opportunities they have to put themselves to the test away from their usual living environments, to measure themselves against an adventure outside the home, and thereby testing their capacity to manage on their own, to experiment with detachment from the family, to live in groups and share the group's behavioral rules.

Finally, courses are also organized to support the adolescents' formal education in cooperation with their schools. This involves formulating tailored teaching programs and the presence of teachers at the semi-residential centre.

3. Clinical study

3.1 Aim

The aim of this study was to analyze the psychopathological manifestations and psychosocial functioning of a sample of 67 adolescents attending the semi-residential service for adolescent psychopathologies at the Neuropsychiatric Unit for Children and Adolescents of the local public health services in Padova (Italy) between 2006 and 2009.

This analysis aimed to assess the efficacy of a multi-professional (educational, psychological, pharmacological) integrated therapeutic intervention, in terms of the patients' clinical progress, psychopathological changes and global psychosocial functioning, 12 months after starting the program.

3.2 Sample

The study sample consisted of 48 males (71.6%) and 19 females (28.4%), aged between 13 and 19 years when they began to attend the semi-residential service, divided into three age groups, i.e. 13-14 (46.3%), 15-16 (41.8%) and 18-19 (11.9%); 29.9% of the sample were attending lower secondary school, 34.3% were at higher secondary school, and 35.8% had abandoned school.

3.3 Materials and methods

The patients' functioning and psychopathology were assessed using the Global Assessment of Functioning (GAF) scale and the Achenbach Youth Self Report 11-18 (YSR), respectively, which were completed at the beginning of the semi-residential treatment and repeated after 12 months.

The GAF (Startup et al., 2002) is a scale used by operators to rate a patient's psychosocial functioning and activities, regardless of the nature of their psychiatric disease. It corresponds to Axis V of the DSM-IV (APA, 1994). The GAF scale comprises 10 levels (further divided into 10 points) and each patient is assigned to a given level on the strength of a scoring system: the higher the score, the better the patient's psychosocial functioning. The levels of functioning are described as it follows: **91 - 100** Superior functioning in a wide range of activities, life's problems never seem to get out of hand, he/she is sought out by others because of his or her many positive qualities. No symptoms. **81 - 90** Absent or minimal symptoms (e.g. mild anxiety before an exam), good functioning in all areas, interested and involved in a wide range of activities, socially effective, generally satisfied with life, no more than everyday problems or concerns (e.g. an occasional argument with family members). **71 - 80** If symptoms are present, they are transient and expectable reactions to psychosocial stressors (e.g. difficulty concentrating after family argument); no more than slight impairment in social, occupational, or school functioning (e.g. temporarily falling behind in schoolwork). **61 - 70** Some mild symptoms (e.g. depressed mood and mild insomnia) OR some difficulty in social, occupational, or school functioning (e.g. occasional truancy, or theft within the household), but generally functioning pretty well, has some meaningful interpersonal relationships. **51 - 60** Moderate symptoms (e.g. flat affect and circumstantial speech, occasional panic attacks) OR moderate difficulty in social, occupational, or school functioning (e.g. few friends, conflicts with peers or co-workers). **41 - 50** Serious symptoms (e.g. suicidal ideation, severe obsessive rituals, frequent shoplifting) OR any serious impairment in social, occupational, or school functioning (e.g. no friends, unable to keep a job). **31 - 40** Some impairment in reality testing or communication (e.g. speech is at times illogical, obscure, or irrelevant) OR major impairment in several areas, such as work or school, family relations, judgment, thinking, or mood (e.g. depressed, avoids friends, neglects family, and is unable to work; child frequently hurts younger children, is defiant at home, and fails at school). **21 - 30** Behavior is considerably influenced by delusions or hallucinations OR serious impairment, in communication or judgment (e.g. sometimes incoherent, acts grossly inappropriately, suicidal preoccupation) OR inability to function in almost all areas (e.g. stays in bed all day, no job, home, or friends) **11 - 20** Some danger of hurting self or others (e.g. suicide attempts without clear expectation of death; frequently violent; manic excitement) OR occasionally fails to maintain minimal personal hygiene (e.g. smears feces) OR gross impairment in communication (e.g. largely incoherent or mute). **1 - 10** Persistent danger of severely hurting self or others (e.g. recurrent violence) OR persistent inability to maintain minimal personal hygiene OR serious suicidal act with clear expectation of death.

The YSR 11-18 (Achenbach, version for 11-18 year-olds) (Achenbach, & Rescorla, 2001) is one of the most commonly used scales for rating juvenile behavior and it is used internationally in the clinical setting and in research. It is in the form of a questionnaire completed by adolescents, and it has been translated and validated for Italians too (Frigerio et al., 2006; Ivanova et al., 2007). The questionnaire yields two profiles: one for competences (activities, social functioning, school performance) and one for behavioral and emotional problems, which can be assessed as "normal", "borderline" or "clinical" on 8 specific syndrome scales. The syndrome scales relating to the various psychopathological pictures are: anxiety/depression, withdrawal, somatization, social problems, thought-related problems, attention problems, aggressive and role-breaking behavior. The problems are grouped into: internalizing problems (anxiety, depression and withdrawal, somatization); externalizing problems (aggressive and role-breaking behavior); and other problems (social problems, thought-related problems, attention problems).

The adolescents' clinical progress was assessed after 12 months by completing the Clinical Global Impressions (CGI) (Guy, 1976) – for the part relating to Global Improvement. This was done by the clinician who had conducted the psycho -diagnostic assessment prior to the adolescents' enrolment on the semi-residential program: patients were judged to have improved clinically when they scored 1-2, to have remained unchanged if they scored 3-5, and to have deteriorated when their score was 6-7.

The Working Alliance Inventory – Observer, Short version (WAI-O-S) was used by an outside observer (a psychologist trainer) to assess the bond between the parents and the therapist, and how much they agree on the action to take and the goals of the therapy. The WAI-O-S has been shown to have a good reliability (r=0.81; Gelfand and DeRubeis, unpublished manuscript), and research has also produced strong support for the reliability of the WAI scales in general, and for their validity (Hanson et al., 2002; Horvath, 1994). The WAI-O-S has been translated into Italian and validated for Italians (Di Giuseppe et al., 1996; Horvath, & Greenberg, 1989; Lingiardi, 2002). This scale consists of 12 items, 10 positively worded and 2 negatively worded, rated on a 7-point Likert-type scale. The items are divided into three subscales of 4 items each. The subscales, based on Bordin's (1979) working alliance theory, are Goal (agreement about goals of therapy; e.g.

"The client and therapist have established a good understanding of the changes that would be good for the client"), Task (agreement about the purposes of the therapy; e.g. "There is agreement on what it is important for the client to work on"), and Bond (the bond between the client and therapist; e.g. "There is mutual trust between the client and therapist"). Given our aim to evaluate parents' capacity to cooperate in the adolescent's treatment, we chose to select the WAI-O-S's *Task* subscale (items 1, 2, 8 and 12). Ranging from a minimum of 0 to a maximum of 28, the ratings were coded as follows: no working alliance (scoring 0-9) , a partial working alliance (10-19) and a good working alliance (20-28). The items were rated considering the parental couple as a *client* asked to become involved in and commit to their child's treatment when the team reported to them on the outcome of the initial assessment procedure and presented its tailored educational-therapeutic project (see section 2.3.1 item 7).

The adolescents' participation was evaluated by the educators, considering certain qualities of the adolescent-educator relationship and the adolescents' participating modalities during the first three months.

After three months of the adolescents attending the day center, the educators filled in four items for each client:

1. General attitude to the activities proposed at the day center: active (a), passive (b), ambivalent or oppositional (c);
2. Mode of talking about his or her self and tackling tests: active (a), passive (b), ambivalent or oppositional (c);
3. Recognition of the existence of an emotional disorder: present (a), indifferent (b), rejected (c);
4. Attitude to the educator: trust (a), indifference (b), mistrust (c).

The patient's participation mode was thus classified as follows: active (prevalence of "a"), passive (prevalence of "b"), ambivalent or oppositional (prevalence of "c"). If two answer modes were seen with the same frequency, the more conservative profile was to be chosen, but no such cases actually occurred.

Compliance with treatment was assessed for each patient according to their adherence to the educational-therapeutic project in terms of their attendance at the center to take part in the educational-pedagogical and clinical activities established in each adolescent's project: adherence to the therapeutic project was judged to be adequate when patients attended 75-100% of their appointments, discontinuous if the percentage was 50-74%, and inadequate if it was less than 50% or the therapeutic intervention was interrupted early.

Statistics: the statistical analysis was conducted using the following variables: gender, age, cultural level of the families of origin, formal education, situation of the parental couple, psychiatric diagnosis (ICD 10), reason for requesting to join the program, attendance at the semi-residential centre, period of stay at the semi-residential centre, adherence to the therapeutic project, working alliance with the parents (WAI-O), type of intervention, mode of participation, principal educational goals, clinical progress (CGI), individual and/or group approach, scores on the syndrome scales in the Achenbach YSR questionnaire, and scores on the GAF scale.

The data collected were input in a database and subsequently processed using the SSPS statistical software, rel. 14; a value of $p < 0.05$ was considered significant. After completing the *frequency analysis*, the *chi square test* was used as a statistical model (calculating the exact value of p) to analyze the gender-related differences in relation to all the above-listed variables. To assess the efficacy of the therapeutic intervention, we used Student's *t-test for paired samples*, comparing the results obtained with the YSR before (T1) versus after the intervention (T2). To compare the results of the GAF assessment between T1 and T2 (T1) we used the *General Linear Model for repeated measures*. The same statistical model was also used to compare the differences in the mean GAF scores between T1 and T2 vis-à-vis the variables of interest, and the most relevant data (interaction effect between GAF and gender, frequency of attendance at the semi-residential center, integration of the therapeutic intervention, and type of intervention).

3.4 Results and discussion
3.4.1 Socio-demographic characteristics of the sample
The sample consisted of 48 males (71.6%) and 19 females (28.4%).

Their *age* at the time of enrolment on the semi-residential program was mainly distributed in the 13-14 year-old (46.3%) and 15-16 year-old (41.8%) age groups, while 11.9% of the adolescents were between 17 and 19 years old. Males and females were equally distributed in the three age groups ($\chi^2 = 1.20$, df = 2, p_{exact} = n.s.).

In our sample, 29.9% of the patients were attending lower middle school, 34.3% were at higher middle school and 35.8% had abandoned school: the reasons this last group was related both to academic difficulties and to major behavioral issues or symptoms of mental illness and isolation that interfered significantly with school attendance. According to the ISTAT survey of 2008, the national rate of adolescents abandoning their education in the first year of high school was 11.1% (ISTAT, 2008).

The drop-out phenomenon in our sample was clearly connected to these adolescents' psychiatric disease and it is also important as a prognostic indicator when considered in terms of the adolescent's psycho-educational growth.

There were no statistically significant differences between males and females as concerned their *school education* ($\chi^2 = .17$, df = 2, p_{exact} = n.s.).

The *cultural level* of the family of origin, judging from the formal education received by each of the parents (lower middle school, high school, university), was mainly medium-to-low: it was low for 32.8% of the sample, medium for 53.7%, and high for only 13.4%. This finding confirms, on the one hand, the trend of previously published studies on the inverse relationship between mental disorders in general and the families' socio-cultural level (Chandra et al., 1993; Flouri et al., 2010; WHO 2004), on the other, it goes to show that the intervention implemented is readily accessible to all, not discriminating between families in economic or cultural terms.

No significant differences emerged between males and females for this variable ($\chi^2 = .30$, df = 2, p_{exact} = n.s.).

In 76.1% of the cases, the families consisted of an intact *parental couple*, while in 23.9% the family was single-parent. No statistically significant differences emerged between males and females for this factor ($\chi^2 = 12$, df = 1, p_{exact} = n.s.).

3.4.2 Main psychopathological signs in our sample of adolescents, their diagnosis and the assessment of their psychosocial functioning
For 40.3% of our patients, the reason for referral to our service was for behavioral problems, 23.9% had affective-relational and family problems, 19.4% had schooling problems, and 16.4% suffered from social isolation. The *reason for requesting the service* varied according to the gender of the sample considered ($\chi^2 = 8.82$, df = 3, p_{exact} = .03): male patients were more

likely to ask for therapeutic intervention for behavioral problems (43.8% of the males vs 31.6% of the females), problems at school (20.8% of the males vs 15.8% of the females) or social isolation (20.8% of the males vs 5.3% of the females), while females were more likely to need to deal with affective-relational problems (14.6% of the males vs 47.4% of the females).

The sample consisted of adolescents who had been attributed a *diagnosis* according to the ICD 10 of psychotic disorders in 25.4% of cases, personality disorders in 34.3% (20.9% of them as a single diagnosis, 13.4% with comorbidities), behavioral disorders in 11.9%, phobias, stress-related and somatoform disorders in 10.4%, mental retardation in 9.0% and affective syndromes in 9.0% (Table 1).

Diagnosis	% (fq)
Psychotic disorders (F20-29)	25.4 (17)
Personality disorders (F60-69)	20.9 (14)
Two comorbid diagnoses (F60-69+ F30-48)	13.4 (9)
Behavioral and emotional disorders (F90-F98)	11.9 (8)
Phobias, stress-related and somatoform disorders (F40-48)	10.4 (7)
Affective disorders (F30-39)	9.0 (6)
Mental retardation, psychological development disorders (F70-89)	9.0 (6)
Total	100.0 (67)

Table 1. ICD 10 diagnoses.

No statistically significant differences emerged between males and females in relation to the diagnosis ICD 10 (χ^2 = 9.72, df = 6, p_{exact} = n.s.).

These data do not confirm the literature on psychopathology in developmental age, in which gender variables are reportedly highly significant; for instance, psychosis, somatization, depression and eating disorders all have a different, gender-related prevalence and incidence (Costello et al., 2006; Frigerio et al., 2009; Kessler & Wang, 2008).

It is well known that problems of aggressive behavior, mental retardation and psychosis are more frequent in males, while eating disorders and internalizing disorders are more common among females.

The scores obtained by our patients in the Achenbach YSR (YSR 11-18) at the baseline assessment were grouped into three clusters, i.e. cluster 1 ("normal") comprises scores in the range of 50 to 64; cluster 2 ("borderline") scores from 65 to 69; and cluster 3 ("pathological") scores from 70 to 100, as recommended in the manual (Achenbach & Rescorla, 2001).

Table 2 shows the percentage of scores obtained at the time of the initial YSR assessment in the three clusters (*normal, borderline* and *pathological*) on the eight syndromes scales. Three questionnaires were not considered because they were incomplete. It is worth noting that half the patients were "borderline" or "pathological" on the subscales for anxious-depressive disorders, social problems, and attention disorders. The same applied to the subscales for social withdrawal.

As concerns the gender-related differences (Table 3), there were no statistically significant differences except for the scales for somatization, anxious-depressive disorders and social problems, where the differences by gender tended towards significance.

YSR syndrome scales	50-64 (normal) % (fq)	65-69 (borderline) % (fq)	70-100 (pathological) % (fq)
Social withdrawal	50.0 (32)	20.3 (13)	29.7 (19)
Somatization	79.7 (51)	15.6 (10)	4.7 (3)
Anxious-depressive disorders	37.5 (24)	26.6 (17)	35.9 (23)
Social problems	39.1 (25)	25.0 (16)	35.9 (23)
Thought-related disorders	73.4 (47)	18.8 (12)	7.8 (5)
Attention disorders	48.4 (31)	29.7 (19)	21.9 (14)
Delinquent behavior	84.4 (54)	10.9 (7)	4.7 (3)
Aggressive behavior	68.8 (44)	14.1 (9)	17.2 (11)

Table 2. YSR 11-18 pretest: percentages and frequencies (for 64 subjects).

In particular, there was a larger proportion of females with somatization and social problems among the "borderline" patients, and the girls prevailed for anxious-depressive disorders and social problems among the "pathological" cases.

YSR syndrome scales	50-64 (normal) % (fq)		65-69 (borderline) % (fq)		70-100 (pathological) % (fq)		χ^2, df, p_{exact}
	Male	Female	Male	Female	Male	Female	
Social withdrawal	52.2 (24)	44.4 (8)	21.7 (10)	16.7 (3)	26.1 (12)	38.9 (7)	1.03, 2, n.s.
Somatization	87.0 (40)	61.1 (11)	8.7 (4)	33.3 (6)	4,3 (2)	5.6 (1)	6.2, 2, .06*
Anxious-depressive disorders	45.7 (21)	16.7 (3)	26.1 12)	27.8 (5)	28.3 (13)	55.6 (10)	5.59, 2, .07*
Social problems	47.8 (22)	16.7 (3)	21.7 (10)	33.3 (6)	30.4 (14)	50.0 (9)	5.29, 2, .08*
Thought-related disorders	78.3 (36)	61.1 (11)	17.4 (8)	22.2 (4)	4.3 (2)	16.7 (3)	3.19, 2, n.s.
Attention disorders	54.3 (25)	33.3 (6)	23.9 (11)	44.4 (8)	21.7 (10)	22.2 (4)	3.02, 2, n.s.
Delinquent behavior	80.4 (37)	94.4 (17)	13.0 (6)	5.6 (1)	6.5 (3)	0 (0)	2.14, 2, n.s.
Aggressive behavior	71.7 (33)	61.1 (11)	10.9 (5)	22.2 (4)	17.4 (8)	16.7 (3)	1.40, 2, n.s.

*Tending towards significance

Table 3. YSR 11-18: comparison between males and females in the three clusters of scores, *normal, borderline* and *pathological* (64 subjects).
To enable their comparison, the percentages of males and females for each syndrome scale were calculated out of the total of the respective subsamples.

In the operators' assessment of global functioning using the GAF scale, the range most often found was 51-60, with 29.9% of the adolescents revealing moderate symptoms, e.g. flat affect and circumstantial speech, occasional panic attacks or moderate difficulties in their social, occupational or school functioning (few friends, conflict with peers, etc.); this was followed by 23.9% of the patients with scores of 41-50 (more severe symptoms e.g. suicidal ideation, severe obsessive rituals, frequent shoplifting or any serious impairment in social, occupational, or school functioning, e.g. no friends, unable to keep a job) and 22.4% in the range of 31-40, with even more severe symptoms (some impairment in reality testing or communication, e.g. speech is at times illogical, obscure, or irrelevant, or major impairment in several areas, such as work or school, family relations, judgment, thinking, or mood, e.g. depressed, avoids friends, neglects family, and is unable to work; child frequently hurts younger children, is defiant at home, and fails at school) (Fig. 1).

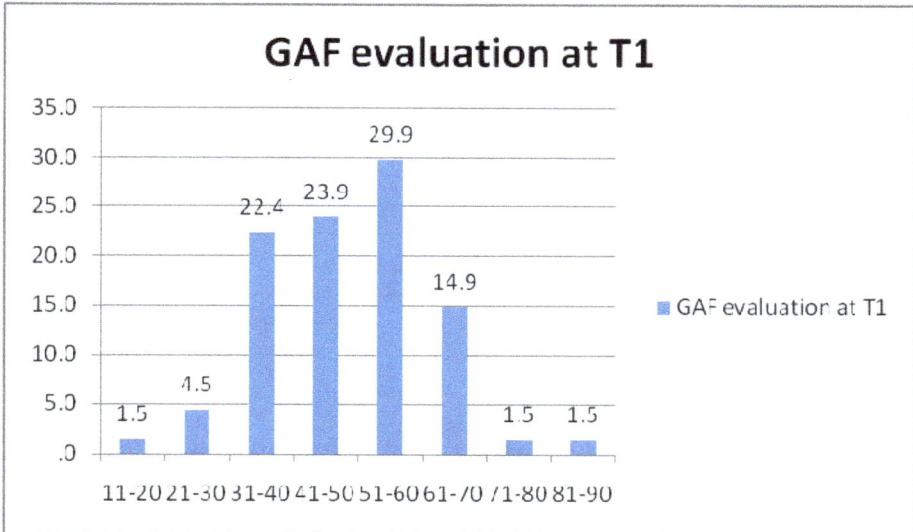

Fig. 1. Percentages of patients on different GAF scoring levels at T1.

3.4.3 Characteristics of the therapeutic project

The main *goals* of the educational-therapeutic project tailored to each patient were to help them achieve autonomy and improve their self-esteem (41.8% of cases) and socialization (29.9% of cases). Support for the family was identified as one of the priorities in 19.4% of cases, support in the adolescents' schooling in 9.0%. No statistically significant differences emerged between males and females for this variable (χ^2 = .22, df = 3, p_{exact} = n.s.).

The majority of the adolescents attended the semi-residential centre for a *period of time* that exceeded three months; 50.7% of them attended for more than nine months (Table 4).

Attendance at the semi-residential centre	% (fq)
<3 months	14.9 (10)
3-9 months	34.3 (23)
>9 months	50.7 (34)
Total	100.0 (67)

Table 4. Period of attendance at the semi-residential centre.

No statistically significant differences emerged between males and females concerning the duration of the treatment (χ^2 = 2.15, df = 2, p_{exact} = n.s.).
Approximately half the adolescents (49.3%) came to the semi-residential centre for 5-15 *hours a week*, 28.4% of them for less than 5 hours a week and 22.4% for more than 15 hours a week.
Their *attendance at the semi-residential centre* varied significantly as a function of gender in the sample considered (χ^2 = 11.88, df = 2, p_{exact} = .002): most of the females attended the centre for less than 5 hours a week (47.4% of the females vs 20.8% of the males), or for more than 15 hours a week (36.8% of the females vs 16.7 of the males), while the majority of the males attended the centre for between 5 and 15 hours a week (62.5% of the males vs 15.8% of the females).
In 23.9% of the cases considered, there was an *unscheduled interruption* of the therapeutic project, within three months of joining the semi-residential centre in 14.9% of them; the difference between males and females was not significant (χ^2 = .09, df = 1, p_{exact} = n.s.).
The *type of therapeutic intervention* for the majority of cases was of the integrated type (73.1%) with no differences between the genders (χ^2 = 1.34, df = 1, p_{exact} = n.s.) (Table 5).

Type of intervention	% (fq)
Mainly educational one	25.4 (17)
Multi-professional integrated	74.6 (50)
Total	100.0 (67)

Table 5. Type of intervention.

In particular, the different psycho-educational therapy proposals are summarized in Table 6, where it is clear that in 41.8% of the cases a multi-professional integrated intervention (educational, psychological and pharmacological) was used, while an integrated educational and psychological intervention was applied in 28.4%, and a mainly educational-pedagogical type of intervention in 24.5%.

Integration of the intervention	% (fq)
Educational	25.4 (17)
Educational and psychological	28.4 (19)
Educational and pharmacological	4.5 (3)
Educational, psychological and pharmacological	41.8 (28)
Total	100.0 (67)

Table 6. Integration of the intervention.

No statistically significant differences emerged between males and females for the integration of the intervention (χ^2 = 2.63, df = 3, p_{exact} = n.s.).
Going into more detail on the therapeutic project, as concerned the *educator-adolescent-group* relationship, there was a prevalence of individual interventions (65.7%) over group interventions (34.3%), with no significant differences between males and females (χ^2 = 2.07, df = 1, p_{exact} = n.s.).
This can be explained in relation to the global usage of the service, characterized by cases of even severe psychiatric illness, for whom a dual relationship may be easier for the individual to tolerate and less risky from the point of view of any break down.

As for the patients' *adherence to their therapeutic project*, this was adequate in the majority of cases (68.7%), while in 17.9% it was discontinuous, and in 13.4% it was inadequate, i.e. the treatment was abandoned ahead of schedule or patients attended less than 50% of their scheduled appointments. There were no gender-related differences for this variable (χ^2 = 1.02, df = 2, p_{exact} = n.s.).

The adolescents' mode of *participation* at the semi-residential centre was judged as active in 46.3% of cases, ambivalent in 29.9%, passive in 14.9% and oppositional in 9.0%, with no gender-related differences (χ^2 = 3.60, df = 3, p_{exact} = n.s.).

The *working alliance with the parents* was generally adequate (53.7%), sometimes partial (35.8%) and occasionally lacking (10.4%). Here again, there were no significant differences between males and females (χ^2 = .49, df = 2, p_{exact} = n.s.).

As for the overall *clinical progress (CGI)* of the sample considered, over the course of 12 months there was an improvement in 56.7% of the cases, while 10.4% of the patients deteriorated; in 32.8% the adolescents' clinical conditions remained unchanged. There were no significant differences between males and females (χ^2 = 3.09; df = 2, p_{exact} = n.s.).

3.4.4 Assessment of the efficacy of the therapeutic intervention

To assess the efficacy of the intervention, we used Students t-test for paired samples to compare the results of the YSR obtained at the baseline (T1) and a year later (T2) (Table 7). For all the domains of the YSR except for thought-related disorders (n.s.) and somatization (which tended towards significance), the patients had significantly lower mean scores at T2.

YSR syndrome scales	T1	T2	t	df	p.
Social withdrawal	1.83	1.49	2.83	58	.006
Somatization	1.27	1.17	1.76	58	.08
Anxious-depressive disorders	2.02	1.49	4.50	58	.000
Social problems	2.02	1.61	3.75	58	.000
Thought-related disorders	1.37	1.34	0.63	58	n.s.
Attention disorders	1.71	1.32	4.16	58	.000
Delinquent behavior	1.22	1.07	2.42	58	.02
Aggressive behavior	1.49	1.22	3.78	58	.000

Table 7. Student's t-test for paired samples comparing YSR scores at T1 and T2.

On the GAF scales too, the operators' mean assessments identified a significant remission of the symptoms, which changed from "severe" at T1 to "moderate" at T2 (Table 8).

	T1	T2	F	df	p
GAF	49,22	57,24	39.74	1	.000

Table 8. General linear model (GLM) on GAF scores obtained at T1 and T2.

Figure 2 shows that higher scores were obtained on the GAF reassessment, with a rightward migration of many of the patients (GAFT2), indicating a significant improvement in their global functioning. In particular, the percentage of patients in the range of 31-40 (which indicates a severely impaired psychosocial functioning) decreased considerably from T1 to T2, while there was a considerable increase in the number of patients judged to have only mild symptoms and a good general functioning (scores 61-70). It is also worth noting that it was only at T2 that some of the patients were judged to have an optimal functioning and no symptoms (scores 91-100).

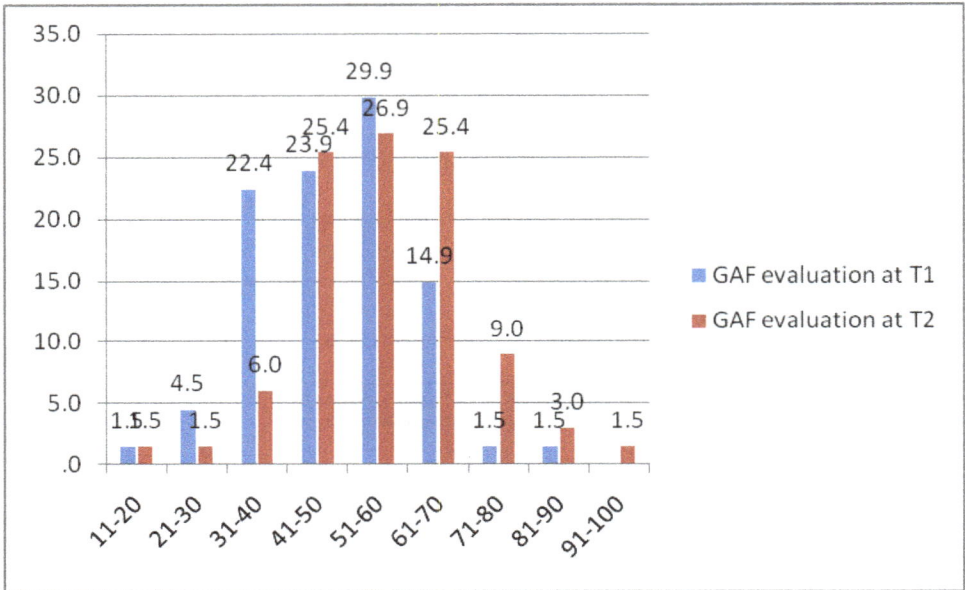

Fig. 2. Percentages of patients in the various ranges of GAF scores at T1 and T2.

The interaction with the time of administration of the GAF (T1 and T2) and the gender-related variables showed a trend towards statistical significance. In fact, according to the operators' assessments, females who started from a more severe assessment at T1 had a greater improvement at T2 (Table 9 and Fig. 3).

Gender	GAF T1	GAF T2	Interaction between GAF and gender		
			F	df	p.
Male	52.46	57.96	3.74	1	.06*
Female	43.58	55.42			

*Tending towards significance

Table 9. General linear model (GLM) for the GAF scales: interaction effect between GAF and gender.

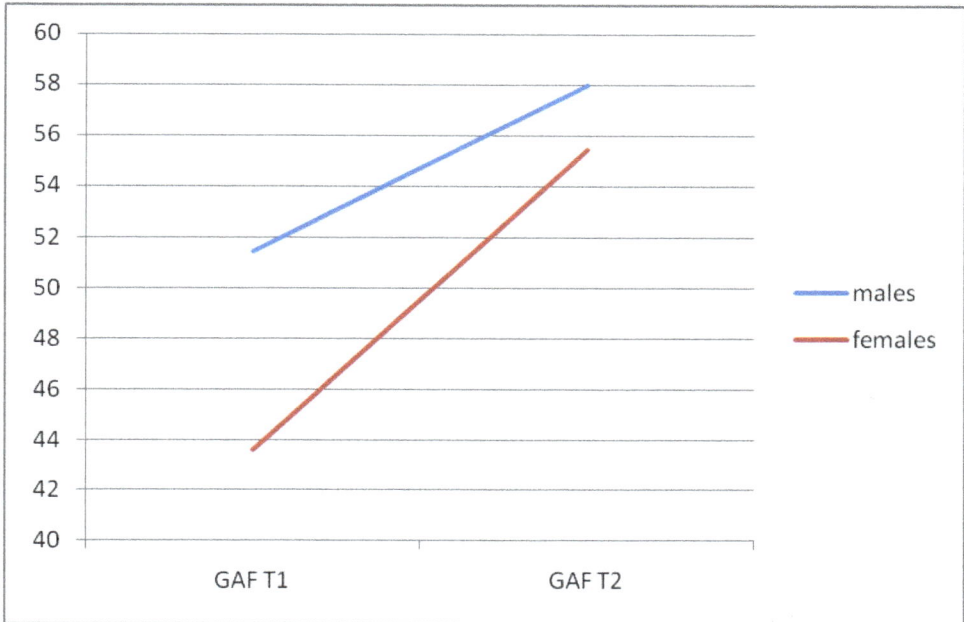

Fig. 3. General linear model (GLM) for the GAF scales: variation in mean GAF scores for males and females at T1 and T2.

The improvements seen in the GAF at T2 correlated with the number of hours the adolescents spent at the semi-residential centre. Table 10 shows a significant interaction between these two variables; although they had the lowest mean scores for the sample at T1, patients who attended the centre for more than 15 hours a week obtained the best improvement in absolute terms at T2. Moreover, the more the number of hours of weekly attendance at the centre increased, the greater the improvement seen in the GAF scores at T2, and this was particularly evident for patients who spent more than 15 hours a week at the centre (Fig. 4).

For multiprofessional intervention to be effective, in adolescent patients requiring treatment for such severe psychopathologies as those identified in our series of patients, naturally takes much longer and a more intensive treatment.

Attendance at the semi-residential centre	GAF T1	GAF T2	Improvement in GAF score (T2-T1)	Interaction between GAF and attendance at the centre		
				F	df	p
1-5 hours a week	51.21	56.21	5.00			
5-15 hours a week	49.48	56.00	6.52	5.25	2	.008
>15 hours a week	46.13	61.27	15.14			

Table 10. General linear model (GLM) for the GAF scores: interaction effect between GAF and attendance at the centre.

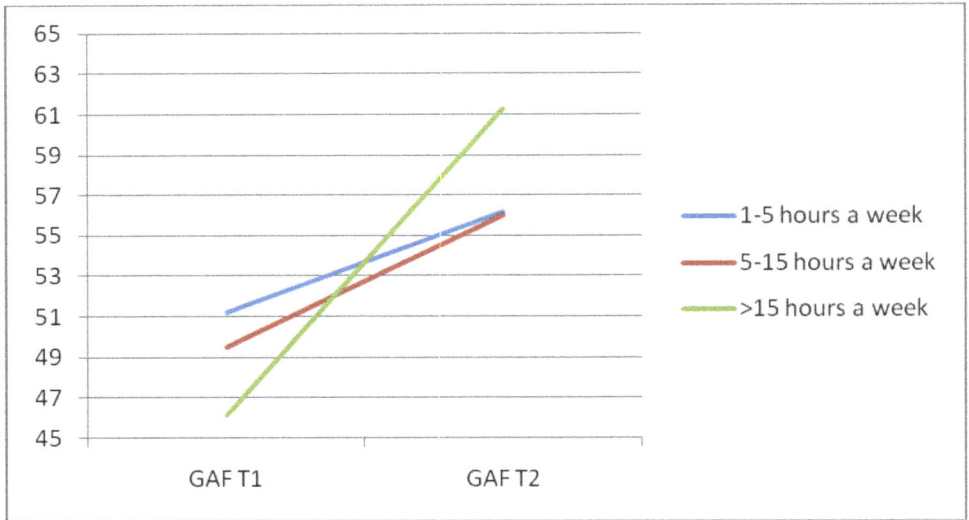

Fig. 4. General linear model (GLM) for the GAF scores: variation in mean GAF scores from T1 to T2 by time spent at the centre.

The interaction between the variation in the GAF scores between T1 and T2 and the type of intervention (mainly one-to-one or multi-professional integrated) was noteworthy, even though it was not statistically significant: the integrated intervention coincided with a greater improvement between T1 and T2 (Table 11 and Fig. 5).

This finding is confirmed in the literature by various studies supporting the greater efficacy of multimodal intervention in this mental health setting. In various different clinical pictures, the validity of a multimodal treatment approach comprising individual psychotherapy, pharmacology and family-based interventions is emphasized and recommended, even though evidence-based findings on the effects of different treatment methods are limited (Gatta et al., 2010a; Herpertz-Dahlmann & Salbach-Andrae, 2009; Masi et al., 2008; Nützel et al., 2005; Reeves & Anthony, 2009; Steiner & Remsing, 2007).

The interactions between the type of intervention (individual or in groups) and the variations in the GAF scores from T1 to T2 was not significant, indicating that both types of intervention are equally effective (Fig. 6).

Integration of interventions	GAF T1	GAF T2	Interaction between GAF and integration of interventions		
			F	df	p
One-to-one	52.72	57.17	2.98	1	.09
Integrated	47.94	57.27			

Table 11. General linear model (GLM) for the GAF scores: interaction effect between GAF scores and integration of interventions.

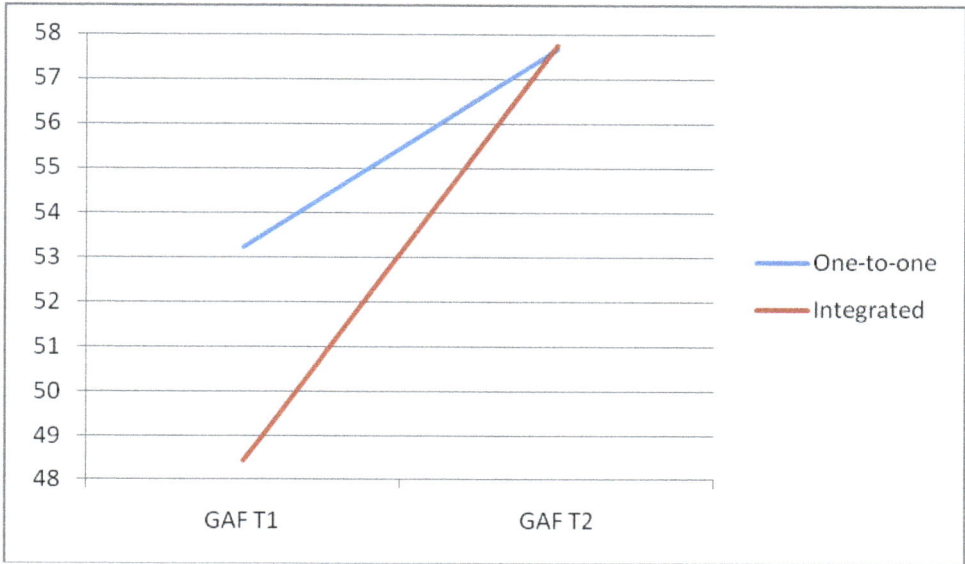

Fig. 5. General linear model (GLM) for the GAF scores: variation in mean GAF scores at T1 and T2 by type of intervention.

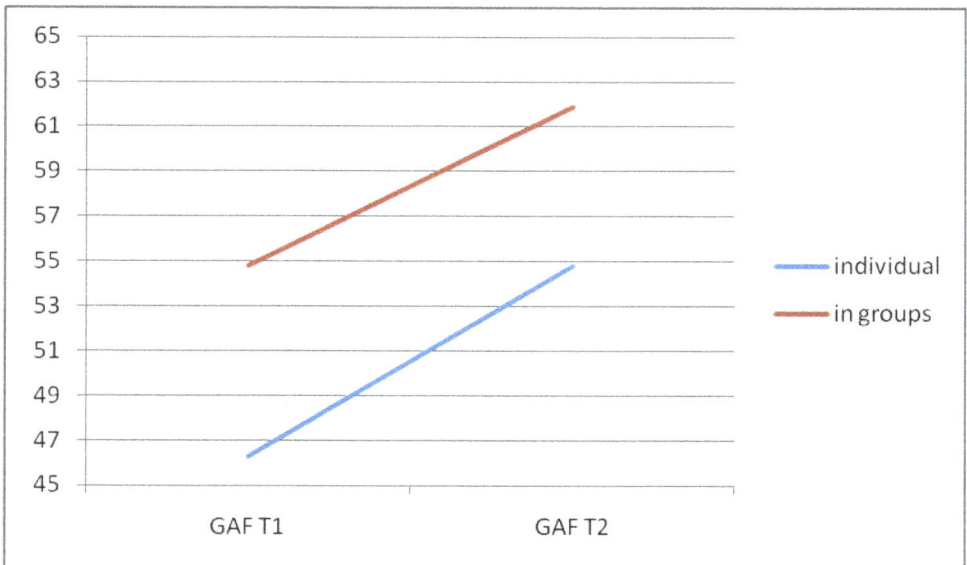

Fig. 6. General linear model (GLM) for the GAF scores: variations in mean GAF scores at T1 and T2 by type of operator-adolescent relationship.

The adolescents' *clinical progress* (improved, unchanged, deteriorated, based on the CGI) was correlated with the *time* spent at the semi-residential centre and a prevalence of patients who deteriorated (71.4%) emerged among those who attended for less than three months (while 13.6% of these patients remained unchanged and 5.3% improved); coinciding with a treatment period of 3-9 months, there were more than 1 in 3 of the patients who improved and another 1 in 3 of those who remained unchanged (36.8% and 36.4%, respectively), as opposed to 14.3% of those whose condition deteriorated. Among those attending for more than nine months, we found a majority of the patients who improved and remained unchanged (57.9% and 50.0%, respectively) and 14.3% of those who deteriorated (χ^2 = 20.51, df = 4, p_{exact} = .001).

In addition, among the patients who abandoned the treatment ahead of schedule we found 71.4% of the adolescents whose condition deteriorated, 13.6% of those who remained unchanged and 21.1% of the patients who improved. On the other hand, among the cases who completed the treatment agreed with the operators, we found a marked prevalence of the patients judged to have remained unchanged or improved (86.4% and 78.9%) as opposed to a minority of those whose condition deteriorated (28.6%) (χ^2 = 10.4, df = 2, p_{exact} = .006).

A study conducted by Luk et al. in 2001 on the drop-outs among young patients accessing mental health services showed that the adolescents who were not compliant were those judged to be less likely to improve at the time of the initial assessment and those whose parents found the treatment less well-organized, which goes to show the importance of parental compliance for patients of developmental age.

As for the relationship between *compliance* and *clinical progress*, an adequate adherence correlated with a positive clinical progress after 12 months. Among those whose compliance was adequate we found 86.8% of the patients who improved, 54.5% of those remaining unchanged and 14.3% of those who deteriorated (χ^2 = 24.64, df = 4, p_{exact} = .000).

A more positive clinical course in the longer term also correlated with a more positive *cooperation with parents* (χ^2 = 10.44, df = 4, p_{exact} = .04) (Table 12)

Working alliance	Clinical progress (CGI)		
	Improved % (fq)	Unchanged % (fq)	Deteriorated % (fq)
Adequate	68.4 (26	36.4 (8)	28.6 (2)
Partial	28.9 (11)	45.5 (10)	42.9 (3)
Absent	2.6 (1)	18.2 (4)	28.6 (2)
Lacking	100.0 (38)	100.0 (22)	100.0 (7)

Table 12. Comparison between the clinical course and the type of cooperation obtained from parents.

The working alliance with parents is an important variable that influences the therapeutic program for adolescents, correlating significantly with the latter's compliance. Among our patients who adhered adequately to the therapeutic project we found a clear majority of parents who also cooperated adequately (86.1%), more than half of the parents who cooperated only partially (54.2%) and only 28.6% of the parents who were uncooperative; on the other hand, among the patients who interrupted their treatment ahead of schedule (although there were only nine instances of this), we found none whose parents had been adequately cooperative (χ^2 = 20.79, df = 4, p_{exact} = .001).

Likewise, among the adolescents who participated actively in the semi-residential project, we found a high percentage of parents who cooperated adequately (63.9%), 25% of those who cooperated only partially, and 28.6% of those who failed to do so (χ^2 = 12.04, df = 6, p_{exact} = .006).

It is worth noting the finding concerning the adolescents' mode of *participation* in the semi-residential activities, which influenced their subsequent clinical progress: those who took an active part had a more positive follow-up assessment on their clinical progress, while those who were oppositional or ambivalent fared less well in the late assessment (Table 13.).

Mode of participation	Clinical progress (CGI)		
	Improved % (fq)	Unchanged % (fq)	Deteriorated % (fq)
active	65.8 (25)	27.3 (6)	.0 (0)
passive	13.2 (5)	22.7 (5)	.0 (0)
oppositional	2.6 (1)	13.6 (3)	28.6 (2)
ambivalent	18.4 (7)	36.4 (8)	71.4 (5)
Total	100.0 (38)	100.0 (22)	100.0 (7)

Table 13. Comparison between clinical progress and the adolescents' mode of participation at the semi-residential centre.

The above results relating to the relationship between compliance with the therapy, participation, alliance with the parents, and the patient's clinical progress are consistent with a number of published studies dealing with these topics.

The alliance with the parents proved to be a sine qua non for undertaking any therapeutic intervention with their children and for this to be successful (Gatta et al., 2005b, 2009b, 2010c, 2011; Marcelli, 2009).

Some authors emphasize that treating young patients it is very important to deal with their parents too (Diamond & Josephson, 2005; Hawley & Weisz, 2005, Nock & Ferriter, 2005; Nock & Kazdin, 2005), particularly when the young patients have behavioral disorders (Kazdin et al., 2006; Schaeffer & Borduin, 2005) like many of the patients attending our semi-residential service. It is also important to consider that a semi-residential intervention enables adolescents to remain in their habitual living environment and consequently demands a certain degree of cooperation on the part of their parents, or at least for the family environment not to be harmful to the adolescent.

It may sometimes be useful to take action on the parents themselves, as emerged from recent research conducted on several patients at our semi-residential service to investigate the influence of direct intervention to modify the parents' perception of their caregiving experience in relation to children with mental disorders (Gatta et al., 2010b): it emerged from our study that paying particular attention, in the course of several meetings, to aspects of the parents' experience and burden can improve their perception of the caregiving experience as well as reinforcing the therapeutic alliance. As in psychotherapy, the alliance can provide a corrective emotional experience sufficient to induce the reprocessing of internalized models relating, in this case, to caregiving. There is a risk of the treatment being abandoned prematurely every time an adolescent is taken into care and this risk increases when the parents take part in and exacerbate the patient's resistances. Moreover, any conflict between the parental couple, previously masked by the attention the pair was paying to the adolescent's problems, may come to the surface and find expression in aggressive projections of each party to the couple on the other. Supportive treatment for the parental couple should therefore be recommended also with a view to protecting their child against the parents' acting out.

As regards the correlation between the alliance with the parents and the adolescents' mode of participation, it is clear once again that one of the variables most capable of influencing the therapeutic process is the parents' cooperation, which is probably an expression of their more global attitude to their growing and increasingly independent child. The children of parents who are cooperative benefit more from the proposed therapy and can invest successfully in the new interpersonal relationships offered by the semi-residential environment, and this leads to higher scores on the scales for social competences. The opposite applies to the children of uncooperative parents, who are unable to invest strongly enough in the relationships offered and promoted in the setting of the centre. This finding reveals all the ambiguity of these adolescents as they oscillate between dependence and independence: their parents' support still seems to be a fundamental condition for them to be able to invest in new relationships outside the family.

Judging from the data emerging from our study, the alliance with the parents seems to be linked to the type of family nucleus involved. Among those with whom an adequate alliance was constructed we found a slight prevalence of adolescents who were the offspring of intact *parental couples* (56.9% intact couples vs 43.8% single-parent families), whole among those with whose parents it was impossible to construct an effective working alliance, we found a marked prevalence of adolescents coming from single-parent families (31.3% single-parent families, 3.9% intact parental couples). This finding can be placed in relation to the lack of a sufficiently supportive family environment, as documented by previous studies, and to the fact that single-parent families have to be seen as a possible factor of risk both for the onset of psychopathologies and for the failure of their treatment (Gatta et al., 2009a, 2009b; Hanington et al., 2011; Manzano et al., 1993).

4. Conclusions

The results relating to our patients' clinical progress after 12 months, the data deriving from administering the YSR and the scores on the GAF scale demonstrate the validity and efficacy, in the approach to adolescents with a mental illness, of a treatment based on an integrated psychological, psychiatric and educational-pedagogical intervention. We were able to reveal the importance of factors such as the active involvement of the adolescents, the parents' compliance with the therapeutic project, and the positivity of a multidisciplinary approach to their taking into care.

In particular, an important factor emerging from our research is the role of the adolescent's active participation. Shared objectives configure in the educational background an area of shared intentionality that succeeds in touching on different levels of change to expect from the therapeutic program, from educational goals that stem from a lack of motivation and interest to relational and even interior goals relating to the adolescent's of growing process of identification (Pasqualotto, 2005). The theoretical premise for each shared process lies in the need for these individuals to regain control of the competences and abilities impaired by their mental illness, thereby reasserting their fundamental rights as citizen in the sense of feeling a part of their affective, relational and productive world (Saraceno, 1995).

The educational-therapeutic experience aims to expand the patient's field of experience and offers new opportunities (see the aims of the service) in which the adolescents can feel an active part, a carrier of change in themselves and in their surrounding environment, not a passive receptor or someone who submits to decisions made by others. In this sense, the adolescents' active participation in their therapeutic project becomes a favorable prognostic factor of a positive clinical evolution because it stimulates the patients' interior resources to contribute to their personal evolutionary process.

Another fundamental point to emphasize and draw attention to is the parents' cooperation: to establish an adequate therapeutic alliance with the parents appears to be a factor fundamental to a successful clinical course. The parents act as a bridge and give us access to the patient, determining which treatments are acceptable at family level, and the intervention can use them as a vehicle in the sense that a change in their representations of their child and of their role as parents, and a change in the parents' attitudes and mode of interacting with their child are all an important stimulus for mobilizing their child's development (Fava Vizziello et al., 1991; Gatta et al., 2010b).

Given the small size of our sample and the psychopathological heterogeneity characterizing our cases, combined with the limited period of follow-up and the paucity of literature on this specific topic, it is still impossible to generalize from our results as concerns the efficacy of this type of treatment. Our findings should therefore be considered as preliminary and need to be confirmed in future by prospective studies on larger, more homogeneous populations, as mentioned elsewhere in the literature (Shepperd et al., 2009; Lamb, 2009).

5. References

Achenbach , T.M. & Rescorla L.A. (2001). *Manual for the ASEBA Schoool-Age Forms and Profiles*. University of Vermont, Research Center for Children, Burlington.

American Psychiatric Association (1994). *Diagnostic and Statistical Manual of Mental Disorders, Axis V*. American Psychiatric Association, Washington, D.C.

Ammaniti, M., Sergi, G. (2002). Diagnosi e valutazione clinica in adolescenza, In: *Manuale di psicopatologia dell'adolescenza*, Ammaniti M., pp. 3-31, Raffaello Cortina, Milano.

Angold, A., Costello, E.J., Farmer, E.M., Burns, B.J.,& Erkanli, A. (1999). Impaired but Undiagnosed *Journal of the American Academy of Child and Adolescent Psychiatry*, 38, pp. 129-137.

Bachmann, M., Bachmann, C., Rief, W. & Mattejat, F. (2008). Efficacy of psychiatric and psychotherapeutic interventions in children and adolescents with psychiatric disorders - A systematic evaluation of meta-analyses and reviews. Part I: Anxiety disorders and depressive disorders. *Z Kinder Jugendpsychiatr Psychother*, 36, 5, pp. 309- 320.

Bachmann, M., Bachmann, C., Rief, W., & Mattejat, F. (2008). Efficacy of psychiatric and psychotherapeutic interventions in children and adolescents with psychiatric disorders - A systematic evaluation of meta-analyses and reviews. Part II: ADHD and conduct disorders. *Z Kinder Jugendpsychiatr Psychother*, 36, 5, pp. 321-333.

Bartels, C.S.J., Dums, A.R., Oxman, T.E., Schneider, L.S., Areán, P.A., Alexopoulos, G.S., & Jeste, D.V. (2004). American Psychiatric Association Evidence-Based Practices. *Geriatric Mental Health Focus*, 2, 268-281.

Bittner, A., Egger, H., Erkanli, A., Costello, E.J., Foley, E., & Angold, A. (2007). What do childhood anxiety disorders predict? *Journal of Child Psychology and Psychiatry*, 48,12, pp. 1174-1183.

Bond, G.R., Drake, R.E., Mueser, K.T, Latimer, E. (2001). Assertive Community Treatment for People with Severe Mental Illness: Critical Ingredients and Impact on Patients. *Disease Management & Health Outcomes*, 9, 3, pp. 141-159.

Chandra, R., Srinivasan, S., Chandrasekaran, R., & Mahadevan, S. (1993). The prevalence of mental disorder in school-age children attending a general paediatric department in southern India. *Acta Psychiatrica Scandinavica*, 87, 3, pp. 192-196.

Connor, D.F., Carlson, G.A., Chang, K.D., Daniolos, P.T., Ferziger, R., Findling, R.L., Hutchinson, J.G., Malone, R.P., Halperin, J.M., Plattner, B., Post, R.M., Reynolds, D.L., Rogers, K.M., Saxena, K., & Steiner, H., Stanford/Howard/AACAP Workgroup on Juvenile Impulsivity and Aggression (2006). Juvenile maladaptive aggression: a review of prevention, treatment, and service configuration and a proposed research agenda. *Journal of Clinical Psychiatry*, 67, 5, pp. 808-820.

Costello, E.J., Egger, H., & Angold, A. (2005). 10-Years research update review: the epidemiology of child and adolescent psychiatric disorders: I. Methods and public health burden. *Journal of the American Academy of Child and Adolescent Psychiatry*, 44, 10, pp. 972-986.

Costello, E. J., Foley, D. L., & Angold, A. (2006). 10-Year Research Update Review: the epidemiology of child and adolescent psychiatric disorders: II. Developmental epidemiology. *Journal of the American Academy of Child and Adolescent Psychiatry*, 45, pp. 8-25.

De Martis D. (1997).L'adolescente nei servizi psichiatrici: un impatto problematico. In Telleschi R., Torre G. *Il primo colloquio con l'adolescente* (II edizione) , Raffaello Cortina Editore, Milano.

Diamond, G., Josephson, A. (2005). Family-based treatment research: a 10-year update. *Journal of American Academy of Child and Adolescent Psychiatry*, 44, 9, 872-887.

Dimigen, G., Del Priore, C., Butler, S., Evans, S., Ferguson, L., & Swan, M.(1999). Psychiatric disorder among children at time of entering local authority care: questionnaire survey. *British Medical Journal*, 11, 319, 675.

Di Giuseppe, R., Linscott, J., & Jilton, R. (1996). Developing the therapeutic alliance in children-adolescent psychotherapy. *Applied & Preventive Psychology*, 5, 2, 85-100.

Fava Vizziello, G., Disnan, G., & Colucci, M.R. (1991). *Genitori psicotici. Percorsi clinici di figli di pazienti psichiatrici,* Bollati Boringhieri Editore, Torino.

Fava Vizziello, G. (2003). Le classificazioni diagnostiche. In Fava Vizziello G. *Psicopatologia dello sviluppo*, Il Mulino, Bologna.

Flouri, E., Mavroveli, S., & Tzavidis, N. (2010). Modeling risks: effects of area deprivation, family socio-economic disadvantage and adverse life events on young children's psychopathology. *Social Psychiatry and Psychiatric Epidemiology*, 45, 6, 611-619.

Fonagy, P., Targett, M., Cottrell, D., Philips, J., & Zarrina, K. (2003). Epidemiologia. In *Psicoterapie per il bambino e per l'adolescente: trattamenti e prove di efficacia*. Il Pensiero Scientifico Editore, Roma

Frigerio, A., Vanzin, L., Pastore, V., Nobile, M., Giorda, R., Marino, C., Molteni, M., Rucci, P., Ammaniti, M., Lucarelli, L., Lenti, C., Walder, M., Martinuzzi, A., Carlet, O., Muratori, F., Milone, A., Zuddas, A., Cavolina, P., Nardocci, F., Rullini, A.,

Morosini P., Polidori, G., & De Girolamo, G. (2006). The Italian preadolescent mental health project (PrISMA): rationale and methods. *International Journal of Methods in Psychiatric Research*, 15, pp. 22–35.

Frigerio, A., Rucci, P., Goodman, R., Ammaniti, M., Carlet, O., Cavolina, P., De Girolamo, G., Lenti, C., Lucarelli, L., Mani, E., Martinuzzi, A., Micali, N., Milone, A., Morosini, P., Muratori, F., Nardocci, F., Pastore,V., Polidori, G., Tullini, A., Vanzin, L., Villa, L., Walder, M., Zuddas, A., & Molteni, M. (2009). Prevalence and correlates of mental disorders among adolescents in Italy: the PrISMA study, *European Child And Adolescent Psychiatry*, 18, pp. 217-226.

Gatta, M., Talamini, A., Ramaglioni, E., Bertossi, E., & Condini A. (2005a). Disturbo comportamentale in adolescenza: un sintomo, molteplici diagnosi. *Giornale Italiano di psicopatologia e psichiatria dell'infanzia e dell'adolescenza*, 12, 2, pp. 95-106.

Gatta, M., Condini, A. (2005b). La relazione di alleanza con i genitori come fattore condizionante l'aderenza al progetto terapeutico e l'evoluzione clinica dell'adolescente con disagio psichico. *Giornale Italiano di psicopatologia e psichiatria dell'infanzia e dell'adolescenza*, 12, 2, pp. 131-142.

Gatta M., Bertossi E., Dal Zotto L., Del Col L., Testa C.P., Battistella P. A. (2009a). Psycho educational intervention for psychiatric adolescents: the experience of a daily service. *Giornale di neuropsichiatria dell'età evolutiva*, 29, 132-153.

Gatta, M., Ramaglioni, E., Lai, J., Svanellini, L., Toldo, I., Del Col, L., Salviato, C., Spoto, A., & Battistella P.A. (2009b). Psychological and behavioral disease during developmental age: the importance of the alliance with parents. *Neuropsychiatric Disease and Treatment*, 5, 541-546.

Gatta, M, Pertile, R., Testa, C.P., Tomadini, P., Perakis, E., & Battistella, P.A. (2010a). Working with adolescents with mental disorders: the efficacy of a multiprofessional intervention. *Health*, 2, 7, 811-818.

Gatta, M., Dal Zotto, L., Nequino, G., Del Col, L., Sorgato, R., Ceranto, G., Testa, C.P., Pertile, R., & Battistella, P.A. (2010b). Parents of adolescent with mental disorder: improving their care giving experience. *Journal of child and family studies*, 20, 4, 478-490.

Gatta, M., Spoto, A., Testa, P., Svanellini, L., Lai, J., Salis, M, De Sauma, M., & Battistella P.A. (2010c). Adolescent's insight within the working alliance: A bridge between diagnostic and psychotherapeutic processes. *Adolescent Health, Medicine and Therapeutics*, 1, 45-52.

Gatta, M., Spoto, A., Svanellini, L., Lai, J., Testa, C.P., & Battistella PA (2011). Alliance with patient and collaboration with parents throughout the psychotherapeutic process with children and adolescents: a pilot study. *Giornale Italiano di Psicopatologia* (ahead of print)

Green, J. (2002). Provvision of Intensive Treatment: Inpatient Units, Day Units and Intensive Outreach. In Rutter M, Taylor E. *Child and Adolescent Psychiatry* (4th edition), Blackwell Science,UK

Guy, W. (1976). CGI: Clinical global impression. In: ECDEU *Assessment manual for psychopharmacology*, Rockville, ED: US Department of Health and Human Services, Public Helath Service, Alcohol Drug Abuse and Mental Health Administration, National Institute of Mental Health Psychopharmacology Research Branch, pp. 217-222.

Hanington, L., Heron, J., Stein, A., & Ramchandani, P. Parental depression and child outcomes - is marital conflict the missing link? *Child Care and Health Development.* 2011 doi: 10.1111/j.1365-2214.2011.01270.x. [Epub ahead of print]

Hanson, W. E., Curry, K. T., & Bandalos, D. L. (2002). Reliability generalization of Working Alliance Inventory scale scores. *Educational and Psychological Measurement, 62,* 4, 659-673.

Hawley, K.M., Weisz, J.R. (2005). Youth versus parent working alliance in usual clinical care: distinctive associations with retention, satisfaction, and treatment outcome. *Journal of Clinical Child and Adolescent Psychology,* 34, 1, 117-128.

Herpertz-Dahlmann, B., & Salbach-Andrae, H. (2009). Overview of treatment modalities in adolescent anorexia nervosa. *Child and Adolescent Psychiatric Clinics of North America,* 18, 1, 131-145.

Hofstra, M.B., Van De Ende, J., & Verhulst, F.C. (2001). Adolescent's self-reported problems as predictors of psychopathology in adulthood: 10 year follow up study. *British Journal of Psychiatry,* 179, 203-209.

Horvath, A.O., & Greenberg, L.S. (1989). Development and validation of the working alliance inventory. *Journal of Counseling Psychology,* 36, 2, 223-233.

Horvath, A. O. (1994). Empirical validation of Bordin's pantheoretical model of the alliance: the Working Alliance Inventory perspective. In: Horvath, A. O., & Greenberg, L. S. *The Working Alliance: Theory, Research, and Practice,* Wiley, New York.

Istituto Nazionale di Statistica (ISTAT) (2008). Istruzione: tasso di abbandono delle scuole superiori. In: Barbieri G A, Cruciani S, Ferrara A, *100 Statistiche per il paese,* 35, 48. CSR, Roma.

Ivanova, M.Y., Achenbach, T.M., Rescorla, L.A., Dumenci, L., Almqvist, F., Bilenberg, N., Bird, H., Broberg, A.G., Dobrean, A., Dopfner, M., Erol, N., Forns, M., Hannesdottir, H., Kanbayashi, Y., Lambert, M.C., Leung, P., Minaei, A., Mulatu, M.S., Novik, T., Oh, K.J., Roussos, A., Sawyer, M., Simsek, Z., Steinhausen, H.C., Weintraub, S., Winkler Metzke, C., Wolanczyk, T., Zilber, N., Zukauskiene, R., & Verhulst, F.C. (2007). The generalizability of the Youth Self-Report syndrome structure in 23 societies. *Journal of Consulting and Clinical Psychologyl,* 75, 5, 729-738.

Jeammet, P. (1980). *Psicopatologia dell'adolescenza* (2004, 3rd edition), Borla Editore, Roma.

Kazdin, A.E., Whitley, M., & Marciano, P.L. (2006). Child-therapist and parent-therapist alliance and therapeutic change in the treatment of children referred for oppositional, aggressive, and antisocial behavior. *Journal of Child Psychology and Psychiatry,* 47, 5, 436-445.

Kessler, R.C., Berglund, P.M.B.A., Demler, O., Jin, R., Merikangas, K.R., & Walters, E.E. (2005). Lifetime prevalence and age of onset distributions of DSM-IV disorders in the national Comorbidity Study Replication. *Archives of General Psychiatry,* 62, 6, 593-602.

Kessler, R.C., Wang, P.S. (2008). The descriptive epidemiology of commonly occurring mental disorders in the United States. *Annual Review of Public Health,* 29, 115-129.

Kim-Cohen, J., Caspi, A., Moffitt, T.E., Harrington, H., Milne, B.J., & Poulton, R. (2003). Prior juvenile diagnoses in adults with mental disorders: Developmental follow-back of a prospective-longitudinal cohort. *Archives of General Psychiatry,* 60, 709-717.

Lamb, C.E. (2009) Alternatives to admission for children and adolescents: providing intensive mental healthcare services at home and in communities: what works? *Current opinion in Psichiatry*, 22, pp. 345-350.

Lingiardi, V. (2002). *L' alleanza terapeutica. Teoria, clinica, ricerca.* Cortina Raffaello, Milano.

Luk, E.S., Staiger, P.K., Mathai, J., Wong, L., Birleson, P., & Adler, R. (2010). Children with persistent conduct problems who dropout of treatment. *European Child & Adolescent Psychiatry*, 10, 28-36.

Manzano, J., Favre, C., Zabala, I., Borella, E., Fischer, W., Gex-Fabry, M., Laufer, D., Seidl, R., & Urban, D. (1993). Continuity and discontinuity of psychopathology: a study of patients examined as children and as adults. II. Childhood antecedents of drug dependent adults. *Schweiz Arch Neurol Psychiatr.* 144, 3, 273-284.

Marcelli, D., Braconnier, A., (1989). *Adolescenza e psicopatologia*, Masson (2006), Milano.

Marcelli, D. (2009). Les traitements psychothérapeutiques et rééducatifs. In Marcelli D. *Enfance et psychopatologie* (8e edition), Elsevier Masson, Issy-lesMoulineaux Cedex.

Masi, G., Milone, A., Manfredi, A., Pari, C., Paziente, A. & Millepiedi, S. (2008). Conduct disorder in referred children and adolescents: Clinical and therapeutic issues. *Comprehensive Psychiatry*, 49, 2, 146-153.

MTA Cooperative Group National Institute of Mental Health (2004). Multimodal Treatment Study of ADHD Follow-up: 24-Month Outcomes of Treatment Strategies for Attention-Deficit/Hyperactivity Disorder. *Pediatrics*, 113, 4, 754-761.

Nock, M.K., Ferriter, C. (2005). Parent management of attendance and adherence in child and adolescent therapy: a conceptual and empirical review. *Clinical Child and Family Psychology Review*, 8, 2, 149-166.

Nock, M.K., Kazdin, A.E. (2005). Randomized controlled trial of a brief intervention for increasing participation in parent management training. *Journal of Consulting and Clinical Psychology*, 73, 5, 872-879.

Nützel, J., Schmid, M., Goldbeck, L., & Fegert, J.M. (2005). Psychiatric support for children and adolescents in residential care in a German sample. *Praxis der Kinder-psychologie und Kinderpsychiatrie*, 54, 8, pp. 627-644.

Palareti, L., Berti, C. (2010). Relational Climate and Effectiveness of Residential Care: Adolescent Perspectives. *Journal of prevention and intervention in the community*, 38, 1, pp. 26 – 40.

Pani R., Biolcati R., Sagliaschi S. (2009). *Psicologia clinica e psicopatologia per l'educazione e la formazione*, Il Mulino, Bologna.

Pasqualotto, L. (2005). I presupposti del lavoro educativo, in Ferrari, F., & Lascioli A. (a cura di), *Operativamente educativi*, Franco Angeli, Milano.

Pazaratz, D. (2001). Theory and Structure of a Day Treatment Program for Adolescents *Residential Treatment for Children& Youth,*Vol. 19(1) pp.29-43

Pazaratz, D. (1996). Teaching a young woman to understand the nature and consequences of her behaviour. *Residential Treatment for Children and Youth*, 14, 1, pp.25-35.

Pissacroia, M. (1998). *Trattato di psicopatologia dell'adolescenza*, Piccin, Padova.

Reeves, G., Anthony, B. (2009). Multimodal treatments versus pharmacotherapy alone in children with psychiatric disorders: implications of access, effectiveness, and contextual treatment. *Paediatric Drugs*, 11, 3, pp.165-9.

Rutter, M., Kim-Cohen, J., & Maughan, B. (2006). Continuities and discontinuities in psychopathology between childhood and adult life. *The journal of Child Psychology and Psychiatry*, 47, 3-4, pp. 276-295.

Saraceno B. (1995). *La fine dell'intrattenimento*, Etaslibri, Milano.

Schaeffer, C.M., & Borduin, C.M. (2005). Long-term follow-up to a randomized clinical trial of multisystemic therapy with serious and violent juvenile offenders. *Journal of Consulting and Clinical Psychology*, 73, 3, pp.445-453.

Shepperd, S., Doll, H., Gowers, S., James, A, Fazel, M., Fitzpatrick, R., & Pollock, J. (2009). Alternatives to inpatient mental health care for children and young people. *Cochrane Database System Review*, 15, 2.

Startup, M., Jackson, M.C., & Bendix, S. (2002). The concurrent validity of the Global Assessment of Functioning (GAF). *British Journal of Clinical Psychology*, 41, 4, pp.417-422.

Steiner, H., & Remsing, L. (2007). Work Group on Quality Issues Practice parameter for the assessment and treatment of children and adolescents with oppositional defiant disorder. *Journal of the American Academy of Child and Adolescent Psychiatry*, 46, 1, pp. 126-141.

Velligan, D.I., Draper, M., Stutes, D., Maples, N., Mintz, J., Tai, S. & Turkington, D. (2009). Multimodal Cognitive Therapy: Combining Treatments That Bypass Cognitive Deficits and Deal With Reasoning and Appraisal Biases. *Schizophrenia Bulletin*, 35, 5, pp. 884-893.

Woolfenden, S.R., Williams, K., Peat, J. (2001). Family and parenting interventions in children and adolescents with conduct disorder and delinquency aged 10-17. *Cochrane Database System Review*. 2001;(2).

WHO (1992). *The ICD-10 Classification of mental and behavioural disorders: clinical descriptions and diagnostic guidelines*. World Health Organization, Geneva.

WHO (2004). *Prevention of Mental Disorders: effective intervention and policy options*. World Health Organization 2004, Geneva.

10

"Mental Health Services are Different": Economic and Policy Effects

Ruth F.G. Williams[1] and D.P. Doessel[2]
[1]*La Trobe School of Economics, La Trobe University*
[2]*School of History, Philosophy, Religion & Classics, The University of Queensland*
Australia

1. Introduction

Health economics, like other applied fields of economic study (such as transport economics, regional and urban economics, international trade), draws on a common body of economic and econometric theory. However some scholars, such as Blaug (1998), argue that health economics involves more than the standard application of the tools in the economists' toolkits. One of his emphases was on the complications arising from the fact that medical practitioners demand health services on behalf of patients, given the imperfect information that patients have about diagnosis and therapy, i.e. the imperfect agency relationship. In addition, he emphasised the difficulties of measuring (and evaluating) health outcomes, as well as the work in defining (and measuring) equity, following Le Grand's (1987) pioneering paper.

But it is Arrow's (1963) seminal article that points out the differences in health care that make economic analysis somewhat difficult. The eleemosynary dimension of the health sector (involving not-for-profit institutions), as well as other factors (such as various dimensions of uncertainty), explain societal responses to the numerous market failures in the health sector. Thus, work in the health sector is somewhat different from economic analysis of the meat industry (Beggs, 1988), the car industry (Madden, 1988) etc.

However, mental health economics is even more difficult than health economics. This point is indicated by the following statement: "Mental health economics is like health economics only more so: uncertainty and variations in treatments are greater; the assumption of patient self-interested behaviour is more dubious; response to financial incentives such as insurance is exacerbated; the social consequences and external costs of illness are more formidable" (Frank & McGuire, 2000, p. 895).

This chapter is concerned with another dimension of "difference" (and difficulty) that exists in the analysis of mental well-being. In general reference to all societies, the following statements are axiomatic: vegetarians do not buy meat for their own consumption; people who do not own cars do not buy petrol; and so forth. Such axiomatic statements cannot be made in the context of mental health sectors. Some people with no clinical mental illness consume mental health services; and simultaneously some other people who have clinical manifestations of mental illness do not consume mental health services for various reasons. The term that can be applied to these two problems is "structural imbalance".

The next section will provide some further background on structural imbalance. Section 3 will elaborate on the economic dimensions of structural imbalance commencing with a 2 x 2 matrix. Enumerating the cells of this matrix forms the basis of empirical work. Section 4 discusses the trends that are exacerbating structural imbalance, and their economic basis. Section 5 discusses various policy matters. The Chapter then provides some qualifications in Section 6 and draws conclusions in Section 7.

2. The economic 'mismatching' tendency of mental health services

The term, structural imbalance, is applied to describe the resource misallocation between "need" and "service use". The problem has been noted in the United States (U.S. Department of Health & Human Services, 1999), Ontario (Canada) (Lin *et al.*, 1996), New Zealand (Oakley Browne & Wells, 2006), and also Australia [Doessel *et al.*, 2010) using cross-sectional data, and in time-series data (Doessel & Williams, 2011)]. The purpose of this Chapter is to describe this particular source of resource misallocation in mental health sectors under health insurance, to present some empirical results, and to discuss policy implications of this structural imbalance.

Resource misallocations of various types are ever-present in any economy and in this sense mental health services are no different; however the structural imbalance in mental health services is "a little different". This mismatch in mental health services is not found in other sectors of the economy, as commented in the introduction above: some people without a mental illness do consume mental health services. It is not suggested here that service use and illness are completely misaligned in mental health sectors. Some people with no current symptoms are prone to relapse and require a "maintenance" approach to therapy (Druss *et al.*, 2007).

It is instructive to note that the connotation of "need" here is epidemiological, i.e. a synonym for "people with a mental illness/disorder" or "people having a diagnosis"; and "non-need" means "people without a mental illness/disorder", i.e. no diagnosis of mental illness. The use of this terminology is not to ignore the perspective of the economic literature on "need", which is but one factor in consumer demand. The term "need" with respect to health has several connotations, and an economic classification is now available (Williams & Doessel, 2011). Note also that an optimal implementation of existing therapies, given the current state of knowledge, is implied in the present study. See Andrews (2006).

The evidence from both time-series and cross-sectional data indicates that the structural imbalance in mental health services is extensive. Given that the economic nature of structural imbalance, and its sources, warrants further investigation, and that appropriate policy approaches have not yet been devised to address the problem, it is appropriate here to begin to fill the lacuna.

3. Economic dimensions and empirical evidence

This Section considers structural imbalance first with the conceptual tool of a 2 x 2 matrix. When "need" and "service utilisation" are cross-classified, structural imbalance can be clearly delineated, and it can be measured. There are four (co-existing) concepts that are relevant to the analysis of this problem. "Unmet need" is a term in clinical use which is applied by Andrews (2000) and Whiteford (2000) to describe non-use of services by someone who has a diagnosable mental illness. See also Cosgrove *et al.* (2008). Andrews (2000) and

Whiteford (2000) applied "met non-need" to the case where some people with no mental disorder consume mental health services. There are two other components to this analysis, met need and unmet non-need. The major proportion of a population is in the "unmet non-need category": people without any illness and not receiving services is of little interest here. "Met need" is the term that applies where people with illness are receiving services. These terms complete the four elements that cross-classify need and service use.

To quantify structural imbalance, several steps are undertaken. The first step involves an exercise in enumerating these four above-mentioned components using the cross-classified population sub-groups of "need" (i.e. presence of mental illness) and "service utilisation" (i.e. consumption of mental health resources). See Table 1. This Table suggests an exercise like the tabular form conceived of by Yerushalmy (1947) in his cross-classification approach for determining the sensitivity and specificity of diagnostic tests in medicine. In this Table, the Total population can be summed by rows that form the final column "Total utilisation" and "Total non-utilisation". The columns can also be summed according to the presence of mental illness i.e. "Total need" and "Total non-need", as indicated by the final row.

A useful technique for depicting structural imbalance is to employ Venn diagrams, as shown in Fig. 1. This figure establishes in a visual manner the polar cases, which serves as a structural framework. Conceiving of the polar cases enables the definition of the extreme or "perfect" cases i.e. "structural balance" and "structural imbalance", which then allows us to measure the degree of structural imbalance. The use of polar cases is often employed in economics such as in the Public Finance literature on pure public goods and pure private goods. This approach is also somewhat like establishing maximum and minimum values of an index, such as the Hirschman-Herfindahl Index, the Gini Index etc. In addition, Venn diagrams are relevant to conceive of resources shortages, as shown in Doessel *et al.* (2010).

Consumption of mental health resources	Presence of mental illness		Totals by row
	Present (MI⁺)	Absent (MI⁻)	
MHR⁺	Cell 1 "met need"	Cell 2 "met non-need"	Total utilisation
MHR⁻	Cell 3 "unmet need"	Cell 4 "unmet non-need"	Total non-utilisation
Totals by column	Total need	Total non-need	Total population

Source Doessel, Williams & Nolan, 2009

Notes MI⁺ Persons with mental illness; MI⁻ Persons without mental illness; MHR⁺ Persons consuming mental health resources; MHR⁻ Persons not consuming mental health resources

Table 1. A 2x2 matrix showing mental illness and consumption of mental health resources

The data on both need and utilisation to implement this conceptual approach, which is indicted above in Table 1 and Fig. 1, are available from the Australian Bureau of Statistics (ABS). The first epidemiological survey by the ABS, *Mental Health and Wellbeing...*, was undertaken in 1997 (ABS, 1998). Another survey was conducted in 2007 (ABS, 2008). Table 2 reproduces the structural imbalance quantified on 1997 data (which were the available data at the time of the study). The numbers in the cells can also be shown as proportions, and these are reproduced in Figure 2. Details are available in Doessel *et al.* (2010).

(a)	(b)
PERFECT CORRESPONDENCE	PERFECT NON-CORRESPONDENCE

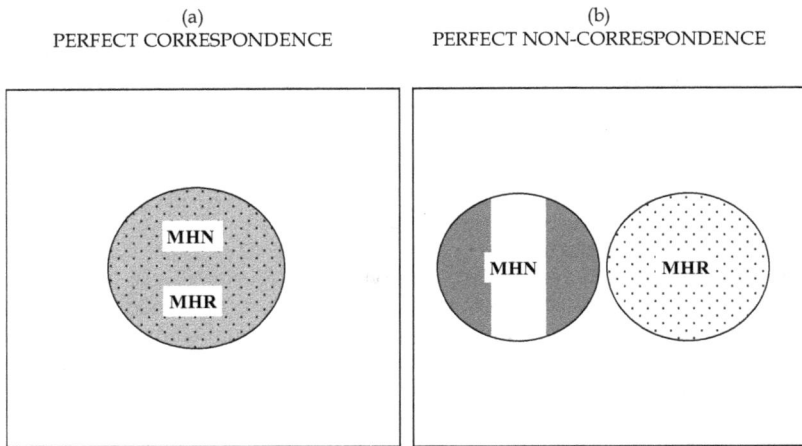

Notes:　MHN: Persons with mental health need
　　　　MHR: Persons consuming mental resources

　　Met Need
　　Unmet Need
　　Met Non-need
　　Unmet Non-need

Fig. 1. Two polar cases: structural balance and structural imbalance in the mental health sector (with sufficient resourcing)

Consumption of mental health resources	Presence of mental illness		Totals by row
	Present (MI⁺) "need"	Absent (MI·) "non-need"	
Consumption MHR⁺	905,600 "met need"	591,600 "met non-need"	1,497,200
Non-consumption MHR⁻	1,477,500 "unmet need"	10,490,100 "unmet non-	11,967,600
Totals by column	2,383,100	11,081,700	13,464,800

Source　Doessel et al. (2010)
Notes　i. The notation is as for Table 1. ii. In this epidemiological study Mental Illness includes Anxiety Disorders (panic disorder, agoraphobia, social phobia, generalised anxiety disorder, obsessive-compulsive disorder and post-traumatic stress disorder), Affective Disorders (depression, dysthymia, mania, hypomania and bipolar affective disorder) as well as Substance Abuse. iii. Mental health services include the following: the services of GPs, psychiatrists, psychologists, nurses, pharmacists, ambulance officers etc. iv. The data employed here relate to Australian adults, i.e. persons 18 years and over, not the total Australian population.

Table 2. Utilisation of "mental health resources" by adults with, and without, mental illness, Australia, 1997

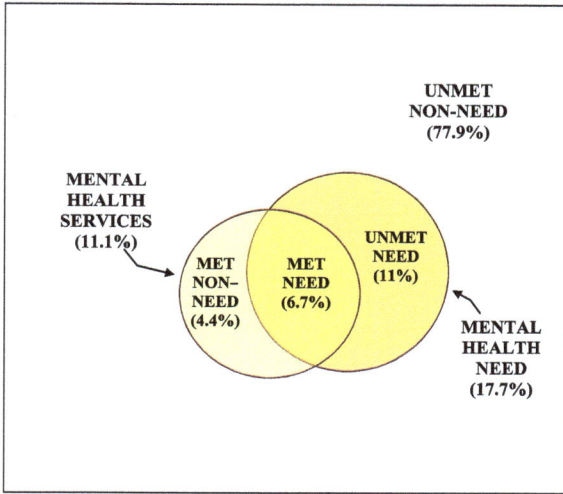

Source Doessel *et al.* (2010)

Fig. 2. Structural Imbalance between the Australian Adult Population with Mental Illness, and the Australian Population Consuming Mental Health Resources, Australia, 1997

Table 3 and Fig. 3 indicate that structural imbalance has a gender-related dimension. The proportions relating to the met non-need and unmet need are not constant across males and females from the 1997 ABS cross-sectional data. Further details are in Doessel *et al.* (2010).

	Male (%)	Female (%)	All Adults (%)
Mental health need	17.4	18.0	17.7
Mental health resources	8.1	14.0	11.1
Met need	5.1	8.3	6.7
Unmet non-need	79.6	76.3	77.9
Unmet need	12.3	9.7	11.0
Met non-need	3.0	5.7	4.4

Source   Doessel *et al.* (2010)
Notes   The relevant denominator for these calculations is male adults, female adults and all adults, respectively.

Table 3. Percentage shares of six categories of mental health/illness to the relevant population, male, female and all adults, Australia, 1997.

Empirical evidence of structural imbalance in Australia's mental health sector is found also in time-series data (Doessel & Williams, 2011). The results of that study determine that the "structural imbalance" is extensive, a result that reflects a sector beset with incomplete information (discussed briefly in Section 3). These results will be summarised here briefly. The research hypothesis in that study is that if there is high correspondence between the people with diagnosed mental disorders, as determined by ABS epidemiological surveys, and the consumers of mental health services, then structural balance exists. It follows that if

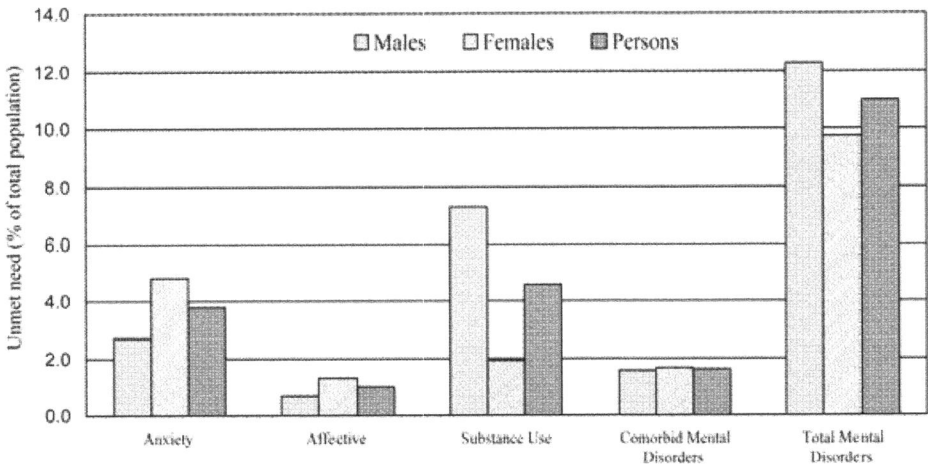

Source   Doessel *et al.* (2010)
Notes   See Fig. 2

Fig. 3. Unmet Need for Four Groups of Mental Disorders and Total Mental Disorders as a Percentage of the Population (Males, Females and Persons), Australia, 1997

there is "correspondence" between the two populations, some measurable characteristic of both groups would be similar. To determine "correspondence", a variable that can be measured in both groups is analysed: the ratio of females to total persons[1], expressed as a percentage. If statistical evidence indicates that the "gender composition" for the available epidemiological data on people with mental disorders is not consistent with the "gender composition" for the available Medicare[2] data on utilisation of mental health services, then we conclude that evidence of structural imbalance exists. The study measures the correspondence of the two above-mentioned ABS (representative sample) epidemiological surveys of mental disorders (ABS, 1998; 2008) and the data that provides an enumeration of consumers of mental health services under Australia's universal health insurance scheme, i.e. Medicare. The results are summarised here briefly.

Table 4 is a summary of the data from the two data-sources and Figs 4, 5 and 6 are reproduced here from the data analysis in Doessel & Williams (2011). The data analysis, involving several steps, will be outlined briefly. First, the data were modelled by applying Ordinary Least Squares regression. Three equations were estimated describing the temporal variation in the data for the three categories of mental health services. A set of fitted values (in which some confidence can be placed) for each of these data sets, were

---

[1] It makes no difference whether the female, or the male, ratio is analysed.

[2] Medicare is Australia's universal, compulsory health insurance scheme. It is financed from general taxation revenue and an ear-marked tax. Medicare enables the payment of subsidies for private fee-for-service medical services (in and out of hospital), the provision of subsidies for private fee-for-service allied services (which, in terms of mental health services, includes psychologists, occupational therapists etc), hospital services to "public patients" at zero prices at "recognised public hospitals", and subsidies for approved pharmaceuticals.

obtained; various extraneous factors associated with modelling these data (seasonal variation, serial correlation etc.) were taken into account, and two dummy variables were inserted for the outliers. Linear equations were found appropriate for all three data sets. We then constructed confidence intervals (CIs) around the fitted values for each of the three data sets. These three Figures depict the comparisons of the gender composition of consumers of three types of mental health services with the gender composition, in percentages, of people with mental disorders. Figure 3 depicts a comparison of the gender composition of consumers of specialist Psychiatry services with the gender composition, in percentages, of people with mental disorders (as determined from the two epidemiological surveys of the prevalence of mental disorders). There are 48 fitted observations depicted in Figure 3 for the time-series data on Psychiatry services from Medicare Australia with 99% upper and lower CIs, and two data points for the 1997 and 2007 epidemiological surveys with their 99% CIs. Figs 4 and 5 present the gender comparison for two other types of service utilisation, the mental health plans prepared by general practitioners (primary care physicians) and allied mental health services. For further details about the statistical estimation and the figures, see Doessel & Williams (2011).

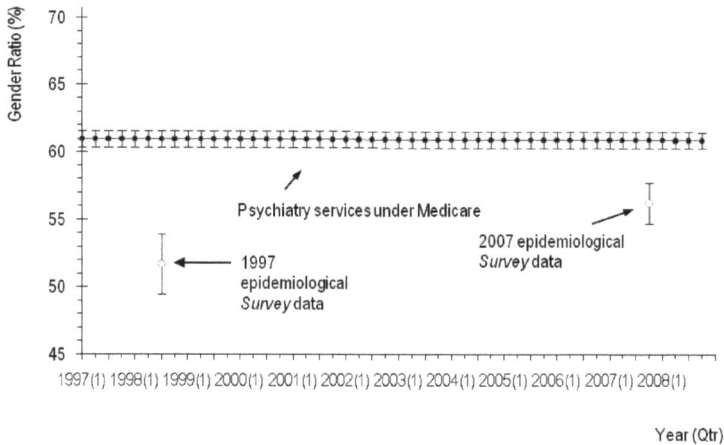

Source   See Doessel & Williams (2011).

Notes   • Point estimates (fitted values) with 99% CI, equation estimated on Medicare data as analysed in Doessel & Williams (2011)
o Point estimates with 99% CI from sample epidemiological survey data, as analysed in Doessel & Williams (2011)

Fig. 4. A Comparison of the Gender Share (Female/Persons) of CIDI-diagnosed Mental Disorders in the 1997 and 2007 Epidemiological Surveys for Australia, and the Gender Share for Specialist Psychiatry Services under Medicare, for 1997(1) to 2008(4).

	Temporal Coverage [b]	Unit of Analysis	No. of Obs.	Mean F/P (%)	Range F/P (%)	SE F/P (%)	SD F/P (%)	95% CIs Upper	95% CIs Lower	99% CIs Upper	99% CIs Lower
Epidemiological Data											
1997 *Survey* (ABS, 1998)	1997	1 year	1	51.7	na	0.8	na	53.3	50.0	53.9	49.5
2007 *Survey* (ABS, 2008)	2007	1 year	1	56.2	na	0.6	na	57.4	55.1	57.7	54.7
Service Utilisation Data											
Specialist Psychiatry Services [a]	1997(1) –2008(4)	Quarters	48	61.0	60.4-61.9	na	0.4	na	na	na	na
GP Preparation of Mental Health Plans [c]	2006(11)–2008(10)	Months	24	65.1	64.1-66.4	na	0.6	na	na	na	na
Allied Mental Health Services [d]	2006(11)–2008(10)	Months	24	69.4	68.7-70.4	na	0.5	na	na	na	na

Source: Doessel & Williams (2011)

Notes: F: females; P: persons; F/P: female-to-persons ratio; SD: standard deviation (for the population-based Medicare data-sets); SE: standard error (for the sample-based ABS epidemiological surveys); CI: confidence interval; na: not applicable.

a. The Psychiatry Items covered by Medicare in this analysis are those listed in Doessel & Williams (2011).

b. The notation in brackets in this column refers either to the relevant quarterly data (March, June, September and December) or to monthly data (Jan., Feb. etc.).

c. The GP Item numbers for the preparation of mental health plans are as follows: 2710, 2712 and 2713.

d. These services are provided by Psychologists, Occupational Therapists and Social Workers. The relevant Allied Health Item numbers are as follows: Psychological Therapy Services (Clinical Psychologists) 80000, 80005, 80010, 80015, 80020; Focussed Psychological Strategies (Registered Psychologists) 80100, 80105, 80110, 80115, 80120; Occupational Therapists 80125, 80130, 80135, 80140, 80145; Social Workers 80150, 80155, 80160, 80165, 80170.

Table 4. Some Characteristics of Two Epidemiological Data Sets and Three Mental Health Service Utilisation Data Sets on Gender Composition (Female-to-Persons Ratio), Australia, 1997-2008

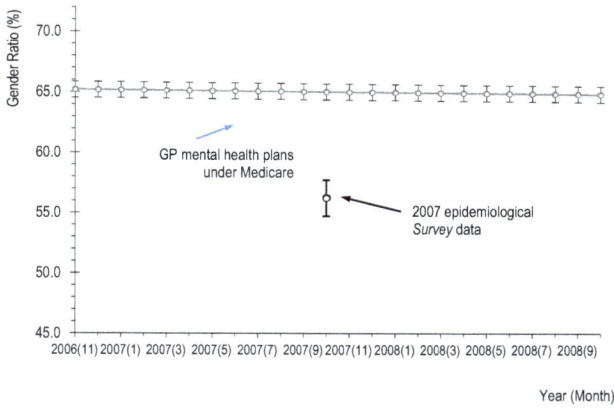

Source   Doessel & Williams (2011)
Notes   See Fig. 4.

Fig. 5. A Comparison of the Gender Share (Female/Persons) of CIDI-diagnosed Mental Disorders in the 2007 Epidemiological Survey for Australia, and the Gender Share for GP-prepared Mental Health Plans under Medicare, for 2006(11) to 2008(10)

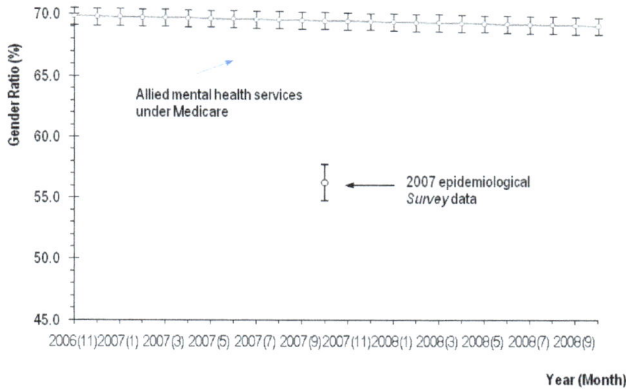

Source   Doessel and Williams (2011)
Notes   See Fig. 4.

Fig. 6. A Comparison of the Gender Share (Female/Persons) of CIDI-diagnosed Mental Disorders in the 2007 Epidemiological Survey for Australia, and the Gender Share for Allied Mental Health Services under Medicare, for 2006(11) to 2008(10).

It is clear from these three figures, indicating the location of the fitted observations and the CIs, that the consumers of the three types of mental health services are statistically different from the people with mental disorders, as determined by a population-based, representative sample survey of adult Australians. Further details are in Doessel & Williams (2011).

Some scholars, e.g. Jorm (2006), contend that unmet need is a "myth" (his term): imperfect data lead to phenomena that are artefacts of "data imperfection". There has been no empirical research reported to substantiate Jorm's assertion.
It is noted earlier that the other main economic problem in mental health is under-resourcing. This is a separate economic problem from structural imbalance, and yet both problems have a similar effect: under-resourcing of the sector also results in some people who need services not being served adequately by the system. For further details, see Doessel *et al.* (2010).

4. The economics of structural imbalance

Several forces underlie structural imbalance and they arise from different sources. The relevant economic analysis is in Williams & Doessel (2010), which gives an economic account of the effect of two trends in the West, one trend being towards the medicalisation of normal sorrows and the other major force relevant to psychiatric diagnosis, the impact of the *DSM-III* innovation. The emphasis in this Section is placed upon **information** and **diagnostic efficacy**. The efficient allocation of resources in mental health depends not only on the use of efficacious therapies, but also on correct diagnosis.

4.1 Two concurrent trends in western countries
The first of the two trends is the medicalisation of normal sorrows. Among those having no clinical mental illness but using mental health services are the "worried well" (Bell, 2005). The growth of the "worried well" is a result of the "depression culture" that has developed in Western society (Horwitz & Wakefield, 2007; Williams, 2009; Williams & Doessel, 2010). Empirical evidence is now available about the "worried well" and related issues (Wagner & Curran, 1984; Horwitz & Wakefield, 2007). Another group comprises some mental health professionals taking an interest in issues other than mental illness, such as managerial performance (Sperry, 1993) and sport (Begel, 1992). Various studies have sought to enumerate the problem of mental health services not being taken up by those in need of services (e.g. Cosgrove *et al.*, 2008; Byles *et al.*, 2011). While these approaches help to indicate a problem of some type, the underlying economic processes need to be elucidated and measured in conceptually appropriate ways. Effective policy responses also can thereby be developed.
The second trend is a widening of the diagnostic net of mental illness which has occurred as a by-product of the paradigm shift brought about after 1980, with the publication of the third revision of the diagnostic manual, the *Diagnostic and Statistical Manual of Mental Disorders*, by the American Psychiatric Association (APA). The third edition and later revisions (APA, 1980, 1987, 1994, 2000) incorporated a major innovation.
A detailed account of the demand-side and supply-side effects of the *DSM-III* innovation in psychiatry is in Williams & Doessel (2010). Figs 7 and 8 tell an abbreviated version of that economic analysis. Although the *DSM-III* has improved the diagnosis of mental illness to some extent (thus lowering the false negative rate), it has also been one mechanism by which the diffusion of some misconceptions associated with mental illness has occurred (Williams, 2009). Using conventional price–quantity space, with a focus on the quantity dimension in this space, Williams & Doessel (2010) consider the impact of the concurrent forces on the false positive rate in the diagnosis of mental illnesses in the West. They show that diagnostic efficacy is relevant to resource allocation in the mental health sector. The

policy implication is that diagnostic practices in the mental health sector need to improve and funding innovation in these practices is of vital importance.

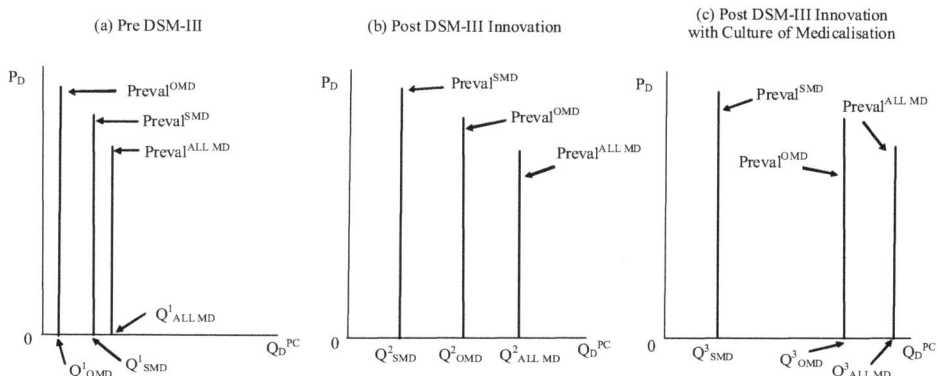

(a) Pre DSM-III   (b) Post DSM-III Innovation   (c) Post DSM-III Innovation with Culture of Medicalisation

P_D Preval^{OMD} Preval^{SMD} Preval$^{ALL MD}$ $Q^1_{ALL MD}$ Q^1_{OMD} Q^1_{SMD} Q_D^{PC}

P_D Preval^{SMD} Preval^{OMD} Preval$^{ALL MD}$ Q^2_{SMD} Q^2_{OMD} $Q^2_{ALL MD}$ Q_D^{PC}

P_D Preval^{SMD} Preval$^{ALL MD}$ Preval^{OMD} Q^3_{SMD} Q^3_{OMD} $Q^3_{ALL MD}$ Q_D^{PC}

Notes Preval^{SMD} is the per capita prevalence of "serious mental disorders", and is constant in the three time periods; Preval^{OMD} is the per capita prevalence of "other mental disorders", and is not constant in the three time periods; Preval$^{ALL MD}$ is the per capita prevalence of "all mental disorders", and is not constant in the three time periods; Preval$^{ALL MD}$ is the sum of Preval^{SMD} and Preval^{OMD}; P_D is the price of a diagnosis of a mental disorder; Q_D^{PC} is the per capita quantity of diagnoses of mental disorders.

Fig. 7. The (Stylised) Per Capita Prevalence of SMD, Other MD and All MD in Three Periods of the Twentieth Century

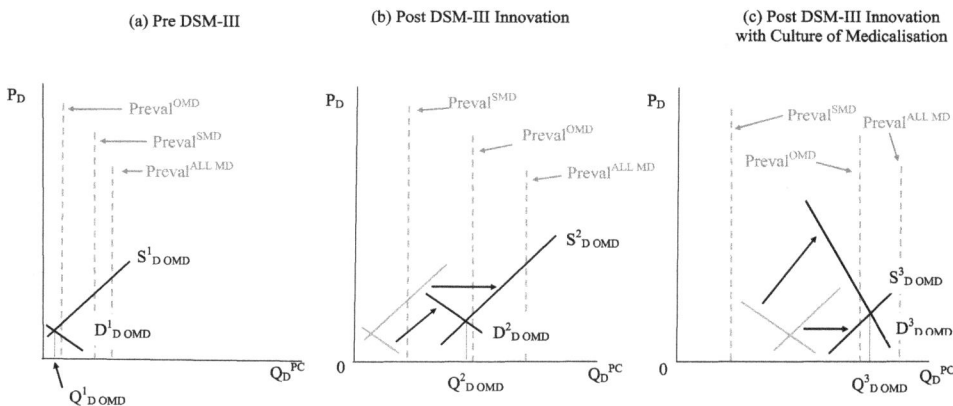

(a) Pre DSM-III   (b) Post DSM-III Innovation   (c) Post DSM-III Innovation with Culture of Medicalisation

P_D Preval^{OMD} Preval^{SMD} Preval$^{ALL MD}$ $S^1_{D OMD}$ $D^1_{D OMD}$ $Q^1_{D OMD}$ Q_D^{PC}

P_D Preval^{SMD} Preval^{OMD} Preval$^{ALL MD}$ $S^2_{D OMD}$ $D^2_{D OMD}$ $Q^2_{D OMD}$ Q_D^{PC}

P_D Preval^{SMD} Preval$^{ALL MD}$ Preval^{OMD} $S^3_{D OMD}$ $D^3_{D OMD}$ $Q^3_{D OMD}$ Q_D^{PC}

Notes See Fig. 7. Note also that the per capita prevalence lines in (a), (b) and (c) are the same per capita prevalence lines indicated in Figure 1. $D^1_{D OMD}$ is the demand curve for per capita diagnoses of other mental disorders in period 1. $S^1_{D OMD}$ is the demand curve for per capita diagnoses of other mental disorders in period 1, and so on.

Fig. 8. A Stylisation of the Markets for Per Capita Diagnoses of Mental Disorders in Three Periods of the Twentieth Century

One way of understanding these matters is in terms of there being a continuum. Fig. 9 illustrates a diagnostic continuum, which conceives of a spectrum from mental illness, mental health to human potential at any point in time. Note that "medicalisation" over time can be shown by enlarging the area of "core mental illness", while performance enhancement can be shown by expanding the boundaries of human potential. The specification of "cut-offs" becomes an important variable in achieving the optimal use of resources. At a very general level, these various societal trends indicate that concepts and practices in psychiatry are influenced by culture.

4.2 Moral hazard

A second aspect of the economics of structural imbalance is the suggestion of moral hazard in the mental health sector. Markets and organisations are both subject to moral hazard. For a review, see Milgrom & Roberts (1992). A very general definition of moral hazard is as follows:

...actions of economic agents in maximising their own utility to the detriment of others, in situations where they do not have to bear the full consequences or, equivalently, do not enjoy the full benefit of their actions... (Kotowitz, 1987, p. 549).

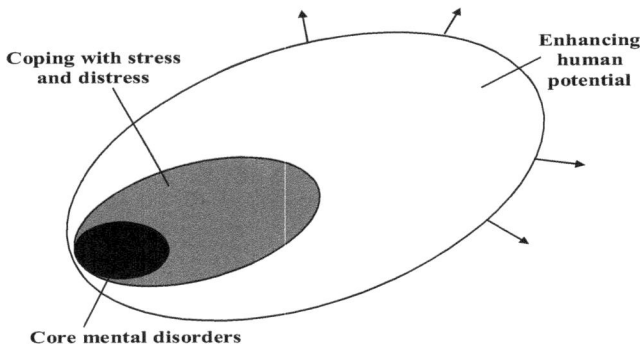

Source: Klerman & Schechter (1981)

Fig. 9. A diagnostic spectrum

Moral hazard is a type of economic behaviour that can occur in markets subject to imperfect information. It is particularly associated with an asymmetry in the distribution of knowledge between the buyer and seller, or a third party insurance carrier. Informational "incompleteness" takes several forms including an asymmetry in the distribution of knowledge in a market or organisation, or factors in the level or quantity of information being uncertain, missing, unavailable, or not yet known (Kotowitz, 1987).

Informational problems are noted in several contexts, e.g. quality uncertainty for various products, such as used cars (Akerlof, 1970), credit (Stiglitz & Weiss, 1981) etc, and in the labour market (Spence, 1974). However, the case of moral hazard described here is rarely, if at all, discussed in the health economics literature, or the general economics literature. Some have argued (e.g. Scitovsky, 1990) that asymmetric information gives scope for second-best contracting. Notwithstanding that case, and also ignoring for now the perspective that moral hazed is so pervasive that one may as well be resigned to it, the general case is that information imperfections lead to inefficiency in resource allocation (Bator, 1958), which suggests an appropriate policy response.

The allocative inefficiency arising from moral hazard in the health sector can require government action. For example, Arrow (1963) argued the case for financing health services by health insurance. Those arguments were highly influential in the introduction of Australia's system of publicly financed, universal medical and hospital insurance (Medicare) (Scotton, 1968; Scotton & Deeble, 1968). In health insurance, the context in which moral hazard is often discussed is that of an insurance carrier having incomplete information about the health status of insured consumers. In such circumstances, the existence of insurance creates incentives for people to behave in an inefficient fashion, by consuming health services beyond the level at which the marginal benefit equals the marginal social cost. This inefficiency is measured by the welfare loss associated with this "extra" consumption (Pauly, 1968).

Moral hazard is usually described in terms of the effect it has on one party in a transaction. But it can also arise for both parties, i.e. both buyer and seller.[3] It could be argued that a multi-dimensional case of moral hazard exists in mental health sectors under insurance: moral hazard can be observed on all sides of transactions in private mental health services, i.e. buyers, sellers, and the insurer as well. A "three-sided" conception of moral hazard in this sector may help to illuminate the source of quite severe resource misallocation in this sector, for which empirical evidence is mounting. Mental health services present a more particular, and complex, sector: specific informational problems associated with mental health issues exist for all three parties to the transactions. On the demand side, consumers may be subject not only to their own incomplete knowledge about health status but misinformation as well. On the supply side, a veil of ignorance exists for the suppliers of mental health services for several reasons. Thirdly, the insurance carrier (say, government) adopts a particular stance on information. If insurance processes do not provide diagnostic information that delivers well-aligned resource allocation, then directing some attention to reforming the processes is relevant. Thus, it is conceivable for moral hazard to develop in these three contexts.

Some reflection indicates that mental health issues are characterised by imperfect information on the part of patients/consumers, mental health professionals and health insurance organisations. Consumers generally do not know what is wrong with them; mental health professionals, in large part, rely on what consumers tell them; and, furthermore, the "state of knowledge" of the aetiology of mental disorders is not perfect. There is an information armamentarium of efficacious therapies available. Also, health insurance carriers are subject to imperfect knowledge.

5. Policy effects

This Section will focus attention on two main policy issues. One issue relates to improving diagnostic efficacy in mental illness. The second point concerns institutional factors. However, to put these points in context, it can be said generally speaking that the adverse

---

[3] This is discussed in Rubin's (1978) study of franchising. The term, double moral hazard, or double-sided moral hazard, was subsequently applied in 1985 to discussions of share-cropping responses to market behaviour (Eswaran & Kotwal, 1985) and product warranties (Cooper & Ross, 1985).

achievements of mental health sectors internationally remain a societal disgrace. The resource insufficiency in these sectors can be alleviated with larger mental health budgets, but structural imbalance cannot be mitigated with more dollars. The misallocation of resources to which this sector is prone may even contribute to the persistent reluctance by governments to provide adequate budgets for people with a mental illness. However, an understanding of structural imbalance is fundamentally important for the economic development of this sector and the improved living standards of mentally ill people who are "in need". The political will to fund mental health sectors adequately is relatively weak, and resourcing waxes and wanes. It is therefore important that the economic causes of structural imbalance are well understood.

The point needs to be emphasised that diagnostic efficacy is not just relevant to treatment; it is relevant also to improving resource allocation in the mental health sector. The quantification of met non-need here provides the evidence that some people without mental disorders are consumers of mental health services. No public policy issue exists if such people fund these services from their own incomes, but if those mental health services are funded either by pooled private health insurance contributions or by partially, or fully, subsidised taxpayer-funded schemes, then there is a policy issue. This issue can be addressed by a requirement that a firm diagnosis of mental disorder is established (by valid psychological instruments) with a further requirement that the (positive) diagnosis so obtained is the pre-condition for receiving subsidised mental health services.

Inefficacy in the diagnostic processes of the mental health sector has two effects: met non-need is being funded; and mentally ill people are receiving inadequate treatment. It means that scarce mental health resources are not put to their highest possible use. Those resources are misallocated, i.e. wasted. There is a vital place for innovation in the diagnostic practices in the mental health sector and also for such innovation to be financed by government.

Institutional factors are specific to the institutional setting of a particular country. This Chapter reflects the economic forces present in **Australia's institutional setting**. In the Australian institutional setting, the major insurance carrier (the government) presently provides little financial incentive for implementing efficacious therapy for mental illness. In the *Medicare Benefits Schedule* (which lists *Schedule* fees for all medical services, and the relevant subsidies), separate diagnostic services of a mental health kind are not listed or subsidised. There are no financial incentives for diagnosis for private mental health services embedded in the Medicare system. Thus, it is correct to hold the view that "throwing more money" at the pre-existing structures may do nothing to address Australia's structural imbalance problem. It is relevant to note that, at the epidemiological level in Australia, diagnostic test instruments are applied i.e. at the population level!

6. Qualifications

There are other issues of concern in Australia's mental health system (Williams & Doessel, 2008). However, the qualifications relating to this Chapter will be mentioned here.

Ideally, a measure of expenditure would be applied in order to measure structural imbalance, but in the absence of such data, we use "people" as a proxy for the ideal concept of expenditure. Further work is also required on the extent to which services are "mismatched" with resources in public mental health services. Those services are also subject to information asymmetries amongst consumers, producers and the government funder. There is mounting anecdotal evidence of public sector mental health services not "meeting" the "unmet need", but whether that phenomenon is due to resource misallocation or to resource shortages in this part of the public sector, or both, is a subject for further research. Also, it is not possible from available data to determine how much "met non-need" is due to the "worried well", and how much is due to those who use government-subsidised services for other reasons (sport, executive performance etc).

Where one "draws the line" between "mental health" and "mental illness" involves treating a continuous variable as discrete; cut-offs need to be implemented. A stylisation of this point is provided in Fig. 9. When "better" epidemiological data become available, sharper depictions of "met non-need" will become available.

The structural imbalance problem analysed here is a different type of problem from the inefficiency arising from the application of inefficacious therapies in this sector. Several large studies of Australian mental health service providers indicate evidence that, even with strong training and support systems, these providers have yet to adopt the concept of fidelity to evidence-based protocols (Deane *et al.*, 2006; Kavanagh *et al.*, 1993). Comparisons undertaken between prescriptions for medications and diagnosis find evidence suggesting the degree of inconsistency or "aberrant prescribing" is not trivial (Dodwell & Esiwe, 2008). Delivering inefficacious treatments, when known efficacious treatments exist, increases the size of the unmet need problem. Expenditures are being incurred for little, or zero, change in mental health status. The relevant conceptual economic framework is in Liebenstein (1966).

7. Conclusion

Some recent Australian studies demonstrate, on cross-sectional data as well as time-series data (albeit less-than-perfect data) that there is extensive structural imbalance for the adult Australian population between those with mental illness and those who use mental health resources. Our analyses of ABS *Mental Health and Wellbeing...* data, summarised here, find that 11 per cent of the adult population are subject to "unmet need" and 4.4 per cent of the adult population are consuming mental health resources despite not having a mental disorder. Those studies find also that the problem of "unmet need" is smaller for females than it is for males, and yet the problem of "met non-need" is larger for females than for males. Considerable differences exist between aggregations of disorders too. Substance Use has, by far, the largest problem of "unmet need", followed by Anxiety Disorders and Affective Disorders. The results suggest that re-allocating the resources used by the "met non-need" (4.6 per cent of the population) to the "unmet need" category (11 per cent of the population) would improve the mental health outcomes of this sector. Although it is imperative that better data are collected, this Chapter provides a benchmark for future exercises in quantifying structural imbalance.

The two sources of structural imbalance discussed in this Chapter are as follows: trends in Western society; and moral hazard. These forces are seldom mentioned in public discourse on mental health issues. In particular, the problem of "met non-need" in Australia, i.e. people with no mental illness consuming mental health resources, is hardly ever discussed. Those discussions are very relevant as they direct attention to the policy implications. Thus, the lack of public discourse is unfortunate. Through time, the self-interested forces underlying "unmet need" and "met non-need" solidify into service delivery practices in the mental health sector.

In general, the moral hazard problem arises from imperfect information, which in turn can lead to an imperfect agency relationship between the patient/consumer and the supplier of services. These informational problems are more severe in the area of mental illness compared to physical illness. In physical medicine, medical professionals have access to a wide range of diagnostic procedures, whether radiology, other imaging technologies (MRI etc), pathology tests and so forth. These diagnostic technologies have the effect of reducing imperfect knowledge in the clinical context. By comparison, diagnosis in mental illness and in mental service delivery is embryonic.

As these problems are not self-correcting, two policy implications will now be outlined in conclusion. First, in order to alleviate the "unmet need", public education and awareness campaigns about mental illnesses and the services available are appropriate responses. Also, the systemic factors that continue to obstruct access to services by those who are mentally ill need addressing. "Unmet need" is alleviated also by imposing reform in this sector: public research funding into developing efficacious therapies that are not just developed, but are applied and adopted as well, and into the financing of efficacious public preventive strategies.

Second, of those people without mental disorders who are consumers of mental health services, it is important to realise that there is no public policy issue if such people fund these services from their own incomes. However, if those mental health services are funded either by pooled private health insurance contributions or by partially, or fully, subsidised taxpayer-funded schemes, then there is a policy issue. It can be addressed by a requirement that a firm diagnosis of mental disorder is established (by valid psychological instruments) with a further requirement that the diagnosis so obtained is the pre-condition for receiving subsidised mental health services.

8. References

Akerlof, George A. 1970, The Market for *"Lemons":* Quality Uncertainty and the Market Mechanism, *The Quarterly Journal of Economics,* Vol.84, No.3, (Aug., 1970), pp. 488-500, ISSN 0033-5533

American Psychiatric Association (1980). Diagnostic and Statistical Manual of Mental Disorders. 3rd Ed. APA, ISBN 089042019X, Washington DC

American Psychiatric Association (1987). Diagnostic and Statistical Manual of Mental Disorders. 3rd Ed., Rev., APA, ISBN 0890420211, Washington DC

American Psychiatric Association (1994). Diagnostic and Statistical Manual of Mental Disorders. 4th Ed., APA, ISBN 890420629 08904220629, Washington DC

American Psychiatric Association (2000). Diagnostic and Statistical Manual of Mental Disorders. 4th — TR Ed., APA, ISBN 0-89042-025-4, Washington DC

Andrews, G. (2000). Meeting the Unmet Need with Disease Management. In: *Unmet Need in Psychiatry: Problems, Resources, Responses,* G. Andrews. & S. Henderson, (Eds), 11-36, Cambridge University Press, ISBN 052166229X, Cambridge, UK

Andrews, J.G. & the Tolkien II Team (2006). *Tolkien II. A Needs Based, Costed Stepped-care Model for Mental Health Services.* World Health Organization Collaborating Centre for Classifications in Mental Health, ISBN 0 9578073 5 X, Sydney

Andrews, G., Issakidis, C. & Carter, G. (2001). Shortfall in Mental Health Utilisation. *British Journal of Psychiatry,* Vol. 179, (Nov., 2001), pp. 417-425, ISSN 1472-1465 0007-1250

Arrow, K.J. (1963). Uncertainty and the Welfare Economics of Medical Care. *The American Economic Review,* Vol.53, No.5, (Dec., 1963), pp. 941-973, ISSN 1944-7981 0002-8282

Australian Bureau of Statistics (1998). *Mental Health and Wellbeing: Profile of Adults, Australia 1997*. Cat. No. 4326.0, ABS, Canberra, Australia.

Australian Bureau of Statistics. (2008). *National Survey of Mental Health and Wellbeing: Summary of Results 2007*, Cat. No. 4326.0, ABS, Canberra, Australia

Bator, F.M. (1958). The Anatomy of Market Failure. *The Quarterly Journal of Economics*, Vol.72, No.3, (Aug., 1958), pp. 351–79, ISSN 1531-4650 0033-5533

Begel, D. (1992). An Overview of Sport Psychiatry. *The American Journal of Psychiatry*, Vol. 149, No.5, (May, 1992), pp. 606-614, ISSN 1535-7228 0002-953X

Beggs, J.J. (1988). Diagnostic Testing in Applied Econometrics. *The Economic Record*, Vol.64, No.185, No.2, (June, 1988), pp. 81-101, ISSN 1475-4932

Bell, G. (2005). *The Worried Well: The Depression Epidemic and the Medicalisation of our Sorrows*, Black Inc, ISBN 1863953817, Melbourne, Australia

Blaug, M. (1998). Where are We Now in British Health Economics? *Health Economics*, Vol.7, Supp.1, (Aug., 1998), pp. S63-S78, ISSN 1099-1050 1057-9230

Byles, J.; Dolja-Gore, X.; Loxton, J.; Parkinson, L. & Stewart Williams, J. (2011). Women's Uptake of *Medicare Benefits Schedule* Mental Health Items for General Practitioners, Psychologists and Other Allied Health Professionals. *Medical Journal of Australia*, Vol.194, No.4, (21 Feb., 2011), pp. 175-179, ISSN 0025-729X

Cooper, R. & Ross, T.W. (1985). Product Warranties and Double Moral Hazard. *Rand Journal of Economics*, Vol.16, No.1, (Spring, 1985), pp. 103-13, ISSN 1756-2171 0741-6261

Cosgrove, E.M.; Yung, A.R.; Killackey E.J.; Buckby, J.A.; Godfrey, K.A.; Stanford, C.A. & McGorry, P. (2008). Met and Unmet Need in Youth Mental Health. *Journal of Mental Health*, Vol.17, No.6, (1 Jan., 2008), pp. 618-628, ISSN 0963-8237

Deane, F. P.; Crowe, T. P.; King, R.; Kavanagh, D. J.; & Oades, L. G. (2006). Challenges in Implementing Evidence-based Practice into Mental Health Services. *Australian Health Review*, Vol.30, No. 3, (Aug., 2006), pp. 305–309, ISSN

Department of Health & Ageing (2007). *Medicare Benefits Schedule, Effective 1 November 2007*, Department of Health & Ageing, ISBN 0642446946, Canberra

Dodwell, D. & Esiwe, C. (2008). Are Prescriptions Consistent with Diagnosis? A Survey of Adult Psychiatry Discharge Notices. *Journal of Mental Health*, Vol.17, No.6, (Dec., 2008), pp.588-593, ISSN 1360-0567

Doessel, D.P. (1986). Medical Diagnosis as a Problem in the Economics of Information. *Information Economics & Policy*, Vol.2, No.1, (March, 1986), pp. 49-68, ISSN 1873-5975

Doessel D.P. & Williams, Ruth F.G. (2011). Resource Misallocation in Australia's Mental Health Sector under Medicare: Evidence from Time-series Data. *Economic Papers*, Vol.30, No.2, (June, 2011), pp. 253-264, ISSN 1759-3441

Doessel D.P., Williams, Ruth F.G. & Nolan, P. (2008). A Central Dilemma in the Mental Health Sector: Structural Imbalance. *Clinical Psychologist*, Vol. 12, No.2, (July, 2008), pp. 57-66, ISSN 1328-4207

Doessel D.P., Williams, Ruth F.G. & Whiteford, H. (2010). Some Empirical Evidence for Australian Mental Health Policy of Resource Insufficiency and Structural Imbalance. *Journal of Mental Health Policy & Economics*, Vol.13, No1.1, (March, 2010), pp.3-12, ISSN 1099-176X

Druss, B.G.; Wang, P.S.; Sampson, N.A.; Olfson, M.; Pincus, H.A.; Wells, K.B.; Kessler, R.C. (2007). Understanding Mental Health Treatment in Persons without Mental Diagnoses: Results from the National Comorbidity Survey Replication. *Archives of*

General Psychiatry, Vol.64, No.10, (Oct., 2007), pp. 1196-1203, ISSN 1538-3636 0003-990X

Eswaran, M. & Kotwal, A. (1985). A Theory of Contractual Structure in Agriculture. *The American Economic Review*, Vol.75, No.3, (June, 1985), pp. 352-67, ISSN 1944-7981 0002-8282

Feinstein, A.R. (1975). Clinical Biostatistics: *XXXI*. On the Sensitivity, Specificity and Discrimination of Diagnostic Tests. *Clinical Pharmacology and Therapeutics*, Vol.17, No.1, (Jan., 1975), pp.104-116, ISBN 1532-6535 0009-9236

Frank, R.G. & McGuire, T.G. (2000). Economics and Mental Health. In: *Handbook of Health Economics Vol. IB*, Elsevier, ISBN 0444504710, Amsterdam, Holland

Hirschleifer, J. & Riley, J.G. (1979). The Analytics of Uncertainty and Information – an Expository Survey. *Journal of Economic Literature*, Vol.*XVII*, No.4, (Dec., 1979), pp. 1375-1421, ISSN 0022-0515

Horwitz, A.V. & Wakefield, J.C. (2007). *The Loss of Sadness: How Psychiatry Transformed Normal Sorrow into Depressive Disorder.* Oxford University Press, ISBN 9780195313048, Oxford, UK

Jablensky, A.; McGrath, J; Herman, H.; Castle, D.; Gureje, O.; Morgan, V. & Korten, A. (1999). *People Living with Psychotic Illness: an Australian Study 1997-98.* Commonwealth Department of Health & Aged Care, ISBN 0 642 36779 5, Canberra, Australia

Jorm, A.F. (2006). National Surveys of Mental Disorders: Are They Researching Scientific Facts or Constructing Useful Myths? *Australian & New Zealand Journal of Psychiatry*, Vol.40, No.10, (Oct., 1978), pp. 830-834, ISSN 1440-1614 0004-8674

Kavanagh, D. J.; Piatkowska, O.; Clark, D.; O'Halloran, P.; Manicavasagar, V.; Rosen, A. *et al.* (1993). Application of Cognitive-behavioural Family Intervention for Schizophrenia in Multi-disciplinary Settings: What Can the Matter Be? *Australian Psychologist*, Vol.28, No.3, (Nov.,1993), pp. 181–188, ISSN 1742-9544

Kessler, R.C.; Andrews ,G.; Mroczel, D.K.;. Escobar,J.I.; Gibbon,M.; Guyer,M.E.; Howes,M.J.; Jin, R.; Vega, W.A.; Walters, E.E.; Wang,P.; Zaslavsky, A.; Zheng, H. (1998). The World Health Organization Composite International Diagnostic Interview Short Form (CIDI-SF). *International Journal of Methods in Psychiatric Research*, Vol.7, No.2, pp.171-185, ISBN 1557-0657 1049-8931

Klerman, G. & Schechter, G. (1981) Ethical Aspects of Drug Treatment. In: *Psychiatric Ethics*, S. Bloch & P. Chodoff, (Eds), Oxford University Press, ISBN 0192611828, Oxford, pp. 117-130

Kotowitz, Y. (1987). Moral Hazard, In: *The New Palgrave: A Dictionary of Economics*, J. Eatwell, M. Milgate & P. Newman, (Eds), 549-551 Macmillan, ISBN 1-56159-197-1, London

Le Grand, J. (1978). The Distribution of Public Expenditure: the Case of Health Care, *Economica*, Vol.45, No.178, (May, 1978), pp. 125-142, ISBN 0013-0427

Leibenstein, H. (1966). Allocative Efficiency *vs* X-efficiency. *The American Economic Review*, Vol.56, No.3, (June, 1966), pp. 392–415, ISSN 1944-7981 0002-8282

Lin, E.; Goering, P.; Offord, D.R.; Campbell D.; Boyle M.H. (1996). The Use of Mental Health Services in Ontario: Epidemiological Findings. *Canadian Journal of* Psychology, Vol.41, No.12, (Dec., 1996), pp. 572-577, ISSN 0008-4255

Madden, G. (1988). An Econometric Model of Australian Automobile Demand: a Segmented Markets Approach. *Economic Analysis & Policy*, Vol.18, No.1 (March, 1988), pp. 53-69, ISSN 0313-5926

Meadows, G.; Burgess, P.; Fossey, E.; Harvey, C. (2000). Perceived Need for Mental Health Care, Findings from the Australian National Survey of Mental Health and Well-being. *Psychological Medicine*, Vol.30, No.3, (8 Sept., 2000), pp. 645-656, ISSN 1469-8978 0033-2917

Meadows, G.; Fossey, E.; Harvey, C.; Burgess, P. (2000). The Assessment of Perceived Need. In: *Unmet Need in Psychiatry: Problems, Resources, Responses*, G. Andrews & S. Henderson, (Eds), 390-398, Cambridge University Press, ISBN 052166229X, Cambridge, UK

Milgrom, P. & Roberts, J. (1992). *Economics, Organization & Management*, Prentice Hall, ISBN 0132246503, Englewood Cliffs, N.J.

Oakley Browne, M.A. & Wells, J.E. (2006). Health Services. In: *Te Rau Hinengaro: The New Zealand Mental Health Survey*, M.A. Oakley Browne *et al.*, (Eds), Ministry of Health, ISBN 0-478-30026-3, Wellington, New Zealand

Parslow, R.A. & Jorm, A.F. (2001). Predictors of Partially Met or Unmet Need Reported by Consumers of Mental Health Services: an Analysis of Data from the Australian National Survey of Mental Health and Wellbeing. *Australian & New Zealand Journal of Psychiatry*, Vol.35, No.4, (Aug., 2000), pp. 455-463, ISSN 1440-1614 0004-8674

Regier, D.A.; Narrow, W.E.; Rupp, A.; Rae, D.S. & Kaelbar, C.T. (2000). The Epidemiology of Mental Disorder Treatment Need: Community Estimates of "Medical Necessity". In: *Unmet Need in Psychiatry: Problems, Resources, Responses* Andrews G. & Henderson S., (Eds), 41-58. Cambridge University Press, ISBN 052166229X, Cambridge, UK

Rubin, P.H. (1978). The Theory of the Firm and the Structure of the Franchise Contract. *The Journal of Law & Economics*, Vol.21, No.1, (Jan., 1978), pp. 223-53, ISSN 1537-5285 0022-2186

Sawyer, M.G.; Arney, F.M.; Baghurst, P.A.; Clark J.J.; Graetz B.W.; Kosky R.J.; Nurcombe B.; Patton G.C.; Prior M.R.; Raphael B.; Rey J.; Whaites L.C. & Zubrick S.R. (2000). *Mental Health of Young People in Australia*. Commonwealth Department of Health an Aged Care, ISBN 0 642 44686 5, Canberra

Scitovsky, T. (1990). The Benefits of Asymmetric Markets. *The Journal of Economic Perspectives*, Vol.4, No.1, (Winter, 1990), pp. 135-134, ISSN 1944-7965 0895-3309

Spence, M. (1974). *Market Signaling*. Harvard University Press, ISBN 0674549902, Cambridge, MA

Sperry L. (1993). Working with Executives: Consulting, Counselling and Coaching. *Individual Psychology: Journal of Adlerian Theory, Research & Practice* Vol.49, No.2, (Fall, 1993), pp. 257-266, ISSN 1522-2527

Stiglitz, J. & Weiss, A. (1981). Credit Rationing in Markets with Imperfect Information. *The American Economic Review*, Vol.71, No.3, (June, 1981), pp. 393–410, ISSN 1944-7981 0002-8282

U.S. Department of Health & Human Services (1999). *Mental Health: A Report of the Surgeon General – Executive Summary*. U.S. Department of Health & Human Services, Substance Abuse and Mental Health Services Administration, Center for Mental

Health Services, National Institutes of Health, National Institute of Mental Health, Rockville, MD, 30.05.2008, Available from http://www.surgeongeneral.gov/library/mentalhealth/home.html.

Vecchio, T.J. (1966). Predictive Value of a Single Diagnostic Test in Unselected Populations. *New England Journal of Medicine*, Vol.274, No.21, (26 May, 1966), pp. 1171-1173, ISSN 1533-4406 0028-4793

Wagner, P.J. & Curran, P. (1984). Health Beliefs and Physician Identified "Worried Well". *Health Psychology*, Vol.3, No.5, pp. 459-474, ISSN 1930-7810 0278-6133 0278-6133 1

Whiteford H. (2000). Unmet Need: a Challenge for Governments. In: *Unmet Need in Psychiatry: Problems, Resources, Responses*, G. Andrews & S. Henderson, (Eds), Cambridge University Press, ISBN 052166229X, Cambridge, UK, pp. 8-10.

Williams, Ruth F.G. (2009). Review Article: Everyday Sorrows are not Mental Disorders: the Clash between Psychiatry and Western Cultural Habits. *Prometheus*, Vol.27, No.1, (March, 2009), pp. 47-70, ISSN 1470-1030 0810-9028

Williams, Ruth F.G. & Doessel, D.P. (2007). The Role of Knowledge Accumulation in Health and Longevity: The Puzzling Case of Suicide. *Prometheus*, Vol.25, No.3, (Sept., 2007), pp. 283-303, ISSN 0810-9028

Williams, Ruth F.G. & Doessel, D.P. (2008), The Australian Mental Health System: an Economic Overview and Some Research Issues. *International Journal of Mental Health Systems*, Vol.2, No. 4, p. 4, Available from www.ijmhs.com/content/2/1/4

Williams, Ruth F.G. & Doessel, D.P. (2010). Psychiatry Interacts with Contemporary Western Views: the *DSM-III* Innovation and its Adverse Effects. *Prometheus*, Vol.28, No.3, (Sept., 2010), pp. 245-266, ISSN 0810-9028

Williams, Ruth F.G. & Doessel, D.P. (2011). *An Economic Classification of "Health Need"*. *International Journal of Social Economics*, Vol.38, No.3, (March, 2011), pp. 291-309, ISSN 1758-6712 0306-8293

Yerushalmy, J. (1947). Statistical Problems in Assessing Methods of Medical Diagnosis, with Special Reference to X-ray Techniques. *Public Health Reports*, Vol.62, No.40, (3 Oct., 1947), pp. 1432-1449, ISSN 1468-2877 0033-3549

11

The Role of Intentional Communities to Support Recovery from Mental Illness

Francesca Pernice-Duca, Wendy Case and Deborah Conrad-Garrisi
Wayne State University,
USA

1. Introduction

Establishing "community" decreases isolation and social stigma and supports both physical and mental well-being (Ralph & Corrigan, 2005) for many individuals marginalized by the consequences of a mental illness. This chapter will focus on the role of intentional *recovery communities* in supporting wellness among people living with mental illness. The chapter will introduce the reader to the concept of recovery from mental illness, a broad variety of approaches designed to facilitate and support recovery as well as recovery oriented environments such as clubhouse programs, peer-run drop-in centers, and peer support groups (e.g., Schizophrenia Anonymous, 12-Step). For example, The FRIENDS program, which is based on the philosophy that social networks evolve from building a strong caring intentional community, has been found to increase and maintain social networks over time to impact overall functioning (Wilson, Flanagan, & Rynders, 1999). Thus, the central values of many peer- based recovery communities recognize that mental health well-being has a direct relationship to the involvement with others. Therapeutic communities constitute an important aspect in the treatment of mental illness and substance abuse disorders. These 'bottom-up' approaches have a long history as adjunctive services to psychotherapy and psychiatry and provide a valuable, if not essential, component for many seeking recovery from mental illness and substance related disorders.

Mental illness can have devastating effects on an individual's family and social relationships. Individuals with chronic or persistent mental illness can experience the loss of support from friends, family or partners, resulting in small or restricted social support resources. Small social support networks have been associated with mental health concerns such as isolation (Brewer, Gadsden, & Scrimshaw, 1994), and an increased likelihood of depression (Lin, Ye, & Ensel, 1999). Poor or inadequate social support networks have also been associated with increased mortality rates among the general population (Berkman, 1995; Berkman, Glass, Brissette, & Seeman, 2000; House, Landis, & Umberson, 1988). One of the earliest research studies on social networks and mental health began with Emile Durkheim's empirical examination on the effects of the lack of social network ties and community integration and the rate of suicide in metropolitan areas (see Durkheim, 2001). Between 1969 and 1985, the interest in social network and mental health research proliferated with over 1,300 published research articles (Biegel, McCardel, & Mendelson, 1985).

Social support networks among people living with severe or chronic mental illness such as schizophrenia, are typically small, and predominately consist of family members or mental health professionals (Davidson, Hoge, Merrill, Rakfeldt, & Griffith, 1995; Goldberg, Rollins, & Lehman, 2003; Hardiman & Segal, 2003; Perese, Getty, & Wooldridge, 2003). Research has shown that small or restricted social networks threaten psychological and emotional well-being (Green, Hayes, Dickinson, Whittaker, & Gilheany, 2002), quality of life (Tempier, Caron, Mercier, & Leouffre, 1998), and increase the likelihood of psychiatric re-hospitalization (Goldberg, Rollins, & Lehman, 2003). Cut-off or estranged family relationships have also been correlated with increased psychological distress and functional impairments (Doane, 1991; Fisk, Rowe, Laub, Calvocoressi, & DeMino, 2000; Froland, Brodsky, Olson, & Stewart, 2000). Individuals living with chronic and persistent mental illness experience functional impairments in daily living skills and social skills. These impairments can negatively impact social opportunities. Traditional medical model approaches continue to view these negative consequences of serious mental illness as inevitable, which can result in a loss of hope, despair, and chronic grief. The notion of recovery from mental illness has received increasing attention in the mental health field in the last decade. Emerging evidence indicates that social network supports play a significant role in the experiences of recovery from mental illness (Corrigan, & Phelan, 2004). State and Federal mental health organizations are beginning to recommend recovery oriented practices in the treatment of mental illness, emphasizing the importance of social ties as an integral part of the recovery process (Hogan, 2003). Longitudinal studies spanning the last 30 years have documented recovery from serious mental illness, such as schizophrenia (DeSisto, Harding, McCormick, Ashikaga & Brooks, 1999; Harding, Brooks, Ashikaga, & Strauss, 1987a; 1987b). These longitudinal studies challenge traditionally held beliefs about chronic mental illness, and provide support for programs that increase social and vocational opportunities.

2. Peer support and recovery communities

The value of peer support is articulated succinctly in the words of John Woodman, a military veteran and resident of the Gordon H. Mansfield Veterans Community in Massachusetts: "[We are] like a band of brothers who have a natural affection for each other. We've seen things nobody should see" (Abrahms, 2011). Those who live with mental illness, addiction, PTSD and other psychiatric health challenges often inherit the burden of isolation, exclusion and stigmatization (Kelly & Gamble, 2005). Limited options for treatment and a mistrust of the system can hamper recovery efforts (Littrell & Beck, 2001), as can cultural bias and cultural-bound resistance to treatment (Landrine, 1992). Studies have shown that the more socially isolated a person is, the more likely he or she is to experience negative outcomes (Stahler, Shipley, Bartelt, DuCette , & Shandler, 1995). Structured social support functions not only to unite individuals in a common social network, but also to provide them with positive social influence. A sense of purpose and the dignity of 'belonging' can serve as the catalyst to motivate an individual toward pro-social behaviors that enhance self-care (Kawachi & Berkman, 2001). Participating in household chores and recreational opportunities can also help clients to become active participants in their lives and recoveries -- making choices and decisions that directly affect their day-to-day existence. This helps them move beyond the conventional treatment model of passively adjusting to their circumstances and into actively engaging with and acknowledging their strengths and limitations (Ridgway, 2001). In addition, peer networks and peer-provided services have been shown to be as effective at relieving symptoms and improving quality of life as non peer-provided support (Solomon, 2004). Paraprofessionals are not only able to relate to those they serve, they have the capability to act as a conduit to mental health providers -- providing trusted support for peers who may be at a lower-functioning stage of recovery.

The *peer principle* is based on the shared experiences and values characterized by mutuality and reciprocity -- that is, peer relationships implies *equality* (Clay, 2005). Peer support services and programs are designed and delivered by people who have both experienced a mental health disorder and/or recovery from a substance use disorder. These services go beyond the traditional treatment setting of the "clinical office" and extend into a community of people seeking to achieve or sustain their recovery. Peer support programs provide individuals with non-hierarchical relationships that support goals and recovery from mental health and/or substance abuse disorders, which is a significant departure from hierarchical relationships often found in the medical model between physicians and their patients. According to mental health services researchers Davidson et al., (2006) defines peer support as support provided to a mental health or substance abuse service recipient, from a peer in recovery working with another peer who is beginning their recovery journey. Peer support, in its purest fashion, involves an "asymmetrical relationship with at least one designated service/support provider and at least one designated support recipient (Davidson, et al., 2006, p.2)."

Peer support also involves social support, such as providing emotional, informational, instrumental, and affiliation support. Emotional peer support involves demonstrating empathy, caring, and bolstering confidence. Informational support includes sharing knowledge and information about community resources, housing supports, parenting classes or information about wellness and recovery. Concrete assistance, such as helping others to accomplish tasks is often referred to as instrumental support, whereas affiliation support links people to others who share similar experiences in mental health and substance use recovery. Affiliation support includes opportunities to socialize, to engage in a 'recovery community' and to acquire a sense of belonging.

Involvement in a peer support program has been positively correlated with higher appraisals of social support, greater involvement in external community activities, and improved quality of life over time (Nelson & Lomotey, 2006). Individuals often report that joining peer support programs provide a sense of belonging, which supplants loneliness and isolation (Clay, 2005, p.13) and offers an opportunity to utilize peer support (Shutt, 2009). However, simply 'being peers' does not automatically translate into 'peer support'. Recipients of peer support describe peer support as an adjustment and developmental process. New members may experience feelings of vulnerability of entering a new community and thus may have an adjustment period before engaging with others (Mead, Hilton & Curtis, 2001). In a qualitative study involving recipients of peer support, this process involves developing trust, withholding information, and connecting with peers who appear to have achieved a higher level of wellness then that of themselves (Coatsworth-Puspoky, Forchuk, & Ward-Griffin, 2006). This may also serve to increase self-esteem and decrease perceived self-stigma of living with a mental illness since connecting with others who are similar to themselves or have achieved a greater level of recovery provide a model for wellness (Verhaeghe, et. al., 2008).

The drive to pursue a greater understanding of the potential for recovery from serious mental illness emerged from consumers of mental health and psychiatric services, public health policies, and data from longitudinal studies. Research suggests that recovery occurs among many people suffering with debilitating psychiatric illnesses (Davidson, et al., 2007; Onken, Craig, Ridgway, Ralph, & Cook, 2007). Recovery has been studied as a subjective experience through qualitative studies (Deegan, 1988; 2003), as well as an objective outcome measuring level of functioning and the absence of symptoms (Harding et al., 1987a).

Subjective accounts have described recovery from mental illness as "reawakening of hope from despair; breaking through denial and achieving understanding and acceptance; moving from withdrawal to engagement and becoming an active participant in life; it is active coping rather than passive adjustment (Beale & Lambric, 1995, p. 5)." Recovery oriented philosophy in mental health has revolutionized service delivery options, including more peer support programs and psychosocial psychiatric rehabilitation.

A crucial part of recovery is the support of a social network of people who believe in the capacities and the strength of the individual challenged or impaired by a psychiatric disability. Family members are often primary caregivers of people living with a serious mental illness and experience the caregiver burden at a higher rate than other types of chronic conditions (Hatfield & Lefley, 1987, 1993). Cross-cultural studies among people living with schizophrenia revealed differences in recovery rates due to familial connections. In Calabrese and Corrigan's (2005) review of the World Health Organization's cross-cultural research on schizophrenia, the author's noted that individuals living in developing countries were 30% more likely to meet recovery criteria from schizophrenia than those living in more industrialized countries like Germany or the United States. The authors contend that cultures in developing countries place greater importance on maintaining family and social relationships and social roles (e.g., teacher, mother, worker), while Western cultures tend to place greater emphasis on autonomy from the nuclear family and de-emphasize the importance of extended family members. The role of the community support movement in the U.S. provided families and former mental hospital patients more opportunities for recovery in the community. The goal of intentional recovery communities, such as clubhouses, is to provide individuals with alternative sources of support and to promote independence and recovery.

The extent to which programs nurture hope has been commonly reported by consumers as encouraging recovery (Young & Ensing, 1999). Successful recovery neither erases traumatizing experiences from memory, nor does it necessarily eliminate symptoms. Rather, successful recovery simply means that the person has adapted to new perspectives of himself and his world (Jacobson & Curtis, 2002; Ridgway, 2001). The experiences of the illness, while still important, are no longer the primary focus of the person's life (Anthony, 1993). The National Consensus Statement on Mental Health Recovery outlines ten components related to the process of recovery which reflect both aspects of the person and recovery environment (U.S. Department of Health and Human Services, 2006). Described as an essential value of the recovery process, *self-direction* is characterized as leading, controlling, or exercising choice over and determining one's own path of recovery by optimizing autonomy, independence, and control of resources. Environments that emphasize *individualized and person-centered* planning provide multiple pathways to the recovery process based on the unique strengths and resiliencies of the consumer. *Empowerment* is described as the authority to choose from a range of treatment and service options as well as to participate in all decisions that will affect the life of the consumer. *Holistic* services encompass important aspects of the consumer's life by recognizing the interplay between mind, body, spirit, and community. This awareness not only pertains to supporting physical and mental health needs, but also to housing issues, employment, education, spirituality, and opportunities for social connection. As part of holistic approaches, the larger community also recognizes it "play[s] a crucial role in creating meaningful opportunities and roles for consumers (U.S. Department of Health and Human Services, 2006)." Recovery services and environments recognize the *non-linear* process of recovery which "is not a step-by step process but one based on continual growth, occasional setbacks, and learning from experience" (U.S. Department of Health and Human Services, 2006)

3. Brief history of development of therapeutic recovery communities

The history of psychiatric hospitalization in the United States supported the notion of very limited social status and obligation and created environments in which the individual's autonomy was stripped away through supervised institutional care, closed and locked psychiatric wards and limiting adult rights and duties (Whitakar, 2002). The deinstitutionalization movement occurred as the result of the passage of several governmental acts (e.g., Barden-Lafollette Act, 1943; National Mental Health Act, 1946) which required federal and state governments to provide rehabilitation and vocational services to individuals with serious mental illness in outpatient treatment centers (Accordino & Hunt, 2001). During the late 1950's numerous studies were conducted by the National Institute of Mental Health (NIMH) and the Joint Commission on Mental Illness and Health that ultimately led to recommendations to increase the understanding of treatment, improve training of professionals, and enhance treatment services for individuals with serious mental illness (Accordino, et al., 2001). The 1960s saw further support of deinstitutionalization as well as protecting the civil rights of individuals with serious mental illness with the passing of the Community Mental Health Act (1963), which supported treatment in least restrictive environments (Accordino et al., 2001). During this time, consumers of mental health services became more vocal and active in the treatment and care they received, thus inspiring a movement in the delivery of psychiatric services to attend to consumer strengths, natural supports, and decrease social isolation (Davidson, et al., 2007; Drake, 2005; Resnick, Fontana, Lehman, & Rosenheck, 2005).

Rationale supporting the development of intentional communities for people living with mental illness stems from a number of psychological and socio-cultural positions, for instance, as pioneers in this area, Fairweather and Onaga (1993) emphasized the developmental incongruences among the statuses of those with mental illness and those without. They note that social rights and obligations increase as humans move from childhood through adolescence and eventually adulthood. In the absence of coming from a family history of wealth and power, most Americans are able to achieve "personal power, increased income, and prestige" through attaining education and skilled employment (Fairweather & Onaga, 1993, p. 4). However, because of deviation from accepted societal norms and behaviors, people living with a mental illness have greater challenges in achieving a socially equitable status in society and following a developmental trajectory comparable to their counterparts without mental illness.

The community support movement of the 1970s ushered in a new era in the treatment of mental illness in the United States. Mental Health services in the era following de-institutionalization have strongly followed a social support framework of intervention, attempting to formalize a model of peer support and increase social contact and engagement by increasing social network resources. During that time, mental health policy in the U.S. utilized informal social networks and support systems as resources for mental health patients transitioning into the community following long-term hospitalization. From a policy and services standpoint, less reliance on formal professional support systems and services helped to contain costs associated with providing a continuum of care. In 1977, the National Institute of Mental Health developed one of the first national initiatives to utilize the social network research and psychosocial rehabilitation services began assisting persons with chronic mental illness with housing, daily living skills, employment and socialization opportunities (Turner & TenHoor, 1978).

As part of the shift from institutional care to community based care, the concept of recovery from a serious mental illness has become a reality for many individuals and their families. However, the social cost of deinstitutionalization resulted in many people returning to homes where they were unwanted or to families who were unable to care for them. To stave off the isolation and stigma often associated with mental illnesses such as Schizophrenia or Bipolar disorder, individuals began congregating and creating support groups to buffer the transition back into society. This resulted in the creation of small communities of support. Today, mental health programs that intentionally bring similar people together to share experiences, provide support, and facilitate skill development are referred to as *intentional recovery communities.* Intentional communities were founded on the principle of consumer-survivors providing mutual support to help each other reintegrate into the community following long-term hospitalization from a serious mental illness. Building an intentional community based on the value of recovery serves as the foundation of the intentional recovery community of the clubhouse (Herman, Onaga, Pernice-Duca, et al., 2005).

Many of the intentional communities found in the U.S. and abroad include the psychosocial rehabilitation model (a.k.a Clubhouse), which acknowledges the influence of the group in hastening recovery from serious mental illness (Pernice-Duca & Onaga, 2009). To date, there are over 300 clubhouse programs worldwide (www.iccd.org). As of 2011, the U.S. Substance Abuse and Mental Health Services Administration (SAMSHA) has listed the Clubhouse Model on the National Registry of Evidence-Based Practices and Programs (NREPP) clubhouses (http://www.nrepp.samhsa.gov/)

4. Intentional recovery communities for addiction and mental illness

4.1 12-step peer support groups

Peer support groups have been in existence for several decades but, by far, the best-known modality is the *12-Step Model* (Alcoholics Anonymous, 2001). Formed under the principal that one alcoholic helping another could bring about lasting change and that "faith without works is dead" (AA: Alcoholics Anonymous, 4th Ed., 2001, pp. 76), the 12-steps of Alcoholics Anonymous have become synonymous with recovery support groups. Started in 1935 by former New York stockbroker Bill Wilson and medical doctor Bob Smith, AA took root in Akron, Ohio after Wilson, an alcoholic struggling against taking a drink while on a business trip, reached out to Smith – an acknowledged alcoholic also battling the disease (Kurtz, 1979). Wilson and Smith employed principals founded by U.S. temperance organizations like the Emmanuel Movement and the Oxford Group as an early blueprint for AA, but it was Wilson's experience with Rowland H., an alcoholic treated by Carl Jung in Zurich, that provided what he described as "the foundation stone upon which our society has been built" (Schoen, 2009, pp. 10). Jung believed that chronic alcoholism was, in essence, a "spiritual thirst (for a) union with god" (Schoen, 2009, pp. 18). In his transmissions with Wilson, Jung invoked the ancient aphorism: *spiritus contra spiritum* which, loosely translated, suggests that one spirit "drives out" the other (Miller & Bogenschutz, 2007, pp. 433). Employing Jung's philosophy, Wilson moved away from the strictly Christian theological underpinnings of the Oxford Group and into a concept that emphasized personal responsibility and an individualized interpretation of a "power greater than ourselves (Alcoholics Anonymous, 2004, p. 59)".

Though recovery, from a 12-Step perspective, is phenomenological (as evidenced by AA sayings like "Recovery is an inside job"), the emphasis is on the power of the group. As the first tradition of AA states: "Personal recovery depends on AA unity" (Alcoholics

Anonymous, 1953, pp. 129). Though 12-Step concepts are still scrutinized by many scientific concerns due to a dearth of empirical evidence (Fiorentine, 1999), they constitute the treatment model of choice in most rehabilitation facilities and serve as the foundation for other self-help groups -- Debtors Anonymous, Overeaters Anonymous and Gamblers Anonymous among them. The largest and most popular program in the world for people wishing to recover from alcoholism (Tongin, Connors and Miller as cited in Barbor & Del Boca, 2010), much of AA's success may rest in its adherence to what has since been described by Irving Yalom as the 12 "therapeutic factors" of group psychotherapy (Yalom & Leszcz, 2005). The group session is seen as information-sharing and, as a process, includes a number of these factors; namely imparting of information, installation of hope, group cohesion, catharsis (sharing has no consequences and can be extremely emotional), imitative behavior (those with long-term sobriety are often revered by peers and their aphorisms passed on to other groups and members), interpersonal learning (the exchange between members that occurs both inside and outside of the group environment) and self-understanding. Perhaps its most salient therapeutic factor is altruism. The essence of the 12th step, which asks that recovering alcoholics "carry the message" to others who still suffer (Alcoholics Anonymous, 4th. Ed., 2004, pp. 60), is an essential part of the process and a key factor in the proliferation of AA and other 12-Step organizations. While there is significant empathy within the fellowship, altruism seems to be the factor that brings about the most lasting change. As the saying goes "We can only keep what we have by giving it away" (personal communications, AA and NA meetings, 1995-2010). With no governing forces and employing only administrative service workers, AA, as an institution, relies solely on the desire of its members to congregate and share their experiences. This intentionality places the responsibility of recovery squarely on the individual, but emphasizes the power of the group in terms of providing support.

4.2 The clubhouse

Approximately 7.5 million Americans belong to as many as 1.5 million self-help groups (Lieberman & Snowden, 1994). Consumers often report joining peer support programs for social support, such as seeing friends, feeling a sense of family, socializing, and exchanging ideas (Mowbray & Tan, 1992). The power and influence social support provides to overall mental well being is not surprising given that humans are a social species meant to live in groups and not in isolation (Weisfeld, 1999). Thus it is apropos that a group of patients that had recently been discharged from a state psychiatric facility banded together to form a support group known as "We are not alone" or WANA. In the 1950's with the assistance of more volunteers, the group became known as the Fountain House which became the template for the development of Clubhouses (Anderson, 1998).

The clubhouse program, which is based on psychosocial psychiatric rehabilitation principles rather than a medical model of treatment, values social relationships and social participation as an active agent of rehabilitation and recovery (Mastboom, 1992). The specific psychiatric rehabilitation environment of the clubhouse is guided by a philosophical orientation reflecting consumer empowerment, competency, community, and recovery (Beard, Propst, & Malamud, 1982;Pernice-Duca, 2009; Warner et al., 1999). These orientations are operationalized in the clubhouse setting through shared decision-making, skill training, and vocational services. The clubhouse program however, can also been described as an exemplary model of the operant-environment (O-E) interaction found in human ecosystems. From this perspective, the social environment creates an atmosphere in which change is possible and interactions within the environment serve to enhance quality of life and hasten the recovery process. However, the O-E interaction is limited and does not explain the humanistic qualities of the social environment. Clubhouses have been designed to increase social connections for individuals with little family or social network ties (Beard, 1992b). Further, they have also been cited as catalysts to recovery in the narratives of clubhouse members (Beard, 1992b; Ely, 1992; Deegan, 1988; Paul, 1992; Peckoff, 1992).

A key component of the Clubhouse psychiatric rehabilitation program is to establish or maintain social relationships. Clubhouses offer individuals opportunities to meet new friends to expand personal networks, as well as to identify themselves as someone other than a person living with mental illness (Macias & Rodican, 1997). Four fundamental principles guide clubhouse programs: (a) the clubhouse belongs to its members, (b) daily attendance is desired and makes a difference to other members, (c) members feel wanted as contributors, and (d) members feel needed (Beard, Propst, & Malamud, 1982). Clubhouse programs offer a range of community supports such as housing assistance, employment training and placement, and self-help resources. The clubhouse model has an egalitarian social structure with members and staff sharing in clubhouse work and decision-making. The central tenet of the clubhouse model is what is known as the "work-ordered day." It mimics a normal workday in that the day begins at 9:00 A.M. and essentially ends at 5:00 P.M., with social activities and support groups occurring after hours. The work-ordered day is designed to provide individuals with a workday structure that incorporates work ethics and social skills needed to prepare one for community reintegration. Clubhouse members work side-by-side along with clubhouse staff, interacting through the work-ordered day activities. Clubhouse participants are referred to as "members," and membership is voluntary.

The clubhouse was designed to address the needs of people living with chronic or persistent mental illness who have encountered losses in social skills, friendships, family connections, and employment (Mastboom, 1992). As a rehabilitation program, clubs assist people in leading more productive, community oriented lives by encouraging skill development within an environment that supports them to meet the demands of daily living, socialization, and employment (Anthony, Cohen, Farkas, & Gagne, 2002).

According to Beard, Propst, & Malmund (1982), social interaction is an important aspect of the program. These authors assert that members "feeling needed" is one of the three core elements of the clubhouse model. Therefore, it is contended that through clubhouse participation, members gain a sense of connection with others, thereby reducing isolation while increasing social ties. Further, members also elicit support from their social support networks and engage in mutually supportive reciprocal interactions with network supports. Clubhouse members make use of the clubhouse model in the purpose of creating change in their lives, specifically in forming significant relationships, promoting educational and employment aspirations and improving one's social life (Norman, 2006). Members adopt the philosophy that the dissimilarities among peers are a resource rather than a limitation. This philosophical and relational attitude has been found to be important in creating a supportive, intentional recovery community.

4.3 Peer-run drop-in centers

Peer-run drop-in centers, or consumer operated services (COPS), are services planned, operated, administered and evaluated by people who have a psychiatric disability (SAMHSA, 1998) or those who utilize mental health services. Peer delivered services are services provided by individuals who identify themselves as having a mental illness and deliver services for the primary purse of helping others with mental illness (Solomon, 2004).

Non-consumers may be involved in the service or program, but their inclusion is within the control of consumers. A primary consumer is a direct recipient of mental health services either public or private. Peer programs are peer-driven, peer-run and peer-operated. They give people choices, decision-making roles, and positions of authority. Successful peer-delivered services are based on the values of equality and respect, encourage active participation by primary consumers, and offer support of consumer autonomy in services delivered. Programs are based on the values of empowerment, self-determination, acceptance and support. Peer support programs and services rely on experiential knowledge gained by the personal experience of having a psychiatric disability.

The President's New Freedom Commission for Mental Health in the U.S. (2003) advocated for a shift in resources to a recovery-based model, including more consumer-run services and programs. The recovery orientation suggests that "adjuncts and alternatives to formal treatment, involvement of self-help groups, and social opportunities at local drop-in centers foster empowerment and provide opportunities for a more meaningful life (Forquer & Knight, pg. 25)." These peer-run programs provide consumers opportunities to learn and share coping skills and strategies and move into more active assistance and away from passive patient roles, and build/or enhance self-esteem, and self confidence. *Peer delivered or consumer-run programs may include* peer-operated drop-in centers, peer-run crises centers, housing programs, peer counseling, peer case-management, advocacy training, and peer support self-help groups.

The peer-operated drop-in center concept originated as a response to the lack of inclusive options in the community. It began as friends helping friends and is based on the value that all individuals deserve to be treated as human beings with rights, respect, and dignity, and to have the opportunity to live their lives in the community. Drop-in centers are a form of peer-support. They are run by primary consumers that provide mutual, social, emotional, and instrumental support to those who share a mental health condition. Drop-in centers have some paid staff and a significant number of volunteers and services are embedded within a formal organization as a freestanding legal entity. The concept of voluntary attendance and participation remains one of the primary attributes of any drop-in center. Drop-in centers serve as an important outreach access point and welcoming place for consumers who want to benefit from peer-delivered services but may choose to not be part of a traditional clinical milieu. Drop-in centers are places that are free from therapy, formal skills training, and clinical supervision. They provide an informal, supportive, intentional community to assist in the recovery process. These recovery experiences may include opportunities to learn and share coping skills and strategies with fellow peers. Peers serve as role models to others with psychiatric disabilities; they are able to navigate through systems and advocate for others who share the disability based on their own experiences. Knowing peers who are successfully coping with their illness leads to more hopefulness and optimism (Saltzer & Liptzin-Shear, 2002).

5. Conclusion

Recovery occurs among many people suffering with serious mental illness (Corrigan & Ralph, 2005; Davidson, et al., 2007; Onken, Craig, Ridgway, Ralph, & Cook, 2007). The drive to pursue a greater understanding of the potential for recovery from serious mental illness emerged from consumers of mental health and psychiatric services, public health policies, and data from longitudinal studies. Also, consumers of mental health services have become more vocal and active in the treatment and care they receive, thus inspiring a movement in the delivery of psychiatric services to attend to consumer strengths, natural supports, and decrease social isolation (Davidson, et al., 2007; Drake, 2005; Resnick, Fontana, Lehman, & Rosenheck, 2005). Psychosocial rehabilitation programs provide numerous services including self-help and mutual-help groups, community residential services, peer run drop-in services, supported education and employment services, and clubhouses (Lucca & Allen, 2001). Research has identified the benefits of many of these programs in providing effective treatment for individuals with serious mental illness. For example, self-help groups have been found to increase social support, and create a sense of belonging, and a sense of empowerment (Hardiman & Segal, 2003). Approximately 7.5 million Americans belong to as many as 1.5 million self-help groups (Lieberman & Snowden, 1994). Consumers often report that joining peer support drop-in centers provide opportunities for social support, such as seeing friends, feeling a sense of family, socializing, and exchanging ideas (Mowbray & Tan, 1992). Identifying with a group may act as a shield in protecting individuals form stigma (Karidi, et al., 2010), improving quality of life and improving social relationships (Schonebaum, et al., 2006).

6. References

Abrahms, S. (July-August, 2011). *Homeless no more.* AARP bulletin, 52(6),12-15.

Accordino, M. P., & Hunt, B. (2001). Family Counseling Training in Rehabilitation Counseling Programs Revisited. *Rehabilitation Education, 15*(3), 255-264.

Alcoholics anonymous (2004). *Alcoholics anonymous* (4th ed.). New York, NY: Alcoholics Anonymous World Services, Inc.

Alcoholics Anonymous (2002). *Twelve steps and twelve traditions.* New York, NY: Alcoholics Anonymous WorldS ervices, Inc.

Anderson, S. (1998). *We are not alone: Fountain House and the development of clubhouse culture.* New York, NY: Fountain House.

Anthony, W. A. (1993). Recovery from mental illness: The guiding vision of the mental health service system in the 1990s. *Psychosocial Rehabilitation Journal, 16*(4), 11-23.

Anthony, W. A., Rogers, E. S., & Farkas, M. (2003). Research on evidence-based practices: Future directions in an era of recovery. *Community Mental Health Journal, 39*(2), 101- 114.

Beard, J. H., Propst, R. N., & Malmund, T. J. (1982). The fountain house model of psychiatric rehabilitation. *Psychosocial Rehabilitation Journal, 5*(1), 1-13.

Beale, V., & Lambric, T. (1995). The recovery concept: Implementation in the mental health system. *Ohio Department of Mental Health,* 1-20, p. 5.

Biegel, D. E., McCardel, E., & Mendelson, S. (1985). *Social networks and mental health: An annotated bibliography.* Beverly Hills, CA: Sage Publications.

Bellack, A.S. (2006). Scientific and consumer models of recovery in schizophrenia: Concordance, contrasts, and implications. *Schizophrenia Bulletin, 32*(3), 432-442.

Berkman, L. F. (1995). The role of social relations in health promotion. *Psychosomatic Medicine, 57*(3), 245-254.

Berkman, L. F., Glass, T., Brissette, I., & Seeman, T. E. (2000). From social integration to health: Durkheim in the new millennium. *Social Science & Medicine, 51*(6), 843-857

Brewer, P., Gadsden, V., & Scrimshaw, K. (1994) The community group network in mental health: A model for social support and community integration. *British Journal of Occupational Therapy, 57*(12), 467-70.

Brissette, I. Cohen, S., & Seeman, T. E. (2000). Measuring social integration and social networks. In S. Cohen, L. Underwood & B. Gottlieb (Eds.), *Support measurements and interventions: A guide for social and health scientists.* NY: Oxford Press.

Calabrese, J. D., & Corrigan, P. W. (2005). Beyond Dementia Praecox: Findings From Long-Term Follow-Up Studies of Schizophrenia. In R. O. Ralph, P. W. Corrigan, R. O. Ralph, P. W. Corrigan (Eds.) , *Recovery in mental illness: Broadening our understanding of wellness* (pp. 63-84). Washington, DC US: American Psychological Association.

Carolan, M. Onaga, E.O., Pernice-Duca, F., & Jimenz, T. (2011). A Place to Be: The Role of Clubhouse in Facilitating Social Support. *Psychiatric Rehabilitation Journal, 35*(2), 125- 132

Clay, S. (2005). About Us: What we have in common. In S.Clay, B. Schell, P. Corrigan, & R. O. Ralph(Eds.) On our own, Together: Peer program for people with mental illness. Vanderbilt University Press.

Caron, J., Tempier, R., Mercier, C., & Leouffre, P. (1998). Components of social support and quality of life in severely mentally ill, low income individuals and a general population group. *Community Mental Health Journal, 34*(5), 459-475.

Coatsworth-Puspoky, R. R., Forchuk, C. C., & Ward-Griffin, C. C. (2006). Peer support relationships: An unexplored interpersonal process in mental health. *Journal of Psychiatric and Mental Health Nursing*, 13(5), 490-497.

Corrigan, P. (2002). Empowerment and serious mental illness: Treatment partnerships and community opportunities. *Psychiatric Quarterly, 73*(3), 217-228.

Corrigan, P.W., Giffort, D., Rashid, F., Leary, M., & Okeke, I. (1999). Recovery as a psychological construct. *Community Mental Health Journal, 35*(3), 231-239.

Corrigan, P.W., & Phelan, S. M. (2004). Social support and recovery in people with serious mental illnesses. *Community Mental Health Journa,l* 40(6), 513-523.

Corrigan, P.W., & Ralph, R.O. (2005) *Recovery in Mental Illness: Broadening Our Understanding of Wellness,* (pp3-17). Washington DC: American Psychological Association, p. 282.

Davidson, L., Borg, M., Marin, I., Topor, A., Mezzina, R., & Sells, D. (2005). Process of recovery in serious mental illness: Findings from a multinational study. *American Journal of Psychiatric Rehabilitation, 8*, 177-201.

Davidson, L., Hoge, M.A., Merrill, M.E., Rakfeldt, J., & Griffith, E.E.H. (1995). The experiences of long-stay inpatients returning to the community. *Psychiatry: Interpersonal and Biological Processes, 58* (2), 122–132.

Davidson, L., O'Connell, M., Tondora, J., Styron, T., & Kangas, K. (2006). The top ten concerns about recovery encountered in mental health system transformation. *Psychiatric Services, 57*(5), 640-645.

Davidson, L., & Roe, D. (2007). Recovery from versus recovery in serios mental illness: One strategy for lessening confusion plaguing recovery. *Journal of Mental Health, 16*(4), 459-470.

Davidson, L., Tondura, J., O'Connell, M., Kirk Jr., T., Rockholz, & Evans, A. (2007). Creating a Recovery-Oriented system of behavioral health care: Moving from concept to reality. *Psychiatric Rehabilitation Journal, 31*(1), 23-31.

Deegan, P. E. (1988). Recovery: The lived experience of rehabilitation. *Psychosocial Rehabilitation Journal, 11*(4), 11–19.

Deegan, G. (2003). Discovering recovery. *Psychiatric Rehabilitation Journal, 26*(4), 368-376.

DeSisto, M., Harding, C. M., McCormick, R. V., Ashikaga, T., & Brooks, G. W. (1995a). The Maine and Vermont three-decade studies of serious mental illness. II. Longitudinal course comparisons. *British Journal of Psychiatry, 167*, 338-342.

Drake, R. E. (2005). How evidence-based practices contribute to community integration: A commentary on Bond et al. *Community Mental Health Journal, 41*(1), 87-90.

Durkheim, E. (2001). Suicide: A study in sociology. In E. S. Shneidman (Ed.) , *Comprehending suicide: Landmarks in 20th–century suicidology* (pp. 33-47). Washington, DC US: American Psychological Association.

Fairweather, G.W. & Onaga, E.O. (1993). Empowering the mentally ill. Austin, TX: Fairweather Publishing.

Fiorentine, R. (1999). After drug treatment: Are 12-step programs effective in maintaining abstinence? *The American Journal of Drug and Alcohol Abuse, 25*(1), 93-116.

Fisk, D., Rowe, M., Laub, D., Calvocoressi, L., & DeMino, K. (2000). Homeless Person With Mental Illness and Their Families: Emerging Issues from Clinical Work. *Families in Society, 81*(4), 351-359.

Forquer, S. and Knight, E. (2001). Managed care: Recovery enhancer or Inhibitor? *Psychiatric Services 52*(1), 25-26.

Froland, C., Brodsky, G., Olson, M., & Stewart, L. (2000). Social support and social adjustments: Implications for mental health professionals. *Community Mental Health Journal, 36*(1), 61-75.

Goldberg, R. W., Rollins, A. L., & Lehman, A. F. (2003). Social network correlates among people with psychiatric disabilities. *Psychiatric Rehabilitation Journal, 26*(4), 393-402.

Green, G., Hayes, C., Dickinson, D., Whittaker, A., & Gilheany, B. (2002). The role and impact of social relationships upon well-being reported by mental health service users: A qualitative study. *Journal of Mental Health, 11*(5), 565-579.

Hardiman, E. R., & Segal, S. P. (2003). Community membership and social networks in mental health self-help agencies. *Psychiatric Rehabilitation Journal, 27*(1), 25-33.

Harding, C. M., Brooks, G. W., Ashikaga, T., & Strauss, J. S. (1987a). The Vermont longitudinal study of persons with severe mental illness: I. Methodology, study sample, and overall status 32 years later. *The American Journal of Psychiatry, 144*(6), 718-726.

Harding, C. M., Brooks, G. W., Ashikaga, T., & Strauss, J. S. (1987b). The Vermont longitudinal study of persons with severe mental illness: II. Long-term outcome of subjects who retrospectively met DSM-III criteria for schizophrenia. *The American Journal of Psychiatry, 144*(6), 727-735.

Hatfield, A. B., & Lefley, H. P. (1993). *Surviving mental illness: Stress, coping and adaptation.* New York, NY: The Guilford Press.

Hatfield, A. B., & Lefley, H. P. (1987). *Families of the mentally ill: Coping and adaptation.* New York, NY: The Guilford Press.

Herman, S. E., Onaga, E., Pernice-Duca, F., Oh, S., & Ferguson, C. (2005). Sense of community in clubhouse programs: Member and staff concepts. *American Journal of Community Psychology, 36*(3/4), 343-356.

Hogan, M. F. (2003). The President's New Freedom Commission: Recommendations to Transform Mental Health Care in America. *Psychiatric Services, 54*(11), 1467-1474.

House, J. S., Landis, K. R., & Umberson, D. (1988). Social relationships and health. *Science, 241,* 540-545.

Karidi, (2010). Perceived social stigma, self-concept, and self-stigmatization of patient with schizophrenia. *Comprehensive psychiatry, 51*(1), 19.

Kawachi, I. & Berkman, L. F. (2001). Social ties and mental health. Journal of Urban Health: Bulletin of the New York Academy of Medicine, 78(3), 458-467.

Kelly, M. & Gamble, C. (2005). Exploring the concept of recovery in schizophrenia. *Journal of Psychiatric Mental and Mental Health Nursing,* 12, 245-251.

Kurtz, E. (1979). Not-god: A history of alcoholics anonymous. Center City, MN: Hazelden Foundation.

Landrine, H. (1992).Clinical implications of cultural differences: The referential versus the indexed self. Clinical Psychology Review, 12, 401-415.

Lieberman, M. A., & Snowden, L. R. (1993). Problems in assessing prevalence and membership characteristics of self-help group participants. *Journal of Applied Behavioral Science, 29,* 166-180.

Lin, N., Ye, X., & Ensel, W. M. (1999). Social support and depressed mood: A structural analysis. *Journal of Health and Social Behavior, 40*(4), 344-359.

Littrell, J. & Bech, E. (2001). Predictors of depression in a sample group of African-American homeless men: Identifying effective coping strategies given varying levels of daily stressors. *Community Mental Health Journal, 37*(1), 15-29.

Macias, C., & Rodican, C. (1997). Coping with recurrent loss in mental illness: Unique aspects of clubhouse communities. *Journal of Personal and Interpersonal Loss, 2,* 205-221.

Mastboom, J. (1992). Forty clubhouses: Model and practices. *Psychosocial Rehabilitation Journal, 16*(2), 9-23.

Mead, S., Hilton, D., & Curtis, L. (2001). Peer support: A theoretical perspective. *Psychiatric Rehabilitation Journal, 25*(2), 134-141.

Miller, W. R., & Bogenshutz, M. P. (2007). Spirituality and addiction. Southern Medical Journal, 100(4), 433-436.

Mowbray, C., & Tan, C. (1992). Evaluation of an innovative consumer run service model: The drop in center. *Innovation and Research, 1*(2), 33–42.

National Institue of Mental Health (2010). Questions and answers of about the national comorbidity survey replication (NCSR) study. Retrieved from http://www.nimh.nih.gov/health/topics/statistics/ncsr-study/questions-and-answers-aboutthenational-comorbidity-survey-replication-ncsr-study.shtml#q8

National Institute of Mental Health. (2010). The Numbers count: Mental disorders in America.Retrieved from: http://www.nimh.nih.gov/health/publications/the-numbers-count-mentaldisorders-in-america/index.shtml#Intro

Nelson G, Lomotey J. (2006). Quantity and quality of participation and outcomes of participation in mental health consumer-run organizations. *Journal of Mental Health* 15(1):63-74.

Norman C. The Fountain House movement, an alternative rehabilitation model for people with mental health problems, members' descriptions of what works. *Scandinavian Journal of Caring Sciences.* 2006;20(2):184–192.

Onken, S. J., Craig, C. M., Ridgway, P., Ralph, R. O., & Cook, J. A. (2007). An analysis of the definitions and elements of recovery: A review of the literature. *Psychiatric Rehabilitation Journal, 31*(1), 9-22.

Perese, E. F., Getty, C., & Wooldridge, P. (2003). Psychosocial club members' characteristics and their readiness to participate in a support group. *Issues in Mental Health Nursing, 24,* 153-174.

Pernice-Duca, F. M. (2008). The structure and quality of social network support among mental   health consumers of clubhouse programs. *Journal of Community Psychology, 36*(7), 929-946.

Pernice-Duca, F., & Onaga, E. (2009). Examining the contribution of social network support to the recovery process among clubhouse members. *American Journal of Psychiatric Rehabilitaion, 12*, 1-30.

Ralph, R. (Ed.), & Corrigan, P. (Ed.). (2005). *Recovery in mental illness: Broadening our understanding of wellness.* Washington, DC US: American Psychological Association. doi:10.1037/10848-000

Resnick, S. G., Fontana, A., Lehman, A. F., & Rosenheck, R. A. (2005). An empirical conceptualization of the recovery orientation. *Schizophrenia Research, 75*(1), 119-128.

Ridgway, P. (2001). ReStorying psychiatric disability: Learning from first person recovery narratives. *Psychiatric Rehabilitation Journal*, 24(4), 335-343.

Salzer, M. S., & Shear, S. (2002). Identifying consumer-provider benefits in evaluations of consumer-delivered services. *Psychiatric Rehabilitation Journal*, 25(3), 281-288.

Schonebaum AD, Boyd JK, & Dudek KJ. (2006). A comparison of competitive employment outcomes for the clubhouse and PACT models. *Psychiatric Services (Washington, D.C.). 57*(10), 1416-20.

Soloman, P. (2004). Peer support/peer provided services underlying processes, benefits and critical ingredients. Psychiatric Rehabilitation Journal, 27(4), 392-401.

Stahler, G. J., Shipley, T. F., Bartelt, D., DuCette, J. P. & Shandler, I. W. (1995). Evaluating alternative treatments for homeless substance-abusing men: Outcomes and predictors of success. Journal of Addictive Diseases. 14(4), 151-167.

Tempier, R., Caron, J., Mercier, C., & Leouffre, P. (1998) Quality of life of severely mentally ill individuals: A comparative study. *Community Mental Health Journal* 34, 477-486

Tongin, J. S., Connors, G. J., & Miller, W. (2010). Treatment matching in alcoholism. In Barbor, T., & Del Boca, F. K. (Eds.), International Research Monographs in the Addictions. New York, Turner, J. C., & TenHoor, W. J. (1978). The NIMH Community Support Program: Pilot approach to a needed social reform. *Schizophrenia Bulletin, 4*(3), 319-348. NY: Cambridge University Press.

Turner, J. C., & TenHoor, W. J. (1978). The NIMH Community Support Program: Pilot approach to a needed social reform. *Schizophrenia Bulletin*, 4(3), 319-348.

U.S. Department of Health and Human Services, Substance Abuse and Mental Health Services Administration, Center for Mental Health Services (2006). *National consensus statement on mental health recovery.* Washington, D.C.

Verhaeghe, M., et. al., (2008). Stigmatization and Self-Esteem of Persons in Recovery from Mental Illness: The Role of Peer Support. *The International Journal of Social Psychiatry* 54 (3), 206-18.

Whitaker, R. (2002). *Mad in America: Bad science, bad medicine, and the enduring mistreatment of the mentally ill.* Cambridge, MA US: Perseus Publishing.

Wilson, M., Flanagan, S., & Rynders, C. (1999). The FRIENDS program: A peer support group model for individuals with a psychiatric disability. *Psychiatric Rehabilitation Journal, 22*(3), 239-247.

Yalom, I. D., & Leszcz, M. (Col). (2005). *The theory and practice of group psychotherapy (5th ed.).* New York, NY US: Basic Books

Young, S. L., & Ensing, L. S. (1999). Exploring recovery from the perspective of people with psychiatric disabilities. *Psychiatric Rehabilitation Journal*, 22(3), 219-231.

12

Irrational Suffering – An Impact of Cognitive Behavioural Therapy on the Depression Level and the Perception of Pain in Cancer Patients

Ewa Wojtyna
University of Silesia in Katowice
Poland

1. Introduction

International Association for the Study of Pain (IASP) provides the definition of pain according to which pain is *an unpleasant sensory and emotional experience associated with actual or potential tissue damage, or described in terms of such damage* (cf. Witte & Stein, 2010). Therefore pain is a phenomenon which extends beyond the somatosensory dimension and its perception is determined by a number of factors, among which mental factors deserve special attention as they can be modified by psychological interventions.

Pain is not always confined to a physical sensation. In the following paper the term 'pain' is reserved for somatic pain. However, the experience of such pain might become a threat to the integrity of the self, which is accompanied by despair. The sensations of this kind will be described as 'suffering'.

2. Pain in cancer patients

Cancer patients commonly experience pain in various stages of their disease. Numerous studies indicate that approximately 1/3 of the patients experience pain in the active stage of their disease, and the proportion rises to 50-78% in the advanced stages of cancer (e.g. Breitbart et al., 2009; Chapman, 2011). Approximately 33% of cancer survivors suffer from a chronic pain syndrome as a result of tissue damage or as a side effect of their treatment (A.W. Burton et al., 2007; van den Beuken-van Everdingen et al., 2007).

A number of factors are responsible for pain experienced by cancer patients. Among the major ones is the development of the disease: tumour compression or infiltration of nerve, plexus and meninges as well as metastases to the bones. Approximately 25% of patients present with pain which is a side effect of radiotherapy, chemotherapy or surgical procedures (Breitbart et al., 2009).

Pain which develops as a result of radiotherapy is caused by skin burns and the reduced blood flow in the irradiated tissues, which may lead to necrosis, neural damage, fibrosis or stenosis. Post-radiotherapy pain occurs not only during the active treatment but also months and even years after the completion of the treatment (cf. Breitbart et al., 2009; A.W. Burton et al., 2007; Colyer, 2003).

Chemotherapy-induced pain is commonly brought on by peripheral neuropathy as well as by the direct damage of the tissue susceptible to chemotherapeutic drugs, such as mucous membrane lining the digestive tract (Visovsky et al., 2007). Such drugs as platinum compounds, vinca alkaloids, taxanes, thalidomide and bortezomid tend to contribute to the development of neuropathy (Armstrong et al., 2005; A.W. Burton et al., 2007).

Pain resulting from the surgical procedures is commonly caused by tissue damage during surgery, scarring, adhesion, lymphoedema, neural damage (e.g. of axillary or intercostobrachial nerves), neuromas or phantom sensations following the amputation of the body part (Breitbart et al., 2009; Chapman, 2011).

3. The psychological aspect of chronic pain in cancer patients

3.1 The consequences of pain for the patient's functioning

Pain, and chronic pain in particular, may have a considerable impact on the patients' quality of life (Breitbart et al., 2009; Cowan, 2011; Wahl et al., 2009). A restriction in mobility and declining physical as well as cognitive functions, especially difficulty concentrating, a sense of powerlessness and helplessness are frequent pain-induced complaints (e.g. Breitbart et al., 2009; Melkumova et al., 2011). Such experiences may lead to the intensification of resignation thoughts and suicidality (Breitbart et al., 2009). Furthermore, the available empirical data confirms the concurrence of insomnia and chronic pain (Goral et al., 2010; Tang et al., 2007). What is more, insomnia may in turn intensify pain sensations. Also pain and insomnia are among major risk factors for suicide (Kutcher & Chehil, 2007).

Apart from physical complaints, other factors contributing to the development of depression are a sense of worthlessness and low self-esteem as well as an impairment of the ability to perform important roles in one's professional and family life, a loss of independence, a sense of meaninglessness and chronic anxiety. Thus it is not surprising that depression is one of the most frequent mental disorders observed among cancer patients. Nearly half of cancer patients suffer from depression and anxiety (cf. Breitbart et al., 2009; Rymaszewska & Dudek, 2009).

Anxiety can be related to the fear of death, of treatment and its side effects, of adverse impact of the disease on the patient's personal, family and professional life, etc. The disorder frequently manifests itself as a generalized anxiety disorder, worrying or generalized future-oriented anxiety. As an unpleasant experience pain may also lead to the development of the fear of future pain or of the intensification of pain to such an extent that it becomes unbearable (Cowan, 2011; Leeuw et al., 2007).

3.2 Pain as a source of chronic stress
3.2.1 Stress and cognitive appraisal

Pain intensifies the patients' level of distress (Zaza & Baine, 2002). Lazarus and Folkman define stress as a *"particular relationship between the person and the environment that is appraised by the person as taxing or exceeding his or her resources and endangering his or her well-being"* (1984, p. 19).

Crucial in this conception is the subject cognitive appraisal of the relationship between an individual and his or her environment, which is seen as the *"process of categorizing an encounter, and its various facets, with respect to its significance for well-being"* (Lazarus & Folkman, 1984, p. 31). This appraisal is a continuous process and embraces the primary appraisal, in which a given situation is recognized as stressful and defined in terms of harm/loss, threat or challenge, and the secondary appraisal, which concerns the possible action which can be taken by an individual in order to resolve the situation. Both these appraisals are linked and occur simultaneously.

According to the cognitive behavioural theories regarding the occurrence of emotions and the generation of activities (e.g. Ellis & Dryden, 2007; Maultsby, 1990), cognitive content informs the person's emotions as well as his or her behaviour. Thus the appraisal of the stressor in the terms of harm/loss is frequently followed by sadness and grief and passive behaviour, threat gives rise to anxiety and escape or erratic behaviours, while challenge may result in a variety of emotions, including positive ones such as hope, which are accompanied by involvement and goal-oriented activities.

3.2.2 Coping

The secondary appraisal in turn enables a person to evaluate his or her own possibilities to act when confronted with a stressor, so that the process of coping can commence. Lazarus and Folkman define coping as *"constantly changing cognitive and behavioural efforts to manage specific external and/or internal demands that are appraised as taxing or exceeding the resources of the person"* (1984, p. 141). Since the appraisal which determines coping is subjective, hence liable to cognitive distortion, coping can be aimed at resolving the problem or at self-regulation of emotions.

Coping itself cannot, however, be equated with the objective adaptability of behaviours. The patient can cope with stress by, for example, following the doctor's recommendations and in so doing reducing the risk of further development of the illness, but, on the other hand, the patient (especially if he or she has a low opinion of their ability to instrumentally resolve the problem) may engage in the activities regarded as unhealthy, such as alcohol consumption, which nevertheless will help them to achieve emotional comfort (cf. Endler, Parker & Summerfeldt, 1998). Finally, chronic stress can be related to the treatment regimen or the changeable course of the disease. Patients suffering from chronic conditions commonly balance between the instrumental and emotion-regulating activities and hence the catalogue of the techniques they employ to cope with stress is subject to change.

At this point the costs of coping must be mentioned, i.e. the loss of resources following the undertaking and continuing the efforts aimed at dealing with the stressful situation. From the perspective of cost assessment it might prove more cost-effective to abandon the efforts and tolerate the stressors rather than undertake an effort to cope with them (cf. Hobfoll, 1998; Schönpflug & Battmann, 1988, as cited in Heszen & Sęk, 2007). In practical terms it means that the patient may choose not to be involved in his or her own treatment, and he or she may experience a sense of hopelessness, reduced activity and lack of motivation to undertake new tasks or challenges.

3.2.3 Neuropsychological aspect of stress

Stress and the ways of coping may also impact on neurophysiological processes related to the reaction to stress: on their intensity, frequency, duration and the reaction patterns. Moreover, chronic sympathetic system and hormonal system arousal may in turn lead to the exhaustion of the body's resources, immune deficiency, and functional – and subsequently structural – disorders of the organs and the systems of the body (cf. Vedhara & Irwin, 2005). Chronic stress leads to the constant activation of the adrenal cortex and the oversecretion of glucocorticosteroids, including cortisol. Although in the case of short-term stress those hormones assist the release of additional energy and help to resolve a difficult situation, in the case of prolonged stress they can cause a number of adverse reactions in the body. For instance chronic hypercortisolemia may contribute to the damage and the atrophy of the hippocampus (Colla et al., 2007; Sapolsky, 2000). In the case of pain neuroimaging tests confirm the presence of dysfunctions and structural alterations of the limbic system and hippocampus, which is the structure that suppresses cortisol secretion (Herbert et al., 2006; Zimmerman et al., 2009). What is more, the hippocampus is the region of the brain where the memories of the context of a given situation and the perception of the stimulus are stored and can be retrieved to help a person to appraise the currently experienced events in a more adequate manner. The damage of the hippocampus contributes to the further increase of the stress level, since the reduction of feedback prevents the effective suppression of hormone secretion from the suprarenal gland while the impairment of memory and dysregulation of affect, the functions normally regulated by the hippocampus, result in the patient seeing his or her life as even more miserable (cf. Wirga & Wojtyna, 2010).

3.3 Psychological factors and pain

The intensity of pain is determined by a number of factors and the size of the damaged tissue is only one of them. Nociceptive stimuli are first modified in the spinal cord through so-called "gate control" (Melzack & Wall, 1965). The interaction of the impulses transmitted by the nerve fibres of various diameter can cause inhibition or intensification of the nociceptive signal. The process is also affected by the impulses coming from the brain. The processes occurring in the central nervous system are of major importance for the chronic pain-related issues.

3.3.1 Anxiety and pain

The perception of pain depends on the level of arousal and emotional state. The level of anxiety is crucial here and the reaction to fear and anxiety manifests itself on several levels:

- physiological – as an activation of the sympathetic system, including faster breathing, the activation of the circulatory system as well as increased muscle tone and reactivity;
- cognitive – as an interpretation of the stimulus as a threat and the appraisal of its consequences;
- behavioural – as activities leading to coping with the threat, including escape and avoidance behaviour.

A number of studies indicate that the level of anxiety is the crucial aspect of coping with pain. The studies concerning chronic pain proved that the catastrophizing of this experience contributes to the reactions which additionally intensify the feeling of pain (e.g. Leeuw et al., 2007; Linton et al., 2000; Mok & Lee, 2008; Nijs et al., 2008). The fear of pain can manifest itself as, for instance, the fear of the feeling of pain itself, the fear of physical activity or movement which can trigger pain or the fear of (re)injury (Leeuw et al., 2007).

Similar phenomena may occur in the case of cancer patients. However, it is not only the fear of pain itself that can contribute to the intensification of sensations of pain, since the physiological symptoms of anxiety, through the increase of muscle tone or intensification of the scanning of one's own body – regardless of the cause of the fear – may also contribute to the alteration of the perception of pain.

3.3.2 Hypervigilance and pain

Pain-related fear may also result in the patient's making an effort to find as much information about the current situation as possible, which leads to so-called hypervigilance: the tendency to scan one's own body and observe its signals. Since the patient's attention is heightened, he or she is likely to notice more disturbing symptoms and perceive the neutral stimuli as painful (cf. Lautenbacher et al., 2010; Rollman, 2009). According to behavioural theories, hypervigilance is reinforced by the patient's relatives and friends, since his or her complaints meet with their attention and care or bring small benefits such as being excused from the chores. From the perspective of cognitive theories, the patient's beliefs concerning the nature of pain and the consequences of his or her disease are of vital importance. The patient may be convinced that pain indicates, for example, the spreading of the cancer and the prompt reaction to even the slightest sensation of pain can help to apply an appropriate procedure and, in consequence, save his or her life. Hypervigilance may also be affected by the vagueness of a painful stimulus. The stimuli whose site and intensity are well defined are less likely to arouse the patient's specific vigilance than the vague ones (e.g. Almay, 1987; Kostarczyk, 2003).

The patient's attitude is of prime importance. The anticipation of suffering contributes to hypervigilance and thus raises the risk of the occurrence and/or intensification of pain (Arntz et al., 1991; Leeuw et al., 2007). On the other hand, the placebo effect represents the opposite phenomenon. It has been demonstrated on numerous occasions that patients who believe in the efficacy of pain treatment feel considerable relief after being given an inert substance (cf. Benedetti, 2009).

3.3.3 Catastrophizing and pain

Another significant factor which may modify painful sensations is catastrophizing, which involves anticipating the worst possible outcome of the symptoms experienced and contributes to appraising the situation as a threat as well as preventing the person from believing in his or her ability to cope with the problem (Leeuw et al., 2007; Nijs et al., 2008; Vowles et al., 2008). Catastrophizing is a cognitive disorder linked to the tendency to anticipate the worst-case scenario and overestimate its probability. It also leads to exaggerating the problems and overlooking positive aspects of the situation such as the availability of useful resources. What lies at the roots of this phenomenon is the patient's previous experiences as well as the assumptions concerning a given disease, in this case, cancer and pain. The assumptions are based on the information from the media, public and cultural sources, books, medical specialists as well as a wide variety of other sources. Therefore the assumptions the patient makes about his or her illness may differ significantly from the objective medical knowledge. A number of studies indicate that catastrophizing is closely linked with the intensification of pain and anxiety (Bishop & Warr, 2003; A.K. Burton et al., 1995), and can even serve as a predictor of the occurrence of pain and the deterioration of the patient's condition, which was demonstrated in the prospective study on back pain (Linton et al., 2000).

3.3.4 Behaviour and pain

The fear of pain is commonly followed by avoidance behaviours (Leeuw et al., 2007). It may lead to, for instance, withdrawal from physical activity, which, in the patient's view, may cause (re)injury or contribute in any way to the intensification of pain. Cancer patients may also avoid certain medical procedures, such as radiotherapy or chemotherapy. In the short term, the patient may feel relief, but in the long term such behaviour will result in the progress of the disease, the consequence of which is the intensification of pain, or it may lead to the decline in the patient's fitness, fatigue and the increased likelihood of injury, which may also contribute to the occurrence of pain in the future.

3.3.5 Beck's model of depression

In the light of the above it is of utmost importance to identify the factors capable of reducing the level of distress, anxiety and depressiveness experienced by cancer patients suffering from chronic pain. Beck's idiosyncratic model of depression can provide a clue here (cf. Beck et al., 1979; Williams, 1997). The model focuses on three aspects. The first one is negative automatic thoughts, which people often take for granted without an in-depth analysis. They bring about mood changes and, as a result, further thoughts and misconceptions arise, which finally leads to the downward spiral of despair. The frequent repetition of such thoughts reinforces them and retains them as patterns in the neural networks of the central nervous system, which increases the risk of clinical depression symptoms in the future (cf. Williams, 1997; Wirga & Wojtyna, 2010).

Another important aspect of Beck's theory is systematic cognitive distortions present in thinking, such as jumping to arbitrary conclusions, excessive generalization, selective disregard, exaggeration, minimization, dichotomous thinking and, finally, personalization involving attributing certain negative characteristics to oneself despite evidence to the contrary (cf. Wiliams, 1997). Such cognitive errors increase the risk of negative automatic thoughts recurrence and contribute to the further mood lowering.

Finally, the third aspect of Beck's model is the depressiogenic cognitive schema. The schema, according to this theory, is a structure which analyses and organizes information coming from the environment and enables a person to promptly identify the meaning of a given stimulus. The schemata are based on an individual's previous experience, and they typically develop over the years. In the case of depression, the schemata involve long-lasting pessimistic attitudes and negative assumptions about oneself, reality and future (Beck et al., 1979; Williams, 1997). Pain and cancer may in this case act as impulses which activate pre-existing schemata.

In conclusion, cognitive content generated in the event of the disease may become the source of stress and mood lowering, which sometimes develops into a clinically diagnosed disorder. Bearing in mind the possibility of systematic cognitive distortions it can be assumed that the individual's emotions and behaviour frequently result from the biased distorted appraisal of the facts. Therefore the emotional-behavioural expression may be inappropriate to the situation.

3.3.6 Cognitive behavioural therapy

Thus if the cognitive approach is adopted, the psychological intervention must be based on the refutation of the cognitive distortions, the construction of the appropriate assessment of the situation and the replacement of the thoughts with more functional ones, conducive to the reduction of suffering (cf. Ellis & Dryden, 2007; Maultsby, 1990). Such interventions are essential for the cognitive behavioural therapy (CBT).

CBT proved very useful in conjunction with oncological treatment (Moorey & Greer, 2002). Numerous studies proved that CBT helps to alleviate pain or reduce the mental components of various somatic complaints, such as pain (Grant & Haverkamp, 1995; Reid et al., 2003), breathlessness (Bredin et al., 1999), nausea and vomiting (cf. Cathcart, 2006). CBT is beneficial in pain treatment as it helps the patient to cope with complaints more effectively, decreases the perception of symptoms and enables the patient to use analgesic medication less frequently or in smaller doses, which in turn may reduce adverse effects of pharmacotherapy (Syrjala et al., 1995). Complementary psychotherapeutic treatment is of particular importance in the case of neuropathic pain, since many patients continue to experience excruciating pain even after the administration of the analgesics. CBT has been shown to be effective in alleviating pain in those patients.

Despite the evidence from the research conducted to date, the current state of knowledge concerning the possible improvement of the cancer patients' quality of life is still inadequate, particularly as far as pain is concerned. Moreover, little is known about the mechanisms which might lead to such improvement.

4. The study

4.1 Aim
The main objectives of the following study were to:
- explore the link between the intensity of irrational beliefs, depressiveness and the severity of pain in cancer patients,
- determine the impact of the cognitive behavioural therapy on the perception of pain in cancer patients.

4.2 Design and subjects
The longitudinal study comprised a pre-test and a post-test after the period of two months. 253 non-terminal cancer patients participated in the study, all of whom were also treated for chronic pain at the Pain Clinic. All the subjects took advantage of the pharmacological assistance provided by the clinic. 128 patients took part in the cognitive behavioural therapy, while others constituted the control group (n=125) and only took advantage of the standard assistance provided by the Pain Clinic. The group allocation was randomized.

4.3 The method of intervention – Rational behavioural therapy
The study employed the cognitive behavioural method known as rational behavioural therapy (Maultsby, 1990). The aim of this method is to isolate the person's beliefs which are chiefly responsible for his or her emotional discomfort. Maultsby proposes that the previously identified beliefs be tested to assess their rationality by means of the rules of healthy (rational) thinking. These rules relate to the following issues:
- *Healthy thinking is based on obvious facts.* Thus this rule aims at exposing cognitive distortions. In order to do that the patient is engaged into a conversation and a so-called camera test is performed ("if this event was captured on film, what would be recorded? Does it conform with your judgement/opinion?"). The weighing pros and cons discussion can also be used. Finally, the behavioural experiments can be utilized, especially those which involve identifying other people's views.
- *Healthy thinking helps protect health and life.* This rule refers to the effects a given way of thinking has on somatic health. The question which proves particularly helpful in this case is whether the thought tested helps to reduce the stress level or intensifies it. It

follows from psychoneuroimmunological knowledge that the prolonged distress will lead to the reduction in immunocompetence (cf. Vedhara & Irwin, 2005). Therefore, a way of thinking which encourages the reduction of distress should be essential for better health.

- *Healthy thinking helps to achieve goals.* This rule relates to the motivational sphere. A healthy way of thinking promotes physical activity. The person who thinks in this way is more motivated to act towards desirable ends.
- *Healthy thinking helps to resolve or avoid unwanted conflicts.* A healthy way of thinking allows the person to maintain desirable relationships with others. It enables the person to cater for his or her own needs and at the same time reduces the risk of undesirable conflicts.
- And finally *healthy thinking helps the person to feel the way he or she wants to feel.* This rule is also known as "a healthy thinking helps to feel better" or "to feel less unwell". It is worth noting at this point that the mood improvement here follows from cognitive content without the use of psychoactive substances.

Thus the rules of healthy thinking relate to the realistic assessment of facts and the appraisal of the effects of a given way of thinking on the most important areas of a person's functioning: physical health, motivational sphere, interpersonal relations and mental health. According to Maultsby a rational way of thinking is characterized by at least three of the above-mentioned rules. The appraisal of the cognitive content is subjective and performed by the patient him- or herself.

The stage of the identification of irrational beliefs is followed by the search for alternative thoughts which concern the same issue but are more adaptive and are correlated with the improvement of the patient's emotional state. The search for alternatives which will conform with the criteria of healthy thinking involves the discussion with the patients. The therapy based on the rules of healthy thinking is the compilation of several classical techniques employed in CBT, such as the "pros and cons" technique, the appraisal of the consequences of thinking or the refutation of cognitive distortions.

The alternative rational thinking is reinforced through daily repetition of healthy thoughts, finding evidence of their truth and by employing the patient's imagination: he or she imagines a desired outcome and a desired emotional and behavioural state resulting from a new way of thinking.

The current study involved the individual therapy consisting of 8 weekly hour-long sessions.

4.4 Study instruments
4.4.1 Depression

The current study used the Polish translation of *Beck Depression Inventory* (*BDI*; Beck et al, 1988, 1996). The inventory can be used to determine the general intensity of depressiveness and the intensity of its following components: affective and somatic symptoms.

The inventory contains 21 questionnaire items. Each item has a set of four possible answer choices, reflecting the range of symptom intensity: from the complete absence of a symptom (value 0) to the clear manifestation (value 3). Thus the total score ranges from 0 to 63, with the higher score indicating more severe depressive symptoms.

The reliability coefficient for *Beck Depression Inventory* was α =0.91, whereas Cronbach's α coefficient for subscales ranged from 0.86 for *Somatic subscale* to 0.96 for *Affective subscale*.

Irrational Suffering – An Impact of Cognitive Behavioural Therapy on the Depression Level and the Perception
of Pain in Cancer Patients
199

4.4.2 Pain intensity

A *Visual Analogue Scale* (VAS) was used to determine the severity of pain. VAS is a simple instrument to measure the patient's subjective assessment of pain severity. The patient is provided with a 100-millimetre line, on which he or she marks the point which represents the severity of pain he or she feels, with the point 0 indicating the complete absence of pain and 100 – the most severe pain imaginable.

4.4.3 Irrational beliefs regarding pain

The study utilized a partly structuralized interview concerning the patient's perception of pain and the possible ways of coping with it. Next the Socratic dialogue was used to find out more details and, as a result, to identify the patient's beliefs concerning pain, which was essential for further therapy. The beliefs were classified as irrational if they were counter-factual (this criterion did not apply to spiritual beliefs) or they failed to conform with at least three of Maultsby's rules of healthy thinking (Maultsby, 1990).

The beliefs were assessed by the patients on the scale of 0 to 100% to determine the strength of the patients' conviction as well as the intensity of the emotional discomfort associated with a given belief. The level of emotional discomfort was marked on the scale of 0 to 100, where 0 indicated composure and 100 the most severe emotional discomfort.

The intensity of irrational beliefs was assessed in two ways. First, the proportion of irrational beliefs was assessed in reference to the total of patient's statements concerning his or her own person identified in the course of the study. Then, in order to estimate the strength of the patient's irrational beliefs, the mean value of the patient's conviction relating to all previously identified irrational cognitive content was calculated.

4.4.4 Catastrophizing

To assess the intensity of catastrophizing with regard to pain the 13-item *Pain Catastrophizing Scale* (PCS; Sullivan et al., 1995) was used. This instrument is used to calculate the general score as well as the score in three subscales: magnification, rumination, and helplessness.

Patients are asked to report how often they experience certain thoughts or feelings while in pain. The answers are marked on the 5-point Likert scale ranging from 0 (*Not at all*) to 4 (*All the time*). Cronbach's α coefficient of reliability for the present study was 0.90.

4.4.5 Demographic data

Demographic data sheet was used to gather information concerning the patients' age, sex, marital status, educational background, professional status, the duration of cancer as well as the patients' specific diagnosis, and the duration for which the patient was registered with the Pain Clinic.

5. Results

The characteristics of the group are presented in table 1.

The pre-test showed no differences in the study variables between the experimental and control groups.

The patients' average score in *Beck Depression Inventory* was 32.57. It is worth noting that as many as 76.1% of the study subjects scored above 13, which, according to the authors of the questionnaire, could be interpreted as a high risk of clinical depression (Beck et al., 1996). 11.45% of the study subjects' score indicated a risk of a major depressive episode.

Characteristics	CBT group n=128	Control group n=125	Total n=253
Age			
Mean	54.12	55.27	54.89
Range	36 - 65	39 - 65	36 - 65
Gender [%]			
Male	47.66	47.20	47.43
Female	52.34	52.80	52.57
Marital status [%]			
Single	1.57	2.4	1.98
Married	71.09	72.8	71.94
Widowed	10.94	9.6	10.27
Divorced/Separated	16.4	15.2	15.81
Educational background [%]			
Elementary	1.56	1.6	1.58
Vocational	35.94	32.0	33.99
Secondary	38.28	40.0	39.13
University	24.22	26.4	25.3
Occupation [%]			
Employed	9.37	8.0	8.69
Unemployed	50.0	53.6	51.78
Housewife	21.88	20.0	20.95
Retired	18.75	18.4	18.58
Duration of cancer [yrs]			
Mean	5.17	5.34	5.21
Range	2 - 11	1 - 9.5	1 - 11
Duration of chronic pain [yrs]			
Mean	1.94	2.01	1.98
Range	0.5 - 6	0.5 - 5.5	0.5 - 6
Pain intensity (VAS)			
Mean	45.26	44.98	45.07
Range	10 - 95	10 - 90	10 - 95
Depression (BDI)			
Mean	33.28	32.01	32.57
Range	3 - 59	2 - 57	2 - 59
Catastrophizing (PCS)			
Total	33.62	33.16	25.31
Magnification	7.07	6.85	6.97
Rumination	12.34	12.01	12.18
Helplessness	14.22	14.28	14.24
Irrational beliefs			
Number (Proportion) [%]	70.11	69.07	69.51
Conviction the beliefs are true [mean]	86.78	88.29	87.33
Level of emotional discomfort [mean]	75.42	74.30	74.87

Table 1. Characteristics of study participants

Examples of statements (strength of conviction)	Cognitive distortions	Healthier alternatives
I can't sleep at all because of the pain (100%)	Exaggeration	*I can sleep a little in spite of the pain.* *I can fall asleep more easily if I concentrate on other things.*
I know that pain is a sign of the advancement of cancer (100%)	Catastrophizing	*Pain is linked to the disease and treatment. It indicates that something has happened to my body, but it does not necessarily mean that something worse is going on. I can work with the doctor to control it.*
Pain destroys my life, I'm going to be a total wreck (80%)	Exaggeration, catastrophizing	*My life goes on in spite of the pain.* *I can still be useful and do a lot of things.*
Even if there is slight relief, I always feel worse later on. I can't do what I want anyway (90%)	Active refutation of positive aspects, dichotomous thinking	*Sometimes I hurt more and sometimes less. When I feel better, I can do something I like or something that I want.* *When I do something nice for myself, I feel even better.* *Perhaps if I engage in something that I like, it will help me to feel better physically.*
When it hurts so much, I know the end is near (90%)	Exaggeration	*I don't know what will happen.* *Pain is just a symptom and I'm alive and I should take advantage of that.*
This pain will never go away. On the contrary, it'll be worse and worse (100%)	Exaggeration, catastrophizing	*I don't know what will happen.* *My pain is sometimes stronger and sometimes not so strong.* *This means that it can be modified One day I might be able to cope with it better than now.*
I've been hurting a little less in the past couple of days, but it's just a lucky chance – it must have been because of the weather (70%)	Minimization	*I don't know why I've been hurting less. But if it's possible, it means that this pain can sometimes be less strong.* *I will find the ways to help me to feel better.* *I will concentrate on the periods when I feel well and try to find out what it is that helps me. It will help me to organize my life better.*
Because of this pain I'm good for nothing (90%)	Generalization, exaggeration	*There are many spheres of life apart from pain. I can still do a lot of things.*
This treatment is pointless – it still hurts like hell. It'd be better to shoot myself or get drunk and never get sober (95%)	Dichotomous thinking	*My treatment helps me to alleviate pain a little, so it is efficient to a certain extent.* *Perhaps in the meantime they will develop a better treatment.* *Rather than worry myself sick, I can concentrate on the present moment.*

Table 2. Patients irrational beliefs concerning pain and their healthier alternatives developed in the course of CBT

The study revealed a variety of irrational cognitive thoughts related to the perception of pain and the possible ways of coping with it. On average as much as 69.51% of statements concerning pain and coping with it identified in the course of the interview were classified as irrational. At the same time the high value of the patients' conviction that their irrational beliefs are true was observed ($M=87.33$; $SD=7.61$). The sample of the patients' statements, with the identification of logical errors and their healthier alternatives, are presented in table 2.

The strong tendency towards catastrophizing and exaggeration of the possible consequences of actual facts is worth noting. Another frequent logical error is dichotomous thinking and generalization, which resulted in the patient's perceiving pain as more severe than it really was.

The analysis of the correlations (Kendall's coefficient tau) demonstrated a positive association between the intensity of irrational beliefs and the level of depressiveness as well as the severity of pain (table 3).

The positive associations between both the level of depressiveness and the intensity of pain on the one hand, and all dimensions of catastrophizing and the proportion of irrational beliefs and the conviction that they are true on the other was demonstrated. It is worth noting, however, that these correlation are stronger in relation to the associations taking into consideration the strength of the patient's conviction that his or her own beliefs are true. Furthermore, it must be stressed that the correlations are stronger for the level of irrational beliefs identified in the interview than for the patients' scores on *Pain Catastrophizing Scale*.

Factor	Pain intensity	Depression		
		Total	Affective symptoms	Somatic symptoms
Catastrophizing				
Total	0.58 $p<0.001$	0.48 $p<0.001$	0.50 $p<0.001$	0.44 $p<0.01$
magnification	0.61 $p<0.001$	0.42 $p<0.01$	0.51 $p<0.001$	0.33 $p<0.05$
rumination	0.57 $p<0.001$	0.45 $p<0.001$	0.46 $p<0.01$	0.43 $p<0.01$
helplessness	0.55 $p<0.001$	0.51 $p<0.001$	0.49 $p<0.001$	0.54 $p<0.001$
Irrational beliefs				
Number	0.74 $p<0.001$	0.65 $p<0.001$	0.70 $p<0.001$	0.61 $p<0.001$
Conviction the beliefs are true	0.77 $p<0.001$	0.69 $p<0.001$	0.72 $p<0.001$	0.66 $p<0.001$
Level of emotional discomfort	0.69 $p<0.001$	0.61 $p<0.001$	0.58 $p<0.001$	0.64 $p<0.001$
Depression				
Total	0.56 $p<0.001$	-	-	-
Affective symptoms	0.55 $p<0.001$			
Somatic symptoms	0.58 $p<0.001$			

Table 3. The correlation between irrational beliefs and depression and the intensification of pain in cancer patients

The final post-test showed significant differences in the study variables between the experimental and control groups. In order to demonstrate the differences resulting from the cognitive behavioural therapy, the analysis of variance with repeated measures (ANOVA) was used (table 4).

Factor	Group	Baseline		Post-test		Source of variance		
		M	SD	M	SD	Group $F(\eta^2)$	Time $F(\eta^2)$	Group x Time $F(\eta^2)$
Pain								
Pain intensity	CBT	45.26	3.12	37.07	2.66	n.s.	6.27* (0.14)	31.54** (0.42)
	Control	44.98	3.37	47.39	3.52			
Depression								
Total	CBT	33.28	5.62	26.85	4.47	n.s.	n.s.	34.61*** (0.47)
	Control	32.01	4.96	33.17	4.63			
Affective symptoms	CBT	12.89	3.13	7.64	2.32	n.s.	n.s.	36.87*** (0.48)
	Control	12.85	2.99	13.01	2.81			
Somatic symptoms	CBT	20.37	3.84	19.22	3.17	n.s.	n.s.	n.s.
	Control	19.92	3.01	20.15	4.22			
Catastrophizing								
Total	CBT	33.62	6.02	22.77	4.68	n.s.	n.s.	43.73*** (0.51)
	Control	33.16	5.72	33.82	5.44			
Magnification	CBT	7.07	1.09	4.88	0.84	n.s.	n.s.	48.25*** (0.54)
	Control	6.85	1.11	6.93	1.45			
Rumination	CBT	12.34	2.75	8.75	1.77	n.s.	5.84* (0.06)	8.51* (0.18)
	Control	12.01	3.02	12.89	2.78			
Helplessness	CBT	14.22	3.17	8.12	1.62	n.s.	n.s.	54.18*** (0.57)
	Control	14.28	3.33	13.99	2.61			
Irrational beliefs								
Number	CBT	70.11	9.23	47.69	6.56	n.s.	6.13* (0.11)	66.04*** (0.71)
	Control	69.07	8.89	76.24	8.64			
Conviction the beliefs are true	CBT	86.78	10.36	68.54	5.87	n.s.	n.s.	64.78*** (0.48)
	Control	88.29	9.90	89.10	8.92			
Level of emotional discomfort	CBT	75.42	6.88	73.13	5.94	n.s.	n.s.	n.s.
	Control	74.30	7.13	75.22	6.86			

Table 4. The impact of cognitive behavioural therapy on the intensity of pain, depressiveness and the irrationality of beliefs
n.s. – not significant; * $p<0.05$ ** $p<0.01$ *** $p<0.001$

The analysis demonstrated the decreased severity of pain, the decreased tendency towards catastrophizing and the less strong conviction that the irrational beliefs are true as well as lower proportion of irrational statements among the patients in the CBT group. Moreover, the intensity of depressive symptoms related to affective component (but not somatic) was also reported to have diminished.

The control group exhibited a small but significant increase in the proportion of irrational beliefs and the intensity of pain, whereas no changes in depressiveness or catastrophizing were observed.

6. Discussion

The results confirm the significance of catastrophizing in the intensification of sensations of pain. At the same time the importance of CBT (restructuring patient's beliefs) for the reduction of depressiveness and the severity of pain was demonstrated. This observation points to the fact that the depressiveness in cancer patients suffering from chronic pain is to a large extent determined by situational rather than endogenous factors. It follows that the pharmacological treatment offered to cancer patients should be complemented by psychotherapy. Furthermore, since the link between the intensity of the irrational beliefs regarding pain and the perceived severity of pain has been established, it appears reasonable to recommend behavioural therapy.

The decrease in the tendency towards catastrophizing helps patients to seek activities which might contribute to the improvement of their quality of life. The healthier alternative thoughts expressed in the course of the therapy included the following: *"I can do a lot in spite of the pain"*; *"Now I can do things I've never had time for"*; *"There are a lot of things in my body that function properly and I can take advantage of that"*; *"Actually I live here and now, in this moment. And the pain which lasts a second can be easily endured"*. The last statement points out the beneficial effect of the shortening of the time (temporal) span to the very short period of time.

The healthier alternatives also included the references to the efficacy of the pain medication. The patients' expectations that the medication will help to alleviate their pain increase the probability of it happening. The phenomenon is similar to the placebo effect. A number of studies (cf. Benedetti, 2009) demonstrated that in the chronic pain treatment the patient's expectations concerning the efficacy of the medication significantly improve his or her general condition. During the 13-week observation of the patients suffering from chronic back pain no significant differences in pain severity were observed between the patients who were administered duloxetine and those given placebo (Skljarevski et al., 2009). A number of studies have found that the administration of placebo reduces the severity of pain in a substantial proportion of patients suffering from chronic pain. It is also reported (Wasan et al., 2006) that the patients who show more severe psychopathological symptoms are more susceptible to the placebo effect with regard to the alleviation of chronic back pain. In the current study the patients exhibited more – although not radically – intense depressive symptoms. Therefore, it can be surmised that they are also particularly susceptible to suggestions concerning the efficacy of pharmacology. In the case of the current study, however, we deal with autosuggestion and actual medication rather than placebo.

Finally, it is worth noting that the condition of the patients was more adequately characterized by the strength of irrationality of beliefs identified in the interview rather than the level of catastrophizing determined on the basis of the questionnaire. This observation should encourage researcher to utilize qualitative methods in preference to paper-pencil tests. It follows from the fact that questionnaires, even those of high accuracy, may provide the indicators of the frequency of symptoms and their severity, but they overlook the significance attached to the symptoms by the patient him- or herself. A questionnaire might fail to cover the issues which, because of their significance for the study subject, will be strongly associated with the phenomenon studied.

7. Conclusions

The study confirms the significance of cognitive content in the perception of pain and the development of depressiveness. By reducing the irrationality of thinking cognitive behavioural therapy can help to improve the mental and somatic functioning of cancer patients suffering from chronic pain. Therefore, the introduction of CBT as an complementary treatment in conjunction with traditional pharmacological treatment is worth considering.

Irrespective of their therapeutic outcomes, the methods of cognitive behavioural interview can be more effective than a questionnaire in isolating those patients to whom psychotherapeutic techniques may be particularly beneficial, as it has been found that the irrational beliefs identified in the interview served as a better predictor of sensations of pain than the catastrophizing tested by means of the questionnaire.

Cognitive restructuring in the patients suffering from chronic pain can help them to avoid unnecessary irrational suffering and alleviate both physical pain and despair.

8. References

Almay, B.G. (1987). Clinical characteristics of patients with idiopathic pain syndromes: Depressive symptomatology and patient pain drawings. *Pain*, Vol. 29, No. 3, 335-346

Armstrong, T., Almadrones, L. & Gilbert, M.R. (2005). Chemotherapy-induced peripheral neuropathy. *Oncology Nursing Forum*, Vol. 32, No. 2, pp. 305-311

Arntz, A., Dreessen, L. & Merckelbach, H. (1991). Attention, not anxiety, influences pain. *Behaviour Research and Therapy*, Vol. 29, No. 1, pp. 41-50

Beck, A.T., Rush, A.J., Shaw, B.F. & Emery, G. (1979). *Cognitive therapy of depression*. Guilford Press, New York

Beck, A.T., Steer, R.A. & Brown, G.K. (1996). *Manual for the BDI-II*. The Psychological Corporation, San Antonio, TX

Beck, A.T., Steer, R.A. & Garbin, M.G. (1988). Psychometric properties of the Beck Depression Inventory: Twenty-five years of evaluation. *Clinical Psychology Review*, Vol. 8, No. 1, pp. 77-100

Benedetti, F. (2009). *Placebo effects*. Oxford University Press, ISBN: 978-0-19-955912-1, Oxford

Bishop, S.R. & Warr, D. (2003). Coping, catastrophizing and chronic pain in breast cancer. *Journal of Behavioural Medicine*, Vol. 26, No. 3, pp. 265-281

Bredin, M., Corner, J., Krishnasamy, M., Plant, H., Bailey, C. & A'Hern, R. (1999). Multicentre randomised controlled trial of nursing intervention for breathlessness in patients with lung cancer. *BMJ*, Vol. 318, No. 7188, pp. 901-904

Breitbart, W., Passik, S.D., Casper, D.J., Starr, T.D. & Rogak, L.J. (2009). Psychiatric aspects of pain management in patients with advanced cancer and AIDS, In: *Handbook of psychiatry in palliative medicine* (2 ed.), Chochinov, H.M. & Breitbart, W. (Eds.)., pp. 384-416, Oxford University Press, ISBN: 978-0-19-530107-6, New York

Burton, A.K., Tillotson, K.M., Main, C.J. & Hollis, S. (1995). Psychosocial predictors of outcome in acute and subchronic low back trouble. *Spine*, Vol. 20, No. 6, pp. 722-728

Burton, A.W., Fanciullo, G.J., Beasley, R.D. & Fisch, M.J. (2007). Chronic pain in the cancer survivor: a new frontier. *Pain Medicine*, Vol. 8, No. 2, pp. 189-198

Cathcart, F. (2006). Psychological distress in patients with advanced cancer. *Clinical Medicine*, Vol. 6, No. 2, pp. 148-50

Chapman, S. (2011). Chronic pain syndromes in cancer survivors. *Nursing Standard*, Vol. 25, No. 21, pp. 35-41

Colla, M., Kronenberg, G., Deuschle, M., Meichel, K., Hagen, T., Bohrer, M. & Heuser, I. (2007). Hippocampal volume reduction and HPA-system activity in major depression. *Journal of Psychiatric Research*, Vol. 41, No. 7, (Oct 2007), pp. 553-560

Colyer, H. (2003). The context of radiotherapy care, In: *Supportive care in radiotherapy*, Faithful, S. & Wells, M. (Eds.), pp. 1-16, Churchill Livingstone, Edinburgh

Cowan, P. (2011). Living with chronic pain. *Quality of Life Research: An International Journal of Quality of Life Aspects of Treatment, Care and Rehabilitation*, Vol. 20, No. 3, pp. 307-308

Ellis, A. & Dryden, W. (2007). *The practice of rational emotive behavior therapy* (2 ed.), Springer Publishing Company, ISBN: 0-8261-5471-9, New York

Endler, N.S., Parker, J.D.A. & Summerfeldt, L.J. (1998). Coping with health problems: developing a reliable and valid multidimensional measure. *Psychological Assessment*, Vol. 10, No. 3, pp. 195-205

Goral, A., Lipsitz, J.D. & Gross, R. (2010). The relationship of chronic pain with and without comorbid psychiatric disorder to sleep disturbance and health care utilization: Results from the Israel National Health Survey. *Journal of Psychosomatic Research*, Vol. 69, No. 5, pp. 449-457

Grant, L.D. & Haverkamp, B.E. (1995). A cognitive-behavioral approach to chronic pain management. *Journal of Counseling & Development*, Vol. 74, No. 1, pp. 25-32

Herbert, J., Goodyer, I.M., Grossman, A.B., Hastings, M.H., de Kloet, E.R., Lightman, S.L., Lupien, S.J., Roozendaal, B. & Seckl, J.R. (2006). Do corticosteroids damage the brain? *Journal of Neuroendocrinology*, Vol. 18, No. 6, pp. 393-411

Heszen, I. & Sęk, H. (2007). *Psychologia zdrowia [Health psychology]*, PWN, Warsaw

Hobfoll, S. (1998). *Stress, culture and community. The psychology and philosophy of stress.* Plenum Press, ISBN: 0306459426, New York and London

Kostarczyk, E. (2003). *Neuropsychologia bólu [Neuropsychology of pain]*. PTPN, Poznań

Kutcher, S. & Chehil, S. (2007). *Suicide risk management. A manual for Health Professionals.* Blackwell Publishing, Oxford

Lautenbacher, S. Huber, C., Schöfer, D., Kunz, M., Parthum, A., Weber, P., Roman, C., Griessinger, N. & Sittl, R. (2010). Attentional and emotional mechanisms related to pain as predictors of chronic postoperative pain: A comparison with other psychological and physiological predictors. *Pain*, Vol. 151, No. 3, pp. 722-731

Lazarus, R. & Folkman, S. (1984). *Stress, appraisal and coping*, Springer-Verlag, New York

Leeuw, M., Goossens, M.E., Linton, S., Crombez, G., Boersma, K. & Vlaeyen, J.W.S. (2007). The fear-avoidance model of musculoskeletal pain: Current state of scientific evidence. *Journal of Behavioral Medicine*, Vol. 30, No. 1, pp. 77-94

Linton, S.J., Buer, N., Vlaeyen, J. & Hellsing, A-L. (2000). Are fear-avoidance beliefs related to the inception of an episode of back pain? A prospective study. *Psychology and Health*, Vol. 14, No. 6, pp. 1051-1059

Maultsby, M.C. (1990). *Rational behavior therapy.* Rational Self-Help Books/I'ACT, ISBN 0-932838-08-1, Appleton

Melkumova, K.A., Podchufarova, E.V. & Yakhno, N.N. (2011). Characteristics of cognitive functions in patients with chronic spinal pain. *Neuroscience and Behavioral Physiology*, Vol. 41, No. 1, pp. 42-46

Melzack, R. & Wall, P.D. (1965). Pain mechanisms: a new theory. *Science*, Vol. 150, No. 699, pp. 971-979.

Mok, L.C. & Lee, I.F-K. (2008). Anxiety, depression and pain intensity in patients with low back pain who are admitted to acute care hospitals. *Journal of Clinical Nursing*, Vol. 17, No. 11, pp. 1471-1480

Moorey, S. & Greer, S. (2002). *Cognitive behaviour therapy for people with cancer.* Oxford University Press, ISBN: 0-19-8508866-2, Oxford

Nijs, J., Van de Putte, K., Louckx, F., Truijen, S. & De Meirleir, K. (2008). Exercise performance and chronic pain in chronic fatigue syndrome: The role of pain catastrophizing. *Pain Medicine*, Vol. 9, No. 8, pp. 1164-1172

Reid, M.C., Otis, J., Barry, L.C. & Kerns, R.D. (2003). Cognitive-behavioral therapy for chronic low back pain in older persons: a preliminary study. *Pain Medicine*, Vol. 4, No. 3, pp. 223-230

Rollman, G.B. (2009). Perspectives on hypervigilance. *Pain*, Vol. 141, No. 3, pp. 183-184

Rymaszewska, J. & Dudek, D. (2009). *Zaburzenia psychiczne w chorobach somatycznych [Mental disorders in the somatic illness]*, Via Medica, ISBN: 978-83-7599-045-4, Gdańsk

Sapolsky, R.M. (2000). Glucocorticoids and hippocampal atrophy in neuropsychiatric disorders. *Archives of General Psychiatry*, Vol. 57, No. 10, pp. 925-935

Skljarevski, V., Ossanna, M., Liu-Seifert, H., Zhang, Q., Chappell, A., Iyengar, S., Detke, M. & Backonja, M. (2009). A double-bind, randomized trial of duloxetine versus placebo in management of chronic low back pain. *European Journal of Neurology*, Vol. 16, No. 9, pp. 1041-1048

Sullivan, M.J.L., Bishop, S. & Pivik, J. (1995). The Pain Catastrophizing Scale: Developmental and validation. *Psychological Assessment*, Vol. 7, No. 4, pp. 524-532

Syrjala, K.L., Donaldson, G.W., Davis, M.W. Kippes, M.E. & Carr, J.E. (1995). Relaxation and imagery and cognitive-behavioral training reduce pain during cancer treatment: a controlled clinical trial. *Pain*, Vol. 6, No. 2, pp. 189-198

Tang, N.K., Wright, K.J. & Salkovskis, P.M. (2007). Prevalence and correlates of clinical insomnia co-occuring with chronic back pain. *Journal of Sleep Research*, Vol. 16, No. 1, pp. 85-95

van den Beuken-van Everdingen, M.H., de Rijke, J.M., Kessels, A.G., Schouten, H.C., van Kleef, M. & Patijn, J. (2007). Prevalence of pain in patients with cancer: a systematic review of the past 40 years. *Annals of Oncology*, Vol. 18, No. 9, pp. 1437-1449.

Vedhara, K. & Irwin, M. (Eds.) (2005). *Human psychoneuroimmunology.* Oxford University Press, ISBN: 0-19-852840-X, Oxford

Visovsky, C., Collins, M., Abbott, L., Aschenbrenner, J. & Hart, C. (2007). Putting evidence into practice: evidence-based interventions for chemotherapy-induced peripheral neuropathy. *Clinical Journal of Oncology Nursing*, Vol. 11, No. 6, pp. 901-913

Vowles, K.E., McCracken, L.M. & Eccleston, C. (2008). Patient functioning and catastrophizing in chronic pain: The mediating effects of acceptance. *Health Psyhology*, Vol. 27, No. 2 (Suppl), pp. S136-S143

Wahl, A.K., Rustøen, T., Rokne, B., Lerdal, A., Knudsen, Ø., Miaskowski, C. & Moum, T. (2009). The complexity of the relationship between chronic pain and quality of life: a study of the general Norwegian population. *Quality of Life Research: An International Journal of Quality of Life Aspects of Treatment, Care and Rehabilitation*, Vol. 18, No. 8, pp. 971-980

Wasan, A.D., Kaptchuk, T.J., Davar, G. & Jamison, R.N. (2006). The association between psychopathology and placebo analgesia in patients with discogenic low back pain. *Pain Medicine*, Vol. 7, No. 3, pp. 217-228

Wiliams, J. M. G. (1997). Depression. In: *Science and practice of cognitive behaviour therapy*, Clark, D.M. & Fairburn C.G. (Eds.), pp.259-284, Oxford University Press, Oxford

Wirga, M. & Wojtyna, E. (2010). Udręki zdrowego umysłu. Neuropsychologia cierpienia [Suffering of healthy mind. Neuropsychology of suffering], In: *Wielowymiarowość cierpienia [Many-sidedness of suffering]*, Binnebesel, J., Błeszyński, J. & Domżał, Z. (Eds.), pp.31-51, Wydawnictwo Naukowe WSEZ, Łódź

Witte, W. & Stein, C. (2010). History, definitions, and contemporary viewpoints. In: *Guide to pain management in low-resource settings*, Kopf, A. & Patel, N.B. (Eds.), pp. 3-7, International Association for the Study of Pain, retrieved from www.iasp-pain.org/AM/Template.cfm?Section=Home&Template=/CM/ContentDisplay.cfm&ContentID=12172

Zaza, C. & Baine, N. (2002). Cancer pain and psychosocial factors: A critical review of the literature. *Journal of Pain and Symptom Management*, Vol. 24, No. 5, pp. 526-542

Zimmerman, M.E., Pan, J.W., Hetherington, H.P., Lipton, M.L., Baigi, K. & Lipton, R.B. (2009). Hippocampal correlates of pain in healthy elderly adults: A pilot study. *Neurology*, Vol. 73, No. 19, pp. 1567-1570

13

Therapeutic Strategies in Schizophrenia

Jacqueline Conway
Team 24, London
England

1. Introduction

Schizophrenia is possibly the most notorious of the mental illnesses and the lack of popular understanding of it, with consequent understandable discomfort upon receipt of the diagnosis, persists to the present day. The evolution of terms to describe what is usually understood by health workers in the UK as *learning disability* is a useful illustration of how mental illness generally has come to be understood. :-

English Mental	*IQ under 20*	*IQ 20-30*		*IQ 50-70*
Deficiency Acts 1913-1927	Idiocy	Imbecility		Feeble-mindedndess
Mental Heath Act,	*IQ 0-50*			*IQ 50-70*
England & Wales 1959	Severe subnormality			subnormality
Mental Heath Act,	*IQ 0-50*			*IQ 50-70*
England & Wales 1983	Severe mental impairment			Mental impairment
	(in both instances, previously popularly known as 'mental handicap').			
ICD-10	*IQ rating under 20*	*IQ 20 - 34*	*IQ 35-49*	*IQ 50-69*
1992	Profound learning disability (LD)	Severe LD	Moderate LD	Mild LD

Fig. 1. Progression of statutory understanding of intellectual impairment in the UK.

....Indeed, any condition which affects neurological or intellectual functioning has progressed through an analogous course of understanding. Epilepsy, which is now known to be an abnormality in cerebral neural transmission, was thought of in earlier times to be perhaps a visitation from God or indicative of shamanic ability. Such lurid explanations are now no longer felt to be appropriate, as more has become known about the underlying pathology. The progression of terms used in the understanding of learning disability is an example of similar development. The progression of understanding of schizophrenia in the 20th century has been aided by inductive appreciation of the *pharmacology* of the illness. This idea will be further considered later on here. Although the progression of knowledge is necessarily contemporaneous on all fronts, public perception of it is undoubtedly affected by the social milieu. Thus, in the progression of understanding of schizophrenia, the first step is that the condition was a result of external forces, such as a result of celestial actions, or of God (in monotheistic cultures). Next, there was an understanding of the importance of direct social factors, such as family and immediate social environment. A reflection upon the psychological effects of these led to the final step in this progression: the role of an affected person's biology. Physiological and ultimately, neurophysiological and biochemical alterations in the disease process are deliberated upon at this final stage of understanding.

Geekie and Read, in 2009, provide an elegant expression of how a *narrative framework* allows a protagonist – such as the affected individual, or society – to *make sense of their experiences*. Thus, in the attempt to understand mental illness, alternative narrative frameworks include:

-   madness as a result of *the whim of the deities* (a view prevalent in ancient Greece, for example)
-   the same disturbances being understood as the result of one's *life experiences or circumstances*
-   " " as a result of *faulty brain chemistry.*

"Within the storytelling framework, we might say that these are all different ways of 'storying' the experience of madness." (1)

...Where "storying" can be understood as placing within a narrative framework in order to make the phenomenon intelligible.

There are, of course, multiple possible narrative frameworks. If one is considering the evolution of understanding of schizophrenia, then theological, sociological and biochemical explanatory modes can all be understood as different types of narrative framework. Each attempts to provide a comprehensive explanation for the disorder. Multiple types of explanation exist for many reasons: cultural factors, which include geographical and temporal contexts, as well as educational ones, are perhaps the most important. In this way, the epistemological foundations of an explanatory mode can be easily understood. The existence of several possible types of explanation should lead to the understanding that each relevant branch of knowledge has a contribution to make to the complete understanding of a subject. Different explanations persist because they are useful in their own contexts: therefore, a complete understanding of a subject involves attending to *all* of the potential reasons underlying it. This is summarised in figure 2 on the following page. As this figure shows, it is possible to understand that all factors which influence a mental illness – for our purposes, schizophrenia – can be appreciated as parts of a unified whole, in which every stage will ultimately affect another stage. The appreciation of this interconnected nature of phenomena allows a clinician to provide a *holistic framework* for management of the disorder, and is especially useful when dealing with the mental illnesses.

Continued...

*The cerebral appreciation of any event can be summarised, in **extremely** simplified terms as:*

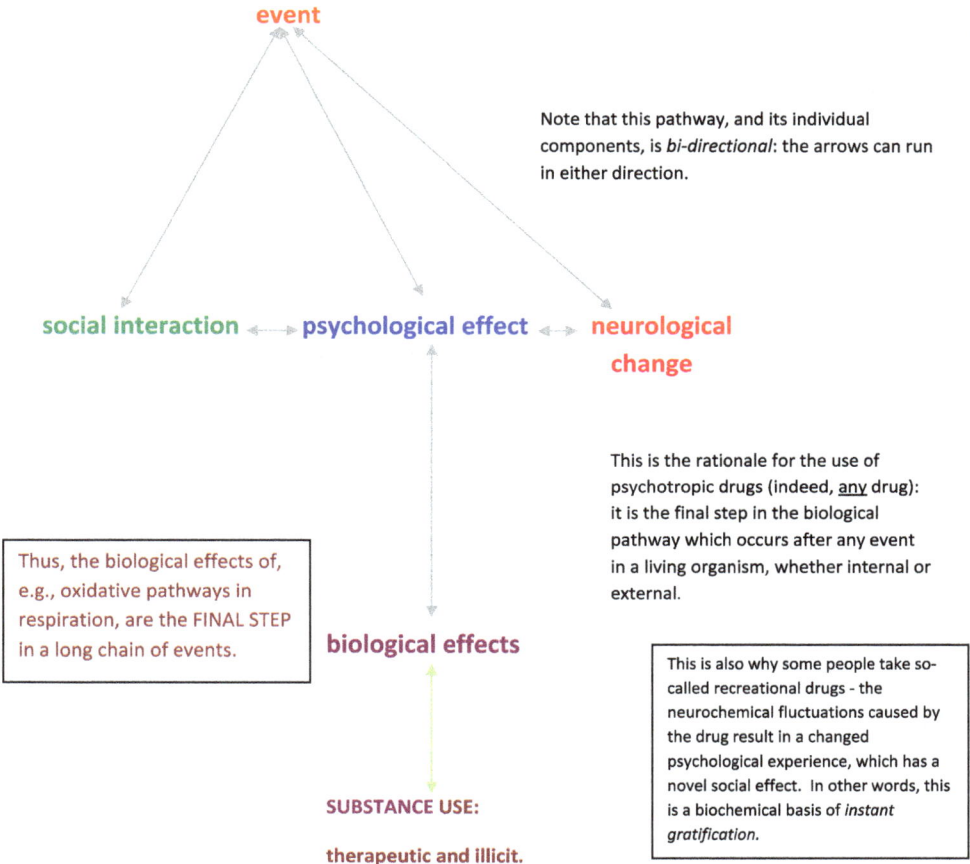

Fig. 2. The interconnected nature of societal, biological and chemical phenomena.

2. Historical overview of the understanding of schizophrenia

Moskovitz and Heim remind us that it is one hundred years since Bleuler originally proposed the concept of the schizophrenic illnesses, in 1911 (2). In their re-appraisal of Eugen Bleuler's original concept of 'Dementia Praecox or the Group of Schizophrenias', it is noted that Bleuler's understanding of this illness was a largely inductive one: he spent a great deal of time with his patients at the Burghölzli institute and his understanding of schizophrenia emerged from this immersive observation. This is reminiscent of modern anthropological fieldwork, and indeed, Bleuler's study was essentially anthropological. This was in marked contrast to the other pioneer of knowledge in schizophrenia, Emil Krapelin. Whereas Bleuler's understanding was 'bottom up' and *inductive,* Krapelin's was 'top down', i.e. theory driven and *deductive.* Both methods of understanding can produce valuable conclusions. The appropriate task to facilitate a complete understanding is to attempt to bring the multiple sets of theories together in a unified and logical whole. Reference to figure 2, on the previous page, can help with this.

Moskovitz and Heim (2) inform us that the term 'schizophrenia' was effectively coined by Bleuler in 1911. It is perfectly possible that some of the rather vivid explanations noted above were similarly previously used to render a phenomenon resembling schizophrenia intelligible, by placing it within a clear narrative framework.

Romme *et al* (3) discuss the case of perhaps one of the most famous voice-hearers in history, St. Jeanne D'Arc [Joan of Arc]. 'Voice-hearing' here refers to a particular subtype of the psychiatric symptom of auditory hallucination. Auditory hallucination – i.e. hearing audible sounds (including intelligible voices either speaking to or about the affected person) in clear consciousness when there is no physical cause for them – *may* be an important symptom of schizophrenia. In schizophrenic illness, there are often associated ideas which make sense of this symptom; these ideas can solidify into unshakeable associated, consequent delusions. Hence, delusions are performing the *storying* function (1), rendering the psychotic phenomena intelligible to the person who is experiencing them.

Romme *et al* discuss how auditory hallucinations, rather than being dismissed out of hand as an indication of psychosis and thus disregarded, can be actively worked with. This validation of the affected person's symptoms is an important element in that person's eventual recovery. There are several alternative explanations for the phenomenon of voice-hearing. A wry aphorism about this is that if you talk to God, you are religious, whereas if God talks to you, you're schizophrenic. As a clinician, I have always noticed that a psychotic person's delusions are reflective of the current temporal context. The cover of the book by Professor Romme and colleagues about voice-hearing and recovery depicts Jeanne D'Arc in battle. She was a French peasant girl who claimed to hear the voice of God calling upon her to free her nation from English domination. This occurred towards the end of the Hundred Years War (1337-1453). Jeanne D'Arc led her compatriots to many important victories as a result of this 'divine guidance'. After her capture, at the age of nineteen in 1431, she was tried and burned at the stake as a witch. Subsequent regal, then ecclesiastical intervention saw her first declared as a martyr and much later, beatified. In the early twentieth century, she was canonized and as St. Jeanne D'Arc, is one of the five patron saints of France (3). This reflects the importance of the cultural context of auditory hallucinations and their interpretation. In fifteenth century Catholic France, 'hearing the voice of God' could reasonably have been understood as a sign of divine communication. Therefore, the 'divine direction' of Joan of Arc to free her nation from the English in the 1420s would have been unsurprising. In late twentieth and twenty-first centuries in rich industrialised countries, a similar phenomenon would be understood as a sign of psychosis which represents an indication for therapy, most usually pharmacological.

It is worthwhile to briefly reflect upon the history of the treatment of people with mental illness. The profound lack of understanding of, and inability to explain, mental illness led to the majority of people affected by it to be excluded from society: indeed, the archaic term for a psychiatrist is *alienist*, which implies involvement with those outside the usual boundaries of society. A few voice-hearers, such as Jeanne D'Arc, have played important historical roles. The vast majority of others, however, together with their affected fellows, were excluded from society. From the seventeenth century onwards, this was often in large lunatic asylums. Medical involvement in such asylums was confined to treating the physical maladies of the residents. It was not until the mid to late eighteenth century that figures such as Pinel in Paris and Chiarugi in Tuscany began to advocate the humane treatment of asylum inmates. Pinel, together with his overseer Pussin at the Bicêtre hospital in Paris introduced compassionate reforms in the management of the patients there (4). Their later contemporary Chiarugi, in Tuscany in 1789, asserted that:

"...it is a supreme moral duty and medical obligation to respect the mental patient as a person" (4).

The foundations of the Italian therapeutic movement known as *Democratic Psychiatry* can be seen here. This sequence of events represented an enormous progression in the care of the mentally ill. Pinel later (in 1801) emphatically advocated for the inclusion of mental disorders as a branch of medicine. As a result, he is regarded as the originator of psychiatry as a medical discipline. Thus, we can say – in light of the earlier remarks here- that Pinel *brought psychiatry into the narrative framework of medicine.*

While the introduction of humane treatment of the mentally ill represented a significant advance on previous approaches, the discovery of effective psychotropic medications was really what 'unlocked the doors of the asylums'. It was not until the discovery of lithium salts as an effective treatment of mania (by Cade in 1949) and the synthesis and subsequent use of chlorpromazine as a major tranquiliser (by Delay and Deniker in 1952) that people who had previously been destined to spend the rest of their lives in asylums could reasonably expect to return to society. Since then, the understanding and development of drug treatments for mental illness has grown apace. The pharmacological appreciation of the nature of schizophrenia began by studying the known chemical effects of the major tranquilisers such as chlorpromazine. Recognition that this drug blocked dopamine receptors - potentially leading to symptoms of iatrogenic Parkinsonism - is what preceded the subsequent explosion of neurochemical understanding of schizophrenia. In this way, by effectively working backwards from the known biochemical effects of a medication, the neuropathology of particular illnesses has come to be appreciated. In other words, inductive reasoning from known psychotropic drug actions led to the understanding of the bases of pathology of these illnesses. Of course, this understanding has continued to grow and some of the consequent latest developments in the neurophysiological field will be considered later on here.

3. Current pharmacological and neurophysiological knowledge about schizophrenia

As indicated above, the first instances of this were arrived at by inductive reasoning about the mechanisms of action of the earliest widely-available psychotropic drugs. In the process of obtaining supplementary information about this knowledge, areas requiring further investigation have, of course, been opened up. Some of these were to further understand the pharmacological mechanisms and some of this work has necessarily explored the underlying neuropathology of schizophrenia. In the process of doing so, further therapeutic avenues became apparent. Miyamoto *et al* (5) wrote a comprehensive review of pharmacological treatments for schizophrenia in 2005. Important work had already been carried out on the detailed neurophysiology and pathology of the disease: in my opinion, the most significant findings were about the importance of sensory gating (6, 7) and of the roles of *excitotoxicity* (8) and *apoptosis* (9) in the presentation of, and progression of this disease. Site-specific dopamine receptor activity can be influenced *either* by (e.g.) interneuronal sensory gating *or* by a simple dose-response effect: in the latter case, a high receptor density implies that low doses of the particular agent will affect that receptor. In contrast, a low receptor density requires a higher dose of binding agent. For example, the second-generation antipsychotic agents sulpride and amisulpiride have differing biological profiles at different doses. These drugs bind to dopamine D2 receptors in the temporal lobe cortex at low doses, conferring their excellent antipsychotic activity. At higher doses, these agents bind to D2 receptors in the corpus striatum, causing difficult extra-pyramidal side effects -again, including iatrogenic Parkinsonian symptoms (5). Therefore, this implies that D2 receptors are at a high density in the temporal cortex, but at a lower density in the striatum, which explains the dose-response effect. At other sites, such as area CA3 of the hippocampus, interneuronal sensory gating is the phenomenon which determines post-synaptic D2 activity (10).

Miyamoto *et al* (5) remind us that for any antipsychotic drug to be clinically effective, it *must* display occupancy of cerebral dopamine D2 receptors. As we have already seen, the particular site of the involved D2 receptor is important. To reiterate, this can be partly determined physiologically (e.g. pre-synaptically), or physically, by the ratio of available drug to available receptor site.

Dopamine receptor blockade was the main mode of action of the first-generation antipsychotic drugs: however, the therapeutic window available for this is extremely narrow. The optimal level of cerebral D2 receptor occupancy classically lies only between 65% to 70%. Below this, there is often no clinical response – although there are a few affected people who *will* show a therapeutic response to very low doses of antipsychotic drug. Above this level of receptor occupancy, symptoms of iatrogenic Parkinsonism, such as tardive dyskinesia, become a real problem. This is further complicated by the fact that chronic treatment with the first-generation ('typical') antipsychotic drugs causes a homeostatic increase of D2 receptors (5). Of course, chronic treatment is the most usual clinical scenario. Ken Steele, a now deceased, well-known advocate of service users' rights in the United States, summarised this succinctly. –

"...Just as a diabetic needs to take insulin to control diabetes, a schizophrenic must remain on medication- each and every day. It's a question of maintenance. ...Schizophrenia is a disease that *can* be controlled, but not yet cured. " (11, original emphasis)

Steele correctly emphasised the chronic nature of pharmacological treatment for schizophrenia. Although he was writing in 2001, the position is unchanged today, some 10 years later: schizophrenia remains "...a disease that *can* be controlled, but not yet cured".

Empirical experience with the first generation of antipsychotic drugs showed that the D2 receptor model clearly could not explain the whole pathological picture of schizophrenia. Work was therefore understandably directed towards trying to find out more about this, because it became apparent that *schizophrenia is not simply a process of excessive dopaminergic activity centred on the cerebral D2 receptors*. In order to further elucidate the neuropathology of schizophrenia, one important branch of work has investigated the role of *sensory gating* in schizophrenia (6, 7, 10, 12). Sensory gating is the process where the conscious mind devotes the majority of its attention to the task which it is directly presented with. Other sensory stimuli are deemed irrelevant while the task in hand is focussed on. A formal definition is given by Potter *et al* (12): ". . . Sensory gating refers to the *pre-attentional* habituation of responses to repeated exposure to the same sensory stimulus." [my emphasis].

A further explanation of this is given by Conway in 2009 (10):

"...Efficient sensory gating allows a person to 'screen out', or ignore background stimuli, such as the noise of a ventilation motor, or traffic outside a window. If the person is unable to do this, as in acute schizophrenia, the now intrusive stimulus may acquire a delusional significance. This is explicable by the pathological cerebral functioning which occurs in schizophrenia: delusions may represent a conscious attempt by the person to comprehend the contemporaneous neurophysiological events in his/her brain. Correctly functioning sensory gating stops the possible misinterpretation of cerebral events."

Javanbakht (7) notes that there is a "...fronto-limbic imbalance..." which he proposes as one of the causes of disrupted sensory gating. I would propose that *excitotoxicity* (8) is perhaps the cause of this imbalance: excitotoxicity represents the consequence of unremitting neuronal stimulation. One result of this is that the content of affected neurones is exhausted and the resultant cellular debris is catabolised by astrocytes. These latter cells are acting, in effect, as cerebral macrophages, clearing the non-functional cellular material produced as a result of *apoptosis* (9). Repeated exacerbations of schizophrenia result in repeated instances of apoptosis, ultimately leading to the cortical (frontal) atrophy typical of chronic schizophrenia. Therefore, a functional fronto-limbic imbalance could be caused by excitotoxic, apoptotic tissue loss in the (pre) frontal cortex. The especially aggressive pathological process which underlies schizophrenia is exemplified by the fact that negative symptoms – which are a possible consequence of cerebral hypofunction caused by actual apoptotic neuronal loss –can be seen in a first attack of schizophrenia (10).

Unremitting cortico-limbic stimulation can be prevented by correctly functioning sensory gating (6, 7, 10, 12, 13). Here, *nicotinic activation,* especially of hippocampal area CA3 (10, 13) will prevent this unremitting stimulation, and its apoptotic consequence (9). The operative nicotinic receptor - the α7 receptor in area CA3 of the hippocampus - (7, 10, 13) desensitises very quickly. Short bursts of nicotinic enhancement, such as that provided by cigarette smoking (10, 13) – or theoretically by nicotine chewing-gum – would, importantly, allow a *transient normalisation of dysfunctional sensory gating.* Therefore, the notoriously heavy cigarette-smoking rate of people with schizophrenia, an attempt at self-medication, (10, 13, 14, 15, 16, 17) might be preventable and thus, important health benefits could be afforded to this vulnerable patient group if the role of nicotinic transmission is remembered (10).

The search for more efficient antipsychotic medication was stimulated, in part, by the experience of the limited efficacy of antipsychotic drugs which had existed hitherto. Certainly the currently available antipsychotic agents represent a great advance on their earlier predecessors, although they are not without difficult side-effects of their own. This simple fact tells us that our understanding of schizophrenia remains incomplete. It was noted above how a relatively simple entity such as dose-response can give an indication about comparative site-specific receptor density. Such working hypotheses can now, fortunately, be confirmed or refuted with the help of powerful neuroimaging techniques such as positron emission tomography (PET scanning), single-photon emission computed tomography (SPECT scanning), or functional magnetic resonance (fMRI) scanning. However, perhaps the most important factor with regard to pharmacological treatments for schizophrenia is to emphasise *the necessity for lifelong continuation of medication* such that the inherent pathology is not allowed to progress. Attention is again drawn to Ken Steele's quote (11): schizophrenia is exactly analogous to diabetes, but the schizophrenic illness process affects the brain.

4. Psychological approaches to the management of schizophrenic illness

Of course, pharmacological treatments are not the only option in schizophrenia. Remembering the importance of holistic treatment – for any illness – one should consider non-medication based adjunctive managements as part of a treatment package. Following on from the statement immediately above, any illness which affects the brain will also consequently affect the mind, thus allowing the possibility of psychological treatments. (This rubric also includes the *social manipulations* employed therapeutically in this illness.) These have proved to be particularly successful in schizophrenia when employed as part of a treatment programme including appropriate pharmacological and social adjustments. Not only does psychological treatment provide a useful adjunct to pharmacological treatment, it has been shown to lower the maintenance medication requirement in this illness (18). In a thoughtful 2004 paper about the efficacy of cognitive behaviour therapy (CBT) for psychotic illness, Tarrier and Wykes performed a meta- analysis of 20 randomised controlled trails of CBT compared to treatment as usual. They found that 14 of these trails had at least "...a small [positive] effect size, and 3 a large [positive] effect size" (18). These authors drew the cautious conclusion that CBT for psychosis was thus able to reduce positive symptoms in schizophrenia (and therefore the need for antipsychotic medication).

A large contributor to this was the effect of *listening to the affected person's symptoms*. The value of listening to symptoms really cannot be overemphasised, principally because of two important issues:

- the validation of an affected person's experience and
- assessment of the current progression of pathology.

Barker *et al* (19) noted that in their study, both the affected people themselves and their immediate social contacts were "not heard by professionals", and their beliefs and opinions about the illness process were discounted. Nine years later, Owens *et al* (20) identified "...an existing dearth of evidence on service users' experiences of mental health services." This implies that subjective experience of the affected person in mental illness continues to be ignored. The importance of listening to symptoms is that they can clearly tell the observer about the likely coincident pathology. The table on the next page is produced from a first-hand account of the progression of schizophrenia (21), which I have correlated with the likely coincident neuropathology.

Thus, one of the most useful features of the psychological approaches to the management of schizophrenia is *validation of the affected person's experience*. As one can see from the following table, by listening to the affected person, a clinician obtains a very clear expression of the likely current pathology. The first-hand effect of *not* listening to an affected person's symptoms is neatly summarised in the following quote, from a mental health academic who had spent twelve months being detained in hospital under the Mental Health Act, with schizophrenia. -

"...My strange religious beliefs were perhaps quite rightly classified as delusional and discounted...*but this left me with the impression that my experiences...were also being discounted...*" (24, my emphasis)

The point made above and in Figure 3, about the importance of listening to the content of hallucinatory voices perhaps reminds us of perhaps how short-sighted this person's clinicians were. As another example of the importance of listening, the testimonial data collected by Barker *et al* is sobering for a therapeutic readership. –

"...They all said the same things: you're hallucinating, they said. I thought: what's caused this? So they said the damaged area of the head, this bit round here [*no indication of area given in transcript*], that's all I was told, really."

Reported subjective experience: verbatim quotes from Snyder (21).	Comment, including when relevant, possible operative neuropathology.
"I developed schizophrenia gradually over a period of nine years, with the most severe symptoms appearing when I was twenty-eight years old."	This puts his probable age of onset at nineteen years old. Late adolescence is the typical age of onset for the schizophrenic illnesses, which require sufficient maturity in the affected neural pathways before the pathology can express itself.
"I cannot think of anything physical or psychological that could have triggered a change in my mental state. I had wonderful, supportive parents, relatives and friends, and I had a wonderful childhood."	The onset of a psychotic illness is, more often than not, triggered by an event which anyone would find severely upsetting. The course of the illness can be further exacerbated by ongoing social or psychological stressors. Mr. Snyder is fortunate in that neither of these apply to him, suggesting that his illness had a very strong neurological basis which, if coupled with the above stressors, may well have been much more severe. This is an example of the genetic heterogeneity of schizophrenic phenotypes.
"Somewhere between the ages of nineteen and twenty-one, I was exposed to the mathematical idea of fractals...I thought I was going to discover some incredible and fabulous mathematical principle that would transform the way we view the universe...Even though I had no evidence to substantiate my self-image, I knew in my heart that I was just like Einstein..."	Here, Mr. Snyder is clearly using a *manic defence* to make sense of his progressive excessive mesolimbic dopaminergic discharge. A manic defence is where the affected person adopts a grandiose explanation for (e.g.) their coincident cerebral pathology. Grandiosity can also be a feature of transient hyperdopaminergia, as seen both in acute schizophrenia and acute mania, or in hypomania.
"At about...twenty-two, I had my first significant paranoid episodes...I started to think about images from horror movies where an insane man breaks into the house and kills everyone...later...I hurt my leg and...feeling very vulnerable ...the nurse might try to infect me with the AIDS virus by injecting me with a tainted needle..."	Here, this gentleman is describing what the progression of hyperdopaminergic discharge feels like. By now he may well have suffered some excitotoxic cell damage (8). However, because he was fortunate in having numerous effective social supports and was well-engaged in treatment, his illness was not allowed to progress to any significant extent and thus it is probable that any excitotoxic cell loss (8) was consequently limited.
"In my second psychotic episode, I experienced for the first time what I can confidently say were auditory and visual hallucinations...At the time, these hallucinations seemed real to me, absolutely real...my family tried to get me medical help. Medications were prescribed, but I	The aggressive nature of the underlying pathology of Mr. Snyder's illness is clearly demonstrated here. The onset of auditory hallucinations may well have been have a consequence of disrupted sensory gating (6,10). The lack of insight, e.g. the lack of acceptance of a psychiatric illness, is common for people affected by severe psychoses. To paraphrase

refused to take them. I didn't believe anything was wrong with me... – those pills were for crazy people!"	Nelson (22), hallucinatory voices and their consequent belief systems are as real and rational to the affected person as the fact that I happen to have two arms and two legs. This is what makes schizophrenia such a problematic illness to treat: like all the mental illnesses, it profoundly alters one's experience of reality. As such, the protagonists' reality at the time has to be actively worked with in order for this person to move forward productively.
"After several months I finally decided to take the medication (Geodon) [=ziprasidone]...I developed a severe case of depression...I wanted to die rather than continue to experience this feeling...At the end of my second year taking Geodon, I began to experience severe akathisia. This unusual type of anxiety is the worst emotional experience I have ever experienced in my entire life..."	Depression is a very common part of the pathological progression of schizophrenia: it's appearance is so common that it may well be an intrinsic consequence of the underlying pathology- possibly due to excitotoxicity (8) caused by apoptosis (9). Akathisia is a type of physical restlessness which is uncontrollable: the affected person has, scatalogically, extremely severe 'ants in their pants'.
"My doctor switched my medication to Zyprexa [=olanzapine], and the akathisia gradually diminished...I now believe that I have fully recovered from schizophrenia, and I realise that my recovery is owed entirely to medication...I did not pursue any type of psychoanalysis. I simply took the medication..."	The idiosyncratic nature of a person's response to treatment is well-demonstrated here. Both ziprasidone and olanzapine are newer antipsychotic medications, which generally have far fewer side effects than their older precursors. In spite of this, ziprasidone – which reputedly has much less tendency to cause weight gain than the commonly-used olanzapine – didn't prove suitable for Mr Snyder. The fact that he "did not pursue any type of psychoanalysis" and still recovered is attributable to this gentleman's excellent social supports. This is in marked contrast to other first-hand accounts, e.g. Steele (11) and Schiller (23): although Mr. Steele was markedly lacking in social support, Mr. Snyder was not. This again indicates the idiosyncratic nature of responses to therapeutic efforts in schizophrenia. A likely explanation is that there is a continuum of severity along the spectrum of schizophrenic illness.

Fig. 3. (above) The probable relationship between symptoms experienced in schizophrenia and causative pathology.

...and:

"...they just didn't want to listen to the patients' side at all: they would make their diagnoses and that was it."

(Both verbatim quotes from Barker *et al* [19]; my addition to first quote.)

...Again, referring especially to the last comment, the success of the psychological managements of schizophrenia, with their essential *validation* of a person's symptoms is unsurprising. As has been stated earlier here, it can clearly be seen that delusions are an attempt by the affected person at storying their experience (1). Another, equally important facet of the psychological approaches is the degree of *empowerment* that they afford the affected person (24). *Education* about the nature of the illness and how an affected person can recognise a potential worsening of symptoms and act to prevent an exacerbation is extremely important. Employment of psychological techniques of management as part of a treatment programme for schizophrenia can render consumption of antipsychotic medication an emphatic choice for the affected person rather than passive compliance- the latter is unfortunately the usual situation.

Psychological treatments for schizophrenia include an array of possibilities (18, 22, 25, 26): cognitive behavioural therapy [in its many variations] personal therapy, psychotherapy [again, with many variations of type] and compliance therapy. All of the psychotherapeutic approaches overlap to some degree. A particularly important ingredient of the psychological therapies for schizophrenia is the degree of empowerment of the affected person: these therapies rely on the agency of the affected person in the maintenance of their own health. As has been indicated above, validation, together with empowerment are two very important contributors to the improvement in, and maintenance of, ego strength. To reiterate an earlier assertion here, the establishment of a robust *therapeutic alliance* between the affected person and the treating team is a significant positive contributor to the eventual success of the treatment. The proven success of methods such as cognitive therapy for schizophrenia is undoubtedly partly attributable to the affected person's experiences being listened to or validated (19, 20, 23). In cognitive therapy, the affected person him/herself becomes the agent of therapeutic change. One facet of cognitive therapy for schizophrenia involves the affected person actively challenging a delusional belief. As an example, it is not uncommon for a person suffering from acute schizophrenia to believe that they are evil. (Hence an acute attack of schizophrenia can include depressive aspects which are experienced as delusional beliefs, or as persecutory hallucinatory voices.) In cognitive therapy, the protagonist would be advised to challenge this psychotic expression of experience by (e.g.) asking the hallucinatory voice to provide evidence for their statement. The affected person is taught how to provide evidence to the contrary. Hence, *dysfunctional thoughts are confronted.* This is the general principle of cognitive therapy, wherever it is used. To pursue this hypothetical example further:

Hallucinatory voice: "You're evil."

Affected person: "No I'm not. I do voluntary work at the local charity shop twice a week and they really like me there."

... and here, the importance of appropriate *social manipulations* as a therapeutic tool becomes evident.

To combat dysfunctional thoughts, as in this example, the person must have enough *ego strength* to be able to do so. This is the aim of the whole treatment package, but especially applies to psychological techniques used in management. The ability to challenge delusional beliefs in cognitive therapy or in psychotherapy for psychosis depends on good ego-strength in the affected person. Therefore, at first glance, it might seem counter-intuitive to employ psychotherapeutic methods in schizophrenia where one of the core pathological features is a disruption of the protagonists' individuality (and thus, by definition, ego-strength). However, in common with all therapies for all illnesses, the aim of treatment is to arrest – or, at the very least, alleviate – the disease process. Psychotherapeutic approaches for schizophrenia centre upon maintaining the affected person's ego-integrity. Psycho-education is thus an immensely important part of the treatment process. If the affected person can understand the need for continued medication and further, if they are able to use psychological techniques to combat a resurgence of symptoms should these arise, the combination is, again immensely empowering. It is thus unsurprising that the eventual dose of maintenance medication can be lowered (18).

Interested readers are referred to the wealth of excellent practical texts for cognitive therapy in schizophrenia, such as Nelson (22). While cognitive therapy has often been successfully used to aid compliance with medication, we have seen here that effective therapy of this kind with a well-engaged service user is known to reduce the required dose of maintenance medication. This is undoubtedly because the affected person can react in a therapeutic manner to the resurgence of symptoms. Other approaches to the presence of hallucinatory voices in schizophrenia include using distraction techniques: some affected people find that listening to music on a personal stereo blocks or drowns out their hallucinatory voices.

As proponents of psychotherapy for the psychoses readily agree, psychotherapy is not a suitable treatment option for everyone affected by schizophrenia. Again, this is perfectly intelligible: while there are treatment approaches which are generally applicable – such as the employment of a drug which has some dopamine D2 antagonism as an antipsychotic measure - each treatment regime must ideally be individually tailored as far as possible. One is referred again to figure 2, to be reminded of the holistic picture in treatment of mental illness. The importance of the holistic picture is emphasised in a review edited by Gleeson, Killackey and Krstev (27): within this review, the assertion is that a therapeutic alliance between proponents of the biochemical and psychodynamic models of schizophrenia is long overdue. Several essays within the review echo this sentiment.

5. Social manipulations in the treatment of schizophrenia

Social and psychological manipulations for illness overlap to a slight degree, most obviously in their therapeutic effects. The theoretical example of combating dysfunctional beliefs in the cognitive treatment of schizophrenia above indicates how important social conditions are. Remembering (from figure 2) that social events produce physiological changes, it is essential to consider a person's social situation when attempting to optimise their functional capacity. Therefore, the affected person must be in a stable and appropriate living situation: the high frequency of serious mental illness in the homeless and vulnerably housed population is testament to the importance of the 'home' situation. While some people with schizophrenia are able, with regular medication and regular clinical review, to maintain paid employment, not everyone is this position is. The usefulness of the attention of a social worker, or similarly qualified professional who has expertise in negotiating fields such as finance, housing and employment, is evident. Active feedback between all specialist practitioners about an affected person is essential: this is the model of the old *Community Mental Health Team* (CMHT) in the UK. The usefulness of this particular model is that a single group of practitioners gets to know the ill person well, and is aware of factors which may alleviate, or aggravate their illness. The current (2011) fragmentation of care in the UK therefore can be potentially unhelpful for the affected person. It is well-recognised that the CMHT can become a surrogate family for the person with a chronic illness such as schizophrenia. In this context, perhaps it is useful to reminisce upon the work of Leff *et al* (28), who described the importance of *expressed emotion* (EE).

EE is understood as the level of critical comments and hostility toward the affected person from a particular carer. Also, the degree of emotional over-involvement of that carer is noted (28, 29). Since these topics were first considered, from the late 1950s onwards, high EE has been repeatedly and reliably shown to be associated with a higher relapse rate of schizophrenia. With the moves towards care in the community of mentally ill people, people with long-term mental illnesses living in residential facilities essentially have statutory replacements for their biological families. Therefore, the principles of EE are similarly applicable. While the degree of EE can be reduced with appropriate staff training, many care personnel in residential facilities are amongst the least trained (29). Previous studies in this area have found that critical personally directed comments towards people with schizophrenia were due to an attribution of dysfunctional behaviours directly to the affected person, rather than to their illness. Psycho-education about the nature and natural history of schizophrenia is therefore a great help for all those closely involved with it: patients, carers and staff members. One of the effects of education is a reduction in EE due to a better understanding of the illness process.

Many of the social aspects of a person's situation are the pragmatic ones, e.g.

- Can they care for themselves independently, or do they need help with tasks such as eating regularly and maintaining personal hygiene?
- Do they have enough money to live on?
- Are they eligible for state benefits?
- Are they able to work, and if so, how does this affect any benefits?
- Do they have secure tenancy of their homes?

One can see that a social worker, or similarly trained professional, is ideally placed to answer these concerns. Remembering the holistic package of treatment which should ideally be provided for the person with schizophrenia, the significant potential reduction in stress makes an important contribution to the maintenance of well-being.

6. Future developments in the treatment of schizophrenia

Unfortunately, constraints of space do not permit a full discussion here of potential future developments in schizophrenia. With respect to future drug developments, the reader is referred to the excellent review by Miyamoto *et al* (5). The pharmacology section above has already mentioned the potential usefulness of nicotinic adjuncts to the treatment of schizophrenia. My particular interest is in the use of substances such as nicotine chewing-gum to provide the short-term enhancement of sensory gating which would normalise the dysfunction seen in schizophrenia (10). The sustained activation of nicotinic receptors such as that provided by nicotine patches is probably unsuitable, because the involved receptors - the α7 nicotinic receptors in the hippocampus- desensitise quickly (13, 30). Galantamine is an α7 ligand which allosterically modulates the receptor to increase neurotransmission (30, 31). The potentiation of nicotinic transmission would therefore be potentially expected to transiently improve the sensory gating deficit intrinsic to schizophrenia and thus improve symptoms (6, 7, 10). The recognition of the importance of nicotinic neurotransmission in schizophrenia has led to the investigation of drugs such as galantamine as potential therapeutic agents for schizophrenia; indeed, symptomatic improvement was seen with the addition of galantamine to the therapeutic regime in two very small samples of patients (29, 30). Enhancement of glutamatergic transmission is another area in which pharmacological effort may be directed in the search for new drug treatments for schizophrenia. Noting the remarks above about the importance of holistic treatments in mental illness, an obvious direction for future treatments in schizophrenia is greater multidisciplinary involvement. Recent legislative changes in the UK, with the amendment of the Mental Health Act 1983 in 2007, pay attention to this. The senior clinician in charge of a service user's treatment used to invariably be the consultant psychiatrist. Under the new Mental Health Act, the person in overall charge of the service user's care is the *responsible clinician* (RC). The RC can be any of the *approved clinicians* (ACs):

- a registered medical practitioner
- a registered mental health nurse (including registered learning disability nurse)
- a registered occupational therapist
- a chartered clinical psychologist, and
- a registered social worker   (32)

The widening of professions eligible for the senior role of responsible clinician is a reflection of greater multidisciplinary involvement in the delivery of care to the service user. Thus, more effort is directed towards holistic care, which is important.

This emphasis provides a useful point at which to close this chapter. One is reminded that especially in the mental illnesses, as in all illness, phenomena are interconnected. In consequence, change at any point on the pathway of causative/therapeutic events can have potential profound effects on all other stages in the pathway.

7. References

[1] Jim Geekie and John Read (2009) *Making Sense of Madness: Contesting the Meaning of Schizophrenia* International Society for the Psychological treatment of Schizophrenia and other psychoses (ISPS) Routledge: London.

[2] Andrew Moskowitz and Gerhard Heim (2011) *Eugen Bleuler's Dementia Praecox or the Group of Schizophrenias (1911): A Centenary Appreciation and Reconsideration* Schizophrenia Bulletin 37 (3):. 471–479.

[3] Prof. Marius Romme, Dr Sandra Escher, Jacqui Dillon, Dr Dirk Corstens, Prof. Mervyn Morris (2009) *Living with Voices: 50 stories of recovery* PCCS Books: Ross-on-Wye, Herefordshire

[4] Pierre Pichot (2000) The *history of psychiatry as a medical speciality* Chapter 1.4 of *New Oxford Textbook of Psychiatry* editor M G Gelder, Juan J López-Ibor Jr., Nancy C Andreasen Oxford University press, New York

[5] S Miyamoto, G E Duncan, C E Marx and J A Lieberman (2005) *Treatments for schizophrenia: a critical review of pharmacology and mechanisms of action of antipsychotic drugs* Molecular Psychiatry 10:79-104.

[6] Lawrence E Adler, Ann Olincy, Merilyne Waldo, Josette G Harris, Jay Griffith, Karen Stevens, Karen Flach, Herbert Nagamoto, Paula Bickford, Sherry Leonard and Robert Freedman (1998) *Schizophrenia, sensory gating and nicotinic receptors* Schizophrenia Bulletin 24(2):189–202.

[7] Arash Javanbakht (2006) *Sensory gating deficits, pattern completion and disturbed fronto-limbic balance, a model for description of hallucinations and delusions in schizophrenia* Medical Hypotheses 67:1173-1184

[8] Deutsch Stephen I, Rosse Richard B, Schwartz Barbara L, Mastropaolo John (2001) *A revised excitotoxic hypothesis of schizophrenia: therapeutic implications* Clinical Neuropharmacology 24(1):43-9.

[9] L. Fredrik Jarskog (2006) *Apoptosis in schizophrenia: pathophysiologic and therapeutic considerations.* Current Opinion in Psychiatry 19(3):307-12.

[10] J L C Conway (2009) *Exogenous nicotine normalises sensory gating in schizophrenia; therapeutic implications* Medical Hypotheses 73: 259-262.

[11] Ken Steele and Claire Berman (2001) *The Day the Voices Stopped (A Memoir of Madness and Hope)* Basic Books: New York.

[12] David Potter, Ann Summerfelt, James Gold, Robert Buchanan (2006) *Review of clinical correlates of P50 sensory gating abnormalities in patients with schizophrenia.* Schizophrenia Bulletin 32(4):692-700.

[13] Dalack Gregory W, Healy Daniel J, Meador-Woodruff James H (1998) *Nicotine dependence in schizophrenia: clinical phenomena and laboratory findings* American Journal of Psychiatry155(11):1490-501.

[14] Ciara Kelly, Robin M. McCreadie (1999) *Smoking habits, current symptoms, and premorbid characteristics of schizophrenia patients in Nithsdale, Scotland* American Journal of Psychiatry 156(11):1751-8.

[15] Hughes JR, Hatsukami DK, Mitchell JE, Dahlgren LA (1986) *Prevalence of smoking among psychiatric outpatients* American Journal of Psychiatry 143:993-7.

[16] Joseph P McEvoy, Shirley Brown (1999) *Smoking in first-episode patients with schizophrenia* American Journal of Psychiatry 156(7):1120-2.

[17] Carol A Tamminga (1999) editor, *Schizophrenia in a molecular age* Review of Psychiatry 18(4):12-4.

[18] Nicholas Tarrier and Til Wykes (2004) *Is there evidence that cognitive behaviour therapy is an effective treatment for schizophrenia? A cautious or cautionary tale?* Behaviour Research and Therapy 42: 1377-1401

[19] Sarah Barker, Tony Lavender and Nicola Morant (2001) *Client and family narratives on schizophrenia* Journal of Mental Health 10, 2: 199-212.

[20] C Owens, D Crone, L Kilgour, W el Ansari (2010) *The place and promotion of well-being in mental health services: a qualitative investigation* Journal of Psychiatric and Mental Health Nursing 17: 1-8.

[21] Kurt Snyder (2006) *Kurt Snyder's Personal Experience with Schizophrenia* Schizophrenia Bulletin 32, 2: 209-211.

[22] Hazel Nelson (1997) *Cognitive Behavioural Therapy with Schizophrenia: A Practice Manual* Nelson Thornes: Cheltenham

[23] Benjamin Gray (2009) *Psychiatry and Oppression: A Personal Account of Compulsory Admission and Medical Treatment* Schizophrenia Bulletin 35 4: 661-663.

[24] Faith B Dickerson and Anthony F Lehman (2006) *Evidence-Based Psychotherapy for Schizophrenia* The Journal of Nervous and Mental Disease 194 1: 3-9.

[25] Wayne S Fenton (2000) *Evolving Perspectives on Individual Psychotherapy for Schizophrenia* Schizophrenia Bulletin 26 1:47-72.

[26] John F M Gleeson, Eóin Killackey and Helen Krstev editors, (2008) *Psychotherapies for the Psychoses: theoretical cultural and social integration* ISPS Routledge: London

[27] Leff J., Kuipers L. & Berkowitz R. (1982) *A controlled trial of intervention in the families of schizophrenic patients* British Journal of Psychiatry 141: 121- 134.

[28] Lucy E Willetts and Julian Leff (1997) *Expressed emotion and schizophrenia: the efficacy of a staff training programme* Journal of Advanced Nursing 26: 1125-1133.

[29] Stephen I. Deutsch, Barbara L. Schwartz, Nina R. Schooler, Richard B. Rosse, John Mastropaolo, and Brooke Gaskins (2008) *First Administration of Cytidine Diphosphocholine and Galantamine in Schizophrenia: A Sustained a7 Nicotinic Agonist Strategy* Clinical Neuropharmacology 31 (1): 34-39.

[30] Emre Bora, Baybars Veznedarolğlu and Bülent Kayahan (2005) *The Effect of Galantamine Added to Clozapine on Cognition of Five Patients With Schizophrenia* Clinical Neuropharmacology 28:139–141).

[31] Tony Zigmond (2011) *A clinician's brief guide to the Mental Health Act* Royal College of Psychiatrists publications: London

14

Mixing Oil and Water: Developing Integrated Treatment for People with the Co-Occurring Disorders of Mental Illness and Addiction

Andrew L. Cherry
University of Oklahoma
Anne & Henry Zarrow School of Social Work,
Tulsa Campus, Tulsa
USA

1. Introduction

This chapter chronicles the shift in scientific assumptions and the ensuing consensus on treating people with a co-occurring mental illness and a substance misuse problem. In this chapter, the term *co-occurring disorder* refers to a person with both a mental illness and a substance use disorder. The paradigm shift and subsequent technology transfer in the fields of addictions and mental health is extremely important for the lessons learned in the effort to integrate the two modalities. There are lessons from the process of moving new ideas based on science into practice. These lessons give us direction for treatment and knowledge transfer in the future. And, finally there is a need to examine critically the underlying flaws that were exposed in the philosophy and practice tradition of both models when they were integrated.

Fundamentally, the attempt to develop and deliver appropriate treatment to persons with a co-occurring disorder illustrates one of the self-correcting mechanisms of science. Unchallenged, clinicians in mental health and substance abuse treatment would have had little motivation to examine the science underlying their practice. In the history of mental health and substance abuse treatment there have been few revolutionary changes in care and treatment that have made life better for people suffering from an addiction or mental illness. Based on a rapidly evolving science and a better understanding of the treatment needs of people with co-occurring disorders, the expectation at the turn of the 21st century was that by integrating the two models, effective treatment could be provided for people with a co-occurring disorder.

Driven by the growing number of persons identified with a co-occurring mental health and substance misuse disorder the *tipping point* had been reached by the mid 1990s. Declared a crisis in the United States, the number of people being identified as having a co-occurring disorder was estimated to be much higher than thought. The higher rates of failure in treatment and repeated treatment episodes were an unnecessary burden on the treatment community, individuals, families of people with co-occurring disorders, and the community in general. In 2002, Charles G. Curie, Administrator of the Substance Abuse and Mental Health Services Administration (SAMHSA) announced that "addressing the needs of persons with co-occurring disorders had become one of the highest priorities for the agency" (Center for Mental Health Services, 2004). The cost in human capital and the financial strain had become unacceptable. Events that followed, especially those predicated on the idea that the two fields of practice should be integrated, revealed a number of strengths and the effectiveness of some approaches; while at the same time exposing ideas and concepts used in both mental health and addiction treatment that are ineffective and harmful.

To begin this exposition on the evolution of knowledge and services for people with a co-occurring disorder, a brief review will examine the cause for the initial growth in awareness, development of consensus, and recommended treatment approaches for people with co-occurring disorders of mental illness and addiction. In the final section of this chapter, based on what we learned trying to combine the two traditions, Integrated Treatment (integrated mental health and addiction treatment interventions) will be deconstructed and an outline for a third treatment technology will be proposed. This proposal will provide a way forward to improve treatment outcomes of people with a co-occurring disorder as well as people with a mental health and addiction disorder.

Motivated by a growing awareness that people with a co-occurring disorder were being underserved, researchers and practitioners in the field of addictionology and mental health finally received support from two major government initiatives in the late 1990s; one in Canada, followed shortly by a major Federal program in the United States managed by SAMHSA. The program in the United States was supported by an infusion of Federal grant money to support a number of state Co-occurring State Incentive Grant (COSIG) projects. The SAMHSA initiative supported integrating the two treatment models. At SAMHSA, the consensus was that collaboration between professionals working in mental health and substance misuse treatment using their different approaches and interventions would complement each other and produce better outcomes for people treated for a co-occurring disorder. Instead, the effort to integrate the two treatment systems revealed flaws in philosophy and concepts in both models that are incompatible and ineffective.

2. A growing consensus

By the late 1970s, clinicians working in the mental health and substance abuse treatment communities were reporting anecdotal evidence of a large number of people who had both a mental illness and an addiction disorder. As research evidence accumulated, concern grew among policy makers, program planners, clinicians and support workers. The concern about the high prevalence of people with co-morbid disorders focused on treatment for these disorders: concerns about effectiveness of the treatment, other support services needed, and the cost of treatment during the lifetime of an individual with a co-occurring disorder. The early studies supported this concern. Evidence from researchers in the field of substance abuse treatment declared that people being treated for an addiction were much more difficult to treat when they presented with depression or anxiety (McLellan & Druley, 1977; Ritzler, Strauss, Vanord, & Kokes, 1977). By the 1980s, practitioners and researchers in mental health were reporting a growing number of other mental health disorders that were made more difficult to treat as a result of a concurrent substance abuse problem (de Leon, 1989).

Two major approaches (parallel and sequential treatment) that were thought to effectively treat people with the co-morbid problems of mental illness and substance abuse began to emerge in the mid 1980s. Although, some mental health programs were making adjustments in the way services were delivered to better treat people with the co-occurring problem of substance abuse in the early 1980s, little in the way of specific programming for people with a co-occurring disorder had been developed. This began to change when a New York State outpatient psychiatric facility in 1984 implemented various interventions from the addiction treatment community, typically interventions used in Treatment Communities (Sciacca, 1991).

The circumstances that created the pressure for these changes involved a constant drumbeat from practitioners and clinicians in both fields, who wanted change and who were challenging the scientific duality of mental illness and addiction. During the 1980s, the chorus of dissenters became louder. Even so, the term 'dual diagnosis' referring to people with the co-morbid disorders of mental illness and addiction did not appear in the subject index of the journal of *Hospital and Community Psychiatry* until 1989. Drake and colleagues, in 1996, argued that naming the disorder was an important event. He points out that when the complexity of a co-occurring disorder was given a simple medical term, interest in problems caused by substance use among people with a mental disorder resulted in "a mandate for recognition and treatment" (Drake, Osher, & Bartels, 1996).

In the 1990s, substance abuse treatment programs were reporting somewhere between 50% and 75% of the people they treated also had a mental health problem. At the same time, mental health programs reported between 20% and 50% of the people they served had a co-occurring problem of substance use or abuse. The major treatment innovation during this period to accommodate people with a co-occurring disorder was from the addiction field where the modified Therapeutic Community (TC) for mentally ill chemical abusers was developed (Sacks, Sacks, De Leon, Bernhardt, & Staines, 1997). The modified TC basically added provisions for residents who needed to take psychotropic medication. On a positive note, it does give addicted people with a mental illness a safe place to stay while they struggled with the transition back to a life without their drug of choice to help modulate their mental illness.

On the mezzo level, an important event occurred in the United States in 1999. In what Kuhn (1962) called a "paradigm shift," in his seminal book, *The Structure of Scientific Revolutions,* a collaboration was established between the National Association of State Alcohol and Drug Abuse Directors (NASADAD) and the National Association of State Mental Health Program Directors (NASMHPD). Their stated purpose was to pursue scientifically based knowledge and treatment for people with a co-occurring disorder (NASMHPD-NASADAD, 1999). This national effort intended to: "foster improvements in treatment," "provide a classification of treatment settings," "reduce the stigma associated with both disorders'" and "increase the acceptance of substance abuse and mental health concerns as a standard part of healthcare information gathering."

Another major push forward came from a series of SAMHSA monograms, *SAMHSA's Report to Congress on the Treatment and Prevention of Co-Occurring Substance Abuse and Mental Disorders (SAMHSA, 2002). The President's New Freedom Commission on Mental Health Final Report(SAMHSA, 2003b); Co-Occurring Disorders: Integrated Dual Disorders Treatment Implementation Resource Kit (SAMHSA, 2003a), and Substance Abuse Treatment for Persons With Co-Occurring Disorders: A Treatment Improvement Protocol – TIP 42(SAMHSA, 2005); Overview Paper 3: Overarching Principles To Address the Needs of Persons With Co-Occurring Disorders* (SAMHSA, 2006a). These and other SAMHSA publications have done much to fill the void caused by the dearth of information on people who experience a co-occurring disorder. This was critical information for program planners, community developers and other decision makers. They were working in an environment where many states and public treatment facilities began trying to retool in an effort to provide more effective services for people admitted with a co-occurring disorder.

In the midst of producing these publications, SAMHSA at a more systems level asked for and received funding from the U.S. Congress to provide Co-Occurring State Incentive Grants (COSIG) to support state efforts to improve treatment for people with co-occurring disorders seeking treatment in their state. These initiative grants provided the following standards for service. Treatment services provided to people with a co-occurring disorder are to be:

1. consumer driven,
2. delivered from an integrated system of care that fosters an equitable distribution of services,
3. the best recovery practices available,
4. welcoming and based on a no wrong door concept (you're in the right place), and
5. culturally competent.

By the late 1990s, there was a consensus among leading experts in the fields of addiction and mental health treatment that sequential treatment (treatment from one provider, than treatment from another) or parallel treatment (treatment by two different providers at the same time) was not an effective and efficient model for with people with a co-occurring disorder (Clement et al., 1993). Instead of improving outcomes for people with a co-occurring disorder, over time the failure rate in treatment for people with a co-occurring disorder remained high. Subsequent research found that sequential and parallel treatment tended to plunge the person seeking treatment into a vicious cycle of treatment failures (Flynn, 2001). These high rates of failure were discouraging to consumers, counselors, and the politicians who had to find a way to pay for expensive and multiple treatment episodes (Cherry, Dillon, Hellman & Barney, 2007).

A consensus slowly formed around the idea that treating people for a co-occurring disorder using a parallel or sequential model of treatment was disjointed and ineffective. Individuals with complex, overlapping conditions were ill-prepared to negotiate disjointed and fragmented systems of care (SAMHSA, 2002). Based on his work, McGovern (2008) reported that as many as 50% of people with a co-occurring disorder never receive concurrent treatment for both disorders."

The implications for a failure to provide effective treatment are far-reaching. By way of an example, individuals with substance use and mental health disorders are highly overrepresented in the criminal justice system. Bureau of Justice Statistics in the United States report 74% of incarcerated individuals have a lifetime prevalence of substance use disorders and 49% report symptoms consistent with a diagnosable mental health condition. This is a rate that far surpasses those found in the general population (Peters, Bartoi & Sherman, 2008).

2.1 The solution: Integrative treatment

The solution, that was proposed, was to integrate the two treatment systems of mental health and substance abuse (Minkoff, 1993). It was believed both problems can be dealt with simultaneously using an integrative approach. Minkoff suggested collaboration between mental health and substance abuse clinicians when treating a person with a co-occurring disorder. The model is based on concomitant treatment, using the concept of treatment stages in treatment planning, and employing interventions derived from the fields of mental health and substance abuse. During the 1990's integrated treatment continued to evolve, and several models of an integrated system of care were delineated (Drake & Mueser, 1996; Lehman & Dixon, 1995; Minkoff, 1991; Solomon, Zimberg, & Shollar, 1993).

Even though leading experts in both fields recommend integrating the two models, there are vital questions that need to be asked. Is an integrative model possible? Can these two traditions with their different philosophies and treatment modalities be combined effectively? And, just to be on the safe side, if neither technology nor a combination of both technologies are effective in treating people with a co-occurring disorder — what other technology is available? Before exploring these questions in more detail, it will be instructive to review a consensus definition of a co-occurring disorder and the numbers; the prevalence rate, and the demographic characteristics of people identified with a co-occurring disorder in the United States.

2.2 What is a co-occurring disorder

The clinical definition of a co-occurring disorder of mental illness and addiction began to take form in the mid-1990s. Roughly defined as the effect of a comorbid mental illness and substance misuse, the effect each has on the other was identified for the primary subgroups among people with a co-occurring disorder.

Researchers and consensus panels made a number of important observations based on assumptions of the day (SAMHSA, 1995; Landry et al., 1991a; Lehman, Myers & Corty, 1989; Meyer, 1986). These researchers and practitioners concluded that behaviors related to substance misuse could mimic psychiatric symptoms and even psychiatric disorders. The effect of substance misuse on the symptomology of a mental illness had also been observed to be related to the type of substance used, the amount of the substance used, and the chronicity of substance misuse. Acute and chronic substance misuse has also been shown to cause a mental illness to emerge or reemerge, and to increase the severity of an existing mental health disorder. Withdrawal from drugs or alcohol, in some people, has also been observed to produce psychiatric symptoms and diagnosable psychiatric disorders. Then again, substance use can have a number of positive benefits for some people with a mental illness. For some people, drugs and alcohol helps manage, reduce and can be used to hide severe psychiatric symptoms.

Among diagnosticians, mainly those who specialize in addiction assessment, psychiatric symptomatology (particularly mild symptoms) are often misidentified as drug-related. If a person presences at intake and reports any substance use in any amount, his or her dysfunctional and maladaptive behaviors, emotional and social problems are all too often attributed to alcohol and drug abuse and dependence. In the same way, a lack of engagement in treatment is often interpreted as an unwillingness to embrace sobriety. This may be an accurate analysis given a specific individual case, however, a person's treatment compliance and participation in a recovery program can also be affected by symptomatology associated with specific psychiatric diagnoses. The negative symptoms associated with schizophrenia, the lack of energy and interest associated with depression, and the fear of new situations associated with anxiety, at times, can make treatment or aftercare participation and compliance too stressful or distressing. The difference is that one interpretation blames the person; the other interpretation can be used to identify interventions to overcome the stress of participation in treatment.

In 2006, a COSIG committee was formed to forge a consensus on an operational definition of a person with a co-occurring disorder. An operational definition was needed so that people with a co-occurring disorder could be identified through screening and assessment. This type of definition would standardize the collection of data and provide a more accurate count of those being identified and treated with a co-occurring disorder. The major mistake with this approach for identifying the operational definition occurred when the committee agreed that the definition should be consistent with the conceptual underpinnings of the COSIG curriculum and training. This makes the definition tautological. The conceptual underpinning for a definition of a co-occurring disorder should be symptom and syndrome not an ideological construct that is a basis for curricula development and training.

The COSIG committee proposed a broad definition and three sub definitions. The committee used standard *Diagnostic and Statistical Manual of Mental Disorders* (DSM) diagnostic criteria as a guide for developing their operational definition. In a broad sense, they suggested that a person with a co-occurring disorder is a person who meets the diagnostic criteria for a major Axis I Mental Disorder or Axis II Personality Disorder (a diagnosis not used in most of the world) and a major Substance Related Disorder. The criteria were fairly specific. Diagnoses of these disorders must occur simultaneously or within a one year time frame of each other. The figure below is a basic diagram of the co-occurring disorder definition, revealing that a portion of this population is accounted for by individuals who simultaneously present with both types of disorders and is also inclusive of individuals who present with both disorders in a relatively close proximity (one year).

Qualifying conditions in rendering diagnoses:

i.   Substance Dependence Disorders that meet criteria for either early or sustained remission can be diagnosed and will be counted toward meeting the diagnostic parameters of the co-occurring disorders definition. Note: Use of controlled environments, drug replacement therapies, or intensive therapies for abstinence maintenance (substance disorder remission) should **not** be counted in the time period for remission. Such instances should be diagnosed as an active disorder and will be counted toward meeting the diagnostic parameters of the co-occurring disorders definition.

ii. Mental Health Disorders that are in remission due to the use of controlled environments, pharmacotherapy, or intensive psychosocial treatments should be diagnosed as the appropriate mental disorder that is in remission; and these disorders will be counted toward meeting the diagnostic parameters of the co-occurring disorders definition. (COSIG Clinical Protocol Committee, 2006, p.1)

2.3 Locus of care by quadrant of severity

Apart from specific diagnoses, when organized by severity of their mental health and substance abuse disorders, individuals with co-occurring disorders fall into one of four broad categories:

Category I. Less severe mental disorder/less severe substance disorder.
Category II. More severe mental disorder/less severe substance disorder.
Category III. Less severe mental disorder/more severe substance disorder.
Category IV. More severe mental disorder/more severe substance disorder.

Based on the severity of an individual's co-occurring disorder, people with co-occurring mental health and substance abuse disorders would receive treatment in one of the following settings:

Setting for Quadrant I. Primary care physicians, community health clinics; no care.
Setting for Quadrant II. Mental Health system (public and private).
Setting for Quadrant III. Substance Abuse system (public and private).
Setting for Quadrant IV. State hospitals, jails, Department of Corrections, forensic units, crisis facilities, and ER's.
Using this schema, a simplified categorization and severity of the co-occurring disorder can be easily matched with the locus of care and treatment. Theoretically, individuals at various stages of recovery from mental health and substance abuse disorders could move back and forth among these categories during the course of their treatment (See Figure 1).

Category III Severe SUD, Mild MI *Locus of Care* Addiction Treatment	Category IV Severe MI, Severe SUD *Locus of Care* Hospitals, Jails, ERs
Category I Mild MI, Mild SUD *Locus of Care* Primary Health Care	Category II Severe MI, Mild SUD *Locus of Care* Mental Health System

Fig. 1. The Four-Quadrant Model

3. The numbers

Epidemiological estimates of the number of people with a co-occurring disorder of mental health and substance misuse have changed over time. Despite the reality that there is a lack of undisputed data on the number of people with co-occurring disorders, there is no dispute about the gravity of the situation. In part, the absence of uniform numbers is related to the lack of knowledge among practitioners about co-occurring disorders and the lack of a universally accepted definition for a co-occurring disorder. Even so, the growing body of epidemiological studies consistently shows that the number of people with a co-occurring disorder is greater than once thought.

In the early 1990's, the prevalence of people in the United States with a mental health disorder, a substance use disorder, or a co-occurring disorder was estimated to be between 28% and 30%. This estimate was based on two epidemiologic surveys, one in the 1980's, the Epidemiologic Catchment Area (ECA) study (Robins & Regier, 1991), and the other, the National Comorbidity Survey (NCS) conducted in the early 1990s (Kessler et al., 1994). These epidemiologic surveys used a standard definition of mental illness found in the *Diagnostic and Statistical Manual of Mental Disorders* (i.e., DSM-III and DSM-IIIR). These surveys estimated that during a one-year period, about 19% of the adults or some 38 to 40 million people had a diagnosable mental disorder. Approximately, 3% had both a mental illness and an addictive disorder; and roughly 6% had an addictive disorder alone (Regier et al., 1993; Kessler et al., 1994).

Studies that followed continued to add to the growing empirical data on the number of people needing treatment for a co-occurring disorder. Research from the substance abuse treatment community suggested that between 50% and 75% of the people they treated also had an obvious mental health problem(s). Mental health researchers studying the co-occurring population in their treatment facilities found between 20% and 50% of the people being treated had a co-occurring problem of substance abuse or dependence (Sacks, Sacks, De Leon, Bernhardt, & Staines, 1997). As epidemiological data from the accumulating studies begins to stabilize, the best estimate in the early years of the 21st century is that about 1 in 4 adults in the United States had been diagnosed with a mental disorder, roughly 58,000,000 people. An estimated 5 million people out of that group of individuals had a co-occurring disorder (Kessler et al., 2005).

These national studies also reported that approximately 50% of people with a severe mental health disorder are also affected by substance misuse. Furthermore, 37% of alcohol abusers and 53% of drug abusers have at least one serious mental illness. Among all the people diagnosed with a mental illness in the United States, an estimated 29% abuse alcohol and drugs (See Figure 2)

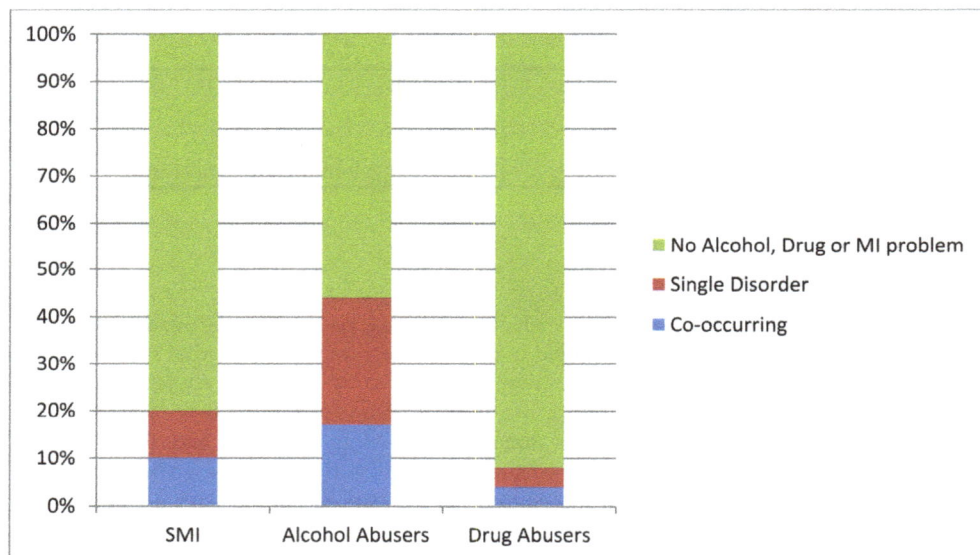

Data compiled from: Robins & Regier, 1991; Kessler et al., 1994; Kessler et al., 2005; CSAT, 2007.

Fig. 2. Prevalence of Alcohol abusers, Drug abusers, Sever Mental Illness (SMI), and Co-occurring disorders in the U.S.

Among individuals with an addictive disorder that lasted at least 12 months, 42.7% reported at least one mental health disorder. Of those who reported a mental health disorder over the previous 12 months also reported at least one addictive disorder. Not surprisingly, the Epidemiologic Catchment Area survey found that people with a severe mental health disorder were at significant risk for developing a substance use disorder during their lifetime. For instance, 47% of people with a schizophrenic disorder also reported a substance misuse disorder. This percentage was over four times higher than what was found in the general population. Among people with a bipolar disorder, 61% had a substance misuse disorder. This percentage was over five times of that found in the general population. Overall, these studies indicate that among individuals experiencing a co-occurring disorder, psychiatric relapse is most often associated with the use of alcohol, marijuana, and cocaine.

Whereas, the most common cause for relapse among people addicted to alcohol or other drugs is the presence of an untreated psychiatric disorder.

3.1 Co-occurring disorders among adolescents

Research since the 1980s indicate that up to 80% of individuals entering publicly funded treatment for substance use disorders have one or more co-occurring psychiatric disorders. Yet only 16% of adults and 26% of adolescents have a co-occurring disorder documented in their intake assessments (Hills, 2007). Adolescents are another important population of individuals with a co-occurring disorder. Children and adolescents were ignored for the most part until the early 1990s. Previously, professional papers and monologues that describe the prevalence of children and adolescents with a co-occurring disorder were based on the rates, behavior, and treatment of co-occurring disorders in adults. Two major epidemiological studies in the early 1990s provided the initial demographic statistics on co-occurring disorders among children and adolescents. The two epidemiological studies, The Epidemiological Catchment Area Study (Robins & Regier, 1991), and the National Comorbidity Survey (Kessler et al., 1994) reported that almost half of adolescents, who were not receiving treatment for a mental health or substance misuse disorder, still met DSM criteria for a substance use disorder and DSM criteria for at least one psychiatric disorder.

In an epidemiological monogram published in the United States, called the New Freedom Commission on Mental Health (SAMHSA, 2003b), it was estimated that more than one in five children (21%) between the ages of 9 and 17 had a diagnosable mental health or substance use disorder associated with at least minimum impairment. An earlier investigation, the Methods for the Epidemiology of Child and Adolescent Mental Disorders (MECA) Study by Shaffer and associates in 1996, found that in many cases, onset of the disorders occurred in children as young as 7 to 11 years of age. Among children in this age group, an estimated 11% experienced significant emotional and behavioral problems at home, at school, and with peers. A smaller number of children and adolescents in this group (5%) experience severe mental health and substance misuse impairment (Shaffer et al., 1996). Institutional settings for children with a co-occurring disorder are a special case. Studies have shown that mental health disorders were higher than expected among children and adolescents who were mired in the child welfare or juvenile justice system. The best numbers (Putnam, 2000) suggest that between 30% and 40% of the children who were in an out-of-home care placement had a serious mental health disorder. In a similar institutional setting, an estimated 70% of children and adolescents in the juvenile justice system in the United States met criteria for one or more mental health disorders

These numbers of adolescents (in these two institutional settings) with a co-occurring disorder indicate a major need for adolescent mental health, substance abuse, or more appropriately services for a co-occurring disorder. These institutions are government entities and agencies created and funded to care for children and adolescents who were removed from the supervision and care of their parents or custodian. These institutions are legally surrogate parents. Subsequently, the expectation is that all children in the care of these institutions who have a co-occurring disorder would receive at least minimal treatment. To the shame of the United States government, only 20% to 25 % receive mental health services. Even among children in these institutions who had insurance, as many as 75% of the children still had unmet mental health service needs (Kataoka, Zhang, & Wells, 2002).

Children and adolescents with substance use disorders fare no better. Use of alcohol and illicit drugs among children and adolescents has been estimated to be around 73% for alcohol and 27% for illicit drugs (SAMHSA, 2003a). By 2004, estimates were suggesting that approximately 1.4 million young people had a substance abuse problem that required treatment, but only 10% of those needing substance abuse treatment actually received any treatment at all (SAMHSA Office of Applied Studies, 2005). Among adolescents in substance abuse treatment, more recent studies have indicated that as many as 50% to 90% can be diagnosed with a co-occurring disorder (Reebye, Moretti, & Lessard, 1995; Roberts & Corcoran, 2005).

For illustration purposes, findings from studies that have focused on adolescent substance use patterns and treatment outcomes, when mental health issues are involved, help describe the complex nature of these comorbid disorders. Researchers studying adolescent substance abuse treatment suggest that there are critical differences between an adolescent in substance abuse treatment with only a substance abuse problem and adolescents with a co-occurring disorder. Children and adolescent with a co-occurring disorder tend to have an earlier onset of substance use, are more frequent users of substances, and can be expected to use substances over a longer period of time. They have increased rates of family, school, and legal problems than their peers, and these emotional and social relationship problems began at an earlier age (Libby, Orton, Stover, & Riggs, 2005; Kessler, Beglund, Demler, Jin & Walters, 2005; Rowe, Liddle, Greenbaum., & Henderson, 2004).

Other studies point to the complexity of treating children and adolescents with a co-occurring disorder at a substance abuse treatment program. These studies report that children and adolescents with a co-occurring disorder are significantly more likely to drop out of substance abuse treatment and have a poor long-term prognosis (Wise, Cuffe, & Fischer, 2001, Crowley et al. 1998). This is very similar to findings among adults who were treated in either a mental health facility or a substance abuse treatment program (SAMHSA, 2005). A common conclusion among practitioners and researchers is that working with adolescents who have a co-occurring disorder is more challenging than working with the child with only a mental health or only a substance abuse disorder (Rowe, Liddle, Greenbaum., & Henderson, 2004). At the beginning of the second decade of the 21st century, our understanding of co-occurring disorders among adolescents is still in its early stages. Much more needs to be done. Effective screening, assessment and effective treatment interventions are still in the future.

3.2 Putting a face on people with a co-occurring disorder

The typology presented here is based on intake data on more than 38,000 adult men and women who were assessed during intake or who were assessed and treated by 28 model agencies and four (4) control agencies between 2005 and 2008 in Oklahoma, U.S.A. This epidemiological study was one component of a state COSIG project to improve services for people with a co-occurring disorder. A focus group of professionals who were actively involved with treating people with a co-occurring disorder were recruited to help validate and refine the typology developed from this data.

To provide adequate treatment and services, knowing the prevailing rate of people with a co-occurring disorder is essential for any behavioral health service system (McGovern, Xie, Segal, Siembab, & Drake, 2006). Agencies need data on the prevalence so as to better allocate scarce resources. This includes, developing clinical and staff trainings on using "best practices" and developing other support services that will reduce the high rates of treatment failure and relapse among people with a co-occurring disorder. Additionally, Drake and others (2005) have asked that research in the future investigate and refine interventions; and, that researchers continue to clarify a typology of people with co-occurring disorders. The following analysis provides a typology of people who were admitted for treatment with an indication of a co-occurring disorder.

3.3 People with a co-occurring disorder differ in many ways

When a clinician meets a person with the co-occurring disorders of mental illness and substance abuse at admission, people with a co-occurring disorder will probably have many of the following characteristics. One of the overarching impressions, based on these data is that people with a co-occurring disorder have more in common with each other than they do with people who seek treatment for only a mental health or an addiction disorder. As a group they are different in many important ways.

There was a difference in the percentage of people identified as having a co-occurring disorder between the model programs (defined as co-occurring treatment capable) and the control programs providing typical treatment. Model Program staff, over three years, identified approximately 38% of their clients as having an indication of a co-occurring disorder. The Control Programs identified discernibly fewer people as having a co-occurring disorder over the same period (average = 22%).

3.3.1 Differences by gender

Over the three years of data collection, there was only a slight change in the gender of those admitted to the model and control programs. As would be expected, there were more males admitted for treatment for a co-occurring disorder than females. Albeit, only slightly more males (52%) than females (48%) were admitted for treatment to the Model Programs. The Control Programs admitted slightly more females (53%) than males (47%). Men tend to be more challenging and defiant in treatment. The comprehensive training in treating people with a co-occurring disorder seems to have reduced staff resistance to treating men with more difficult behavioral problems.

3.3.2 Differences in age

There was no meaningful difference in age among people with a co-occurring disorder, and only a slight difference in the age of males and females. As a group, the age of men in this sample was approximately 36.5 years of age. Females with an indication of a co-occurring disorder were slightly younger (35 years of age). This appears to be a stable characteristic of people with a co-occurring disorder admitted to treatment in Oklahoma.

3.3.3 Difference in education

Education is important because one needs a minimal level of education to able to benefit from most treatment models. In these data, there was no significant difference in education between males with an indication of a co-occurring disorder and males without an indication of a co-occurring disorder. Women, however, with an indication of a co-occurring disorder had slightly less education than women without an indication of a co-occurring disorder. Educational levels tend to be a stable characteristic. Among men there is no significant difference in education. Conversely, women with a co-occurring disorder had slightly less education than women without an indication of a co-occurring disorder.

3.3.4 Difference in income

Income can be a determinant in treatment effectiveness. The average yearly reported income for all men ($7,358, U.S, Dollars) admitted to treatment was slightly higher than all women ($6,562, U.S, Dollars) admitted for treatment. The per capita income in the community where these people with a co-occurring disorder resided in 2008 was $38,415, U.S. Dollars. Clearly, co-occurring disorders that reach a level of severity that need treatment sorely interferes with an individual's ability to support themselves or a family.

3.3.5 Differences in homelessness

When a co-occurring disorder is so severe it interferes with one's ability to earn a living the repercussions can be devastating. Both men and women with an indication of a co-occurring disorder are at risk of becoming homeless. In this sample, 8% of people entering a treatment facility were homeless. Of the 6,300 people who were homeless, 2,960 (47%) of the homeless were individuals with an indication of a co-occurring disorder. Of these homeless individuals with an indication of a co-occurring disorder, 65% were male and 35% were female. About half of the homeless individuals entering treatment will have a co-occurring disorder. Men with an indication of a co-occurring disorder who are homeless will outnumber women who are homeless with a co-occurring disorder by 2 to 1. More intense case management services will be needed when a person with a co-occurring disorder enters treatment as a homeless person.

3.3.6 Differences in admission status

Admission status is important when designing a treatment plan in mental health and substance abuse treatment. In this study, the group of people with a co-occurring disorder had significantly *fewer* 'voluntary admissions' among men and women with an indication of a co-occurring disorder than people admitted for treatment without a co-occurring disorder. More men and women with an indication of a co-occurring disorder were admitted by 'court commitment.' More men and women with an indication of a co-occurring disorder were also admitted with 'emergency detention orders' (See Table 1).

Voluntary Admissions	NO COD	COD
Men	64%	34%
Women	75%	25%
Civil Commitment	NO COD	COD
Men	45%	55%
Women	70%	30%
Emergency Detention	NO COD	COD
Men	47%	53%
Women	60%	40%

Table 1. Admission Status

One can expect fewer men and women with an indication of a co-occurring disorder to be admitted voluntarily. Both men and women with an indication of a co-occurring disorder are likely to be admitted with some form of detention order. Both men and women with an indication of a co-occurring disorder are more likely to come into treatment as a result of legal intervention.

3.3.7 Difference in domestic violence

There was no significant difference among women diagnosed with a co-occurring disorder and women with only a mental health or addiction disorder in terms of domestic violence. Over 44% of women admitted for treatment in any facility where data was gathered reported having a history of domestic violence. Over 10% of women in this sample reported being battered while pregnant. Among the women on which we have data, 3.5% reported that they were the perpetrator of the domestic violence that they were involved in.

Among women admitted for treatment during the four years of this study, the rate of domestic violence tended to be similar year after year. The number of women reporting a history of domestic violence was stable over the four years of this study. As well, the number of women reported being battered while pregnant also remained stable over the four years of this study. In the professional literature researchers assert that domestic violence rates are higher among women with a mental illness or any substance misuse disorder than among women without significant behavioral problems. In the U.S. population at large, over their lifetime, 25% of women experience domestic violence (Tjaden, & Thoennes, 2000). The findings about the extent of domestic violence, in this study, are in line with the professional literature. In this study, domestic violence was over 50% higher among women entering treatment than women in the general population.

3.3.8 Difference in arrest history

A history of being jailed for behavior related to a mental illness or addiction is slightly more common for people admitted to treatment for a co-occurring disorder than people with only a mental illness or an addiction. Men and women with an indication of a co-occurring disorder were arrested more often 30 days before admission (2% were arrested) than men and women with *no* indication of a co-occurring disorder (1.2%).

3.3.9 Difference in people identified with a serious mental illness

At admission 66% of adult men and 68% of adult women in this sample were assessed as being seriously mentally ill. At discharge, 64% of adult men and 67% of adult women were assessed as still being seriously mentally ill. Within this group of women assessed as having a serious mental illness, 29% were also identified as having a co-occurring disorder. This is a ratio of 1 to 3.4 or 1 woman with an indication of a co-occurring disorder for every 3.4 women assessed as having a serious mental illness. n this group of men with a serious mental illness 41% also had an indication of a co-occurring disorder. This is a ratio of 1 to 2.4 or 1 man with an indication of a co-occurring disorder for every 2.4 men identified as seriously mentally ill.

3.3.10 Difference in GAF scores

The Global Assessment of Functioning (GAF) scale used in the mental health field is a numeric scale where zero (0) indicates the poorest level of functioning and 100 equals the highest possible level of functioning. It is a common behavioral health scale used by mental health clinicians and physicians in the United States. In the DSM-IV TR, it is described as a subjective scale to rate the social, occupational, and psychological functioning of adults. The range of scores reflects how well one is meeting various problems-in-living.

Men and women in this sample identified as having a co-occurring disorder were given significantly lower/worse GAF scores than men or women with *no* indication of a co-occurring disorder. At discharge, nonetheless, there was no significant difference in the GAF score between people with an indication of a co-occurring disorder and those with *no* indication of a co-occurring disorder. This finding implies that, at least while in treatment, people with a co-occurring disorder (based on the judgment of clinicians) improved significantly.

The average GAF score for a person with no indication of a co-occurring disorder was significantly higher; the person was healthier (No COD GAF = 47, COD GAF = 41). At discharge, there was little or no difference in the GAF score between people with an indication of a co-occurring disorder and those with *no* indication of a co-occurring disorder (No COD GAF = 50.72, COD GAF = 49.45).

3.3.11 Differential DSM-IV TR diagnosis by discharge type and gender

Substance Use Spectrum Disorder: Over the four years of the study, on average 60% of men and women with an Axis I diagnosis of a substance use spectrum disorder completed treatment, while 18% left Against Clinical Advice (ACA).

Psychoses Spectrum Disorder: Approximately 68% of men and women with a psychoses spectrum disorder completed treatment. About 12% left ACA.

Mood Spectrum Disorder: In this group of men and women with an Axis I diagnosis of a mood spectrum disorder, 55% completed treatment; 20% left ACA.

Anxiety Spectrum Disorder: Among the men with an Axis I diagnosis of anxiety spectrum disorder: 22% completed treatment; 40% left ACA; 15% were administratively discharged. Women with an Axis I diagnosis of anxiety spectrum disorder did slightly worse in treatment; 20% completed treatment, but 44% left ACA.

Undeniably, the people in this treatment sample seeking mental health or substance abuse treatment and who were diagnosed with an anxiety spectrum disorder, were failing in treatment. This could be an anomaly, but the emotional and financial burden on both the individual and society is unacceptable. There is a critical need to investigate treatment effectiveness and outcomes of people in other settings who seek treatment for an anxiety spectrum disorder.

3.3.12 Discharge type among people with a co-occurring disorder and without a co-occurring disorder

Notwithstanding, the reality that completion of treatment at a treatment facility does not ensure long-term recovery; as well, leaving treatment ACA does not ensure relapse and readmission, men and women with an indication of a co-occurring disorder in this study tended to complete treatment more often and leave less often ACA.

Both men and women with an indication of a co-occurring disorder completed treatment significantly more often and left treatment ACA less often than people with no indication of a co-occurring disorder. These findings defy conventional wisdom and the impression of many practitioners and researchers that people with a co-occurring disorder are more difficult to treat than people with a single disorder of mental illness or addiction. In fact, both conditions may be accurate. People with a co-occurring disorder that enter treatment are serious about obtaining treatment for their disorders and so they persist in treatment and do complete treatment hoping that they will be able to overcome their mental health disorder and addiction. Despite their efforts, however, treatment for co-occurring disorders is less than effective and long-term positive outcomes tend to be dismal at best and harmful at worst (See Table 2).

Discharge Type	Completed Treatment	Left ACA
Men No COD	44%	30%
Men COD	62%	16%
Women No COD	38%	35%
Women COD	58%	20%

Table 2. Discharge Status

4. Moving science to service

Moving scientific discoveries to service, in a way that is sustainable, is more about changing the organization than it is about the science or the services provided. To describe how these scientific discoveries made their way into practice, the COSIG project, a SAMHSA initiative carried out in the United States between 2002 and 2011 can be used as a case study. In this construct, a logical role for a federal agency like SAMHSA is designing and funding programs to move *science to service*. The Annapolis Coalition report on the Behavioral Health Workforce, in the Executive Summary of that report (published by SAMHSA) entitled, *An Action Plan for Behavioral Health Workforce Development* delineated the problems caused by the 10 year lag time between the validation of an intervention and its use in the field (Hoge, et al. 2007).

To conceptualizing the *why* and *how* changes occurred, we begin with the knowledge that the COSIG Project was designed as an intentional change effort with specific goals and objectives. These goals and objectives were linked to measures and preferred outcomes that could be used and compared to observed changes. Moreover, using this approach, it was also possible to identify the tools (events, activities, and initiatives) used by the implementation teams in their attempt to make changes in these complex, large organizational systems and agencies that provide mental health and addiction treatment services.

In 2002, SAMHSA released a landmark report to Congress on Co-occurring Disorders that suggested a model of *integrated services and treatment* that was showing unprecedented success in the treatment of people with co-occurring disorders. The report and the subsequent money appropriated by Congress set the stage for the SAMHSA program called COSIG. The Congressional appropriation was used to provide funding, leadership, and support for state efforts. The COSIG project provided a one-time grant to fund States that wanted to develop or enhance their infrastructure to increase their state's capacity to provide accessible, effective, comprehensive, coordinated/integrated, and *evidence-based treatment* services to persons with co-occurring substance abuse and mental health disorders. The COSIG project was funded for 10 years (2002-2011) (Center for Substance Abuse Treatment, 2007).

4.1 Definition of evidence-based treatment

Practices and treatments in behavioral health that have been shown empirically to have statistically significant better outcomes are identified as Evidence-based Practice (EBP) and Evidence-based Treatment (EBT). For the professional organizations of behavioral health practitioners (e.g., American Psychological Association, the American Occupational Therapy

Association, American Nurses Association, the American Physical Therapists Association, and comparable organizations internationally) have made EBP not just a recommendation, but a practice requirement based on ethical principles.

Opponents of designating EBP interventions as the only acceptable standard for professional practice argue that all hard scientific evidence may not be applicable in real life. Knowing what a tested medication can do is entirely different from knowing what method works with an individual with a behavioral health issue. Treatment effectiveness depends on a host of ancillary factors, not the least of which is therapist's style, personality, and training (Thomas & Pring, 2004).

As demonstrated in this instance, moving science to service is a complex and laborious process. Changing large and even small organizations can be difficult, problematic, and even awkward. By nature, organizational change creates anomie within the organization. One of the responses to anomie (caused by the threat of change) is resistance from staff and administrators. Resistance to change from clinicians can be countered by presenting the science behind the need to change. Much more difficult, is resistance among administrators and bureaucrats. Although it sounds crude, more money and threat of job loss are the primary motivators for administrators and bureaucrats. If resistance cannot be assuaged, efforts to make positive changes will likely fail.

A metaphor that might help in understand how change occurs in large institutions such as SAMHSA and state health departments (as well as other government institutions, corporations and conglomerates, universities, and mega non-profit corporations) come from watching supertankers (Ultra-Large Crude Oil Carriers that weigh-in at 625,000 tons when full) navigate the Atlantic Ocean off the coast of Florida. Fundamentally, these institutions are indistinguishable from supertankers in terms of the energy and time it takes for them to make a significant course change. A friend whose fishing boat went down between South Florida and the Bahamas told of seeing one of these monster tankers coming toward his life boat. As it approached, the crew of the supertanker who had spotted him waved and shouted to him words he could not understand over the noise of the tanker. As it passed by, without even slowing down, he told me that he thought they had probably radioed the Coast Guard. As the supertanker disappeared over the horizon he said he began to lose hope of being rescued; he was only a speck in the ocean somewhere in the vast Bahamas triangle. He could not figure out why the crew of the supertanker had not stopped to pick him up. Then several hours later he again saw a supertanker coming from the other direction. It was the same tanker coming back for him. It had taken hours for the tanker to slowdown and miles of ocean for it to "come about". At a speed of about five knots it slowed enough to pick him up. Several hours later, after another slow looping turn, the tanker was back on course. It takes an excruciatingly long time to change course on these supertankers or in large institutions.

5. International co-occurring initiatives

While there was a concerted effort in the United States to develop and implement services for people with a co-occurring disorder, parallel initiatives were going on internationally. Even though, research and program development had a great deal more funding in the United States, countries around the world developed manuals, reports, and resource materials with recommendations for assessing and treating people with a co-occurring disorder. By the year 2000, funders and program planners globally had recognized that the number of people with co-occurring disorders was much larger than they had thought and that treatment failure rates were extremely high. This was especially true in countries where mental health and substance abuse treatment costs were a substantial part of the national GDP. As the evidence grew about the rate of treatment, failure among people with a co-occurring disorder, the excessive and often wasted cost of treatment became a widespread political concern.

To make the point about the international response to the findings from epidemiological studies in different countries that the number of people with a co-occurring disorder was larger than had been known, events in Australia, Canada, and the United Kingdom will be briefly reviewed. What becomes evident from an international perspective is the scientific process was used by each country to study the problem. First, the majority of countries did an epidemiological study to identify the number of people who needed treatment. After establishing the need, groups of experts were organized to identify and recommend effective treatment approaches.

5.1 Australia

Early on, Australia was studying prevalence rates for people with a co-occurring disorder served by a vibrant addiction and mental health treatment community (Croton, 2004). In 2001, researchers also collected data on the overall prevalence of any mental health, substance use, and co-occurring disorder found among inmates in Australian prisons, one of the first studies of its kind. The prevalence of inmates with a mental disorder was 42.7%. The prevalence rate for any substance misuse disorder was 55.3%. With the exception of alcohol use disorders, women inmates had higher rates than men of mental illness and substance use disorders. The prevalence of a co-occurring mental illness and substance use disorders in the previous 12 months was 29% (46% among women vs. 25% among men). There was a significant association between cannabis use disorders and psychosis in men, but not women. There was also a significant association between affective disorders and co-occurring alcohol use disorders in women but not men (Butler, Indig, Allnutt & Mamoon, 2011).

In Australia, alcohol and drug treatment services and mental health services are administered and funded separately. Similar to organizational structure in other countries, separate funding lines provided little or no incentive for collaboration between the two groups of service providers. Previous national initiatives and funding schemas had attempted to minimize barriers to treatment and build strong partnerships between substance abuse treatment and mental health treatment practitioners. Nevertheless, a report by the Australian Institute of health and welfare in 2005 reported that despite previous efforts, people with comorbidity were still not being well served in Australia.

In the 2003–04 Federal Budget, the Australian Government allocated funding for the development of the National Comorbidity Initiative to improve service coordination and treatment outcomes for people with coexisting mental health and substance misuse disorders. One priority area for action under this initiative was to improve data systems and methods of collecting data within the alcohol and drug treatment facilities, and mental health agencies in Australia (AIHW, 2005).

5.2 Canada

When researchers and experts in mental health and substance abuse treatment in Canada realized that a large segment of the treatment population in both sectors had a co-occurring disorder, the next issue was to examine treatment outcomes. As suspected, neither mental health treatment nor substance abuse treatment facilities in Canada provided optimum treatment. Supported by this information, attention turned to the treatment community's capacity to providing co-occurring services.

In 2000, the Canadian Minister of Health authorized Health Canada, a department of the Minister of Health, to form a working group and select a panel of experts from across Canada to synthesize best practice guidelines for providing treatment and services to people with a co-occurring disorder. The Canadian department was responding to the growing recognition that parallel or sequential treatment (treatment at two different facilities; one providing mental health services and the other providing substance abuse treatment) had failed. The panel of experts who identified best practices for this Canadian publication, recommend integrated treatment (integrated mental health and addiction treatment approaches) as a best practice in the treatment and care provided people with a co-occurring disorder (Centre for Addiction and Mental Health, 2002). It was a major step forward when the Canadian Minister of Health, in 2002, published the results of the work of the expert panel in the form of a monogram of resource materials and best practice assessment and treatment approaches that could be used to improve treatment and services for Canadians with a co-occurring disorder.

In the monogram entitled, *Best Practices: Concurrent Mental Health and Substance Use Disorders* (Centre for Addiction and Mental Health), research findings to that point were updated and synthesized, and specific recommendations were made for screening, assessment, and treatment in an effort to improve treatment outcomes for people with a co-occurring disorder. A national inventory of specialized concurrent disorders programs, entitled *National Program Inventory - Concurrent Mental Health and Substance Use Disorders* was also developed and published as a companion document. The monogram was written for managers and staff of mental health, substance abuse and integrated mental health and substance abuse service agencies. In addition, it provided micro level information and recommendations that practitioners in the community who were tasked with providing quality service to people presenting with concurrent mental health and substance use disorders could use in their practice (Centre for Addiction and Mental Health, 2002).

5.3 United Kingdom

Little was known in the United Kingdom about the prevalence of people with co-occurring disorders in 1997 when Virgo and associates (2001) set out to establish the baseline numbers. Inspired by research conducted in the United States (e.g., Kessler et al. 1996; Regier et al. 1990) up to that point, British studies had been limited to inner city London or to small groups of seriously mentally ill individuals. Moreover, the focus of the studies was on substance misuse and consumption rather than on prevalence or consequences (Menezes, 1996). This non-metropolitan United Kingdom study conducted by Virgo and associates was the first to establish the lifetime and point prevalence of substance abuse and dependence among all current seriously mentally ill patients of all branches of the National Health Services (NHS) Trust, not just those with psychosis.

The number of NHS patients with co-occurring disorders, at the time, was slightly smaller in this United Kingdom study than previously reported in the United States. Nonetheless, the findings related to consequences and characteristics of those with a co-occurring disorder were similar to that reported in the United States. In this study, 12% of the NHS patients were identified with an adult mental illness, 12% met criteria for a substance abuse or dependence disorder, and 20% of those surveyed presenting with a serious mental illness were identified as having a co-occurring disorder. These percentages vary, however, depending on the service sector of NHS. The lowest percentage of those identified with a co-occurring disorder (10%) was found among people receiving rehabilitative services. Taking into consideration the need for rehabilitative services among people with a co-occurring disorder, 10% seems to be rather low. On the acute wards, the percentage of people with a co-occurring disorder was as high as 41%. Compared to other patients in the study, those with a co-occurring disorder were younger, were more often male, lived in less stable accommodations, were unemployed, and had more than one psychiatric diagnosis. They tended to report more crises in their life, more abuse by others, were a greater risk to themselves and others, and reported more alcohol and drug involvement. The drugs of abuse reported by co-occurring patients identified as having an adult mental health disorder were alcohol and cannabis. In the group of patients being treated for addiction, who are also identified as having a co-occurring problem, the preferred drugs were heroin and alcohol with a co-occurring depression (Virgo et al., 2001).

Once the prevalence rate among NHS patients was determined, research to identify the best approaches for training mental health teams to treat people with a co-occurring disorder began in the late 1990s. The result of this combined effort was the Pan-London Dissemination Project. This program was a "train the trainer" initiative designed to disseminate information on assessing and treating people with co-occurring disorders (Croton, 2004).

They were also similar initiatives and efforts in other countries to address the needs of their citizens with a co-occurring disorder. Informed by the extensive research in the United States, Germany (Hintz & Mann, 2006), Russia (Mathew et al., 2010), New Zealand (Scott et al., 2008) and other countries followed a similar path in their efforts to provide effective treatment and services for their people struggling with the co-occurring disorders of mental illness and addiction.

6. What if the two fields of practice are NOT compatible

In the history of science there are few if any examples of convenient solutions that were effective and efficient. Programmatically, Integrated Treatment was the easiest next step after Parallel and Sequential treatment models failed to improve outcomes for people with a co-occurring disorder. The fallacy or inconvenient truth in the way integrated treatment was conceptualized (as many practitioners pointed out on a blog called the *dualdx* listserv in 2006-07) the consensus among experts who focused on co-occurring disorders was that the treatment interventions from both treatment traditions were compatible — capable of existing or performing in a harmonious way with one another.

This is a critical assumption. What if the two treatment models are not compatible? What if they work in opposition when combined? What if integrating the two models of treatment is like trying to merge two partly dysfunctional systems? What if philosophically we are trying to do the equivalent of mixing oil and water? What if parallel and sequential treatment failed not because of the specific timing of deployment of the treatment types, but because they work one against the other when combined? For illustration purposes, what if the two treatment approaches are like many medications that cannot be taken together. These possibilities create a dilemma for clinicians, program developers, and funders. If neither technology nor a combination of both technologies are effective in treating people with a co-occurring disorder — what other technology is available?

The answer to the first question, in my view, is that the two treatment modalities are not compatible and they cannot be integrated effectively unless treatment philosophies and policies in both fields are willing to change. Neither field has developed a set of treatment interventions sufficient to recommend either of them in whole.

The answer to the last question — rather than integrate the two systems of mental health and addiction treatment *in whole*, I would argue that an applied research approach be used to carefully select the best components from each field and weave them into a new and third technology. Pursuit of a synthesis of the best practice components in and of itself would go a long way in the development of a more effective and efficient treatment modality. During this process, it will be critical to identify best practices treatment approaches, interventions, and techniques that work and promote wellness for people in treatment. It will also be critical to identify, consciously discard, and then disseminate information on treatment and services that are ineffective, inefficient, and/or produce poor outcomes. Clinicians in the Behavioral Health related fields should be held responsible for disclosing information about their interventions in the same way that drug companies are supposed to reveal the side effects and negative outcomes of the treatments they sell.

To start this process, I recommend that clinicians discard the *paternalistic attitudes* endemic in mental health treatment (e.g., Angell, 2006; Sowers, 2005; Lefley, 1998). I also recommend that the *punitive approach* also referred to as the *conformational approach* that has been one of the distinguishing characteristics of substance abuse treatment be discarded as brutish because it does not meet the standards that define *best practices* (e.g., Quinn, Bodenhamer-Davis, & Koch, 2004; Dongier, 2005).

6.1 Paternalism is NOT Treatment

Clinicians in the field of mental health for the most part have a paternalistic orientation toward their "patients." They are trained in subtle ways to see a person with a mental illness as totally and permanently disabled. Moreover, paternalism among clinicians has a long and rich history.

Clinicians and mental health programs with a paternalistic orientation have few and limited expectations of people with a mental illness, other than the *patient* following the "doctor's orders" and being compliant (Sowers, 2005). By way of example, the perception of permanent disability is so ingrained the science and knowledge of mental health that the concept of *recovery* (a major part of the treatment for addiction) was not included into the mental health model of treatment until after mid-2005.

The hebetude that results from paternalism in mental health gone awry is a legacy of our past. When paternalism was the core of the clinical response to mental illness, people with a mental illness were locked away in mega mental hospitals in the United States for their care and protection. This approach to care and treatment, often referred to in modern times as milieu therapy, caused a secondary disorder where the resulting mental and physical lethargy was accurately named, "institutionalization" (Lamb & Oliphant, 1978).

The attitude of those in the mental health treatment community after the 1840's in the United States was that they were responsible for the *care* and treatment of people with a mental illness. In fact, the charge to the Superintendents of American Asylums in the late 1800s was to care for the physical and mental needs of those with a mental illness and to protect the public (Hurd, 1916).

This "care model" resulted in *institutional behavior*. Institutionalization is an adaptive behavior by people to survive in a situation where pervasive institutional controls result in the mental, emotional, and behavioral characteristics of learned helplessness (Lunt, 2004). Institutionalization of people with a mental disorder became ubiquitous after the American public asylum movement (started in the 1840s) degenerated into mega public mental hospitals where patient management, administration, and financial concerns replaced treatment and rehabilitation.

In the second half of the 20th Century, the attitude of many mental health practitioners toward patients and clients has been shaped by an illness perspective (Beers, 1909; Sowers, 2005). Cynical in nature, in part because of the legal pressure as a result of the "deinstitutionalization movement" in the 1970s, the "illness perspective" rationale went something like, 'Even though most people with a mental illness would be better off in a hospital, it does not mean that he or she has to be confined to a hospital to receive treatment.' Today practitioners are in agreement that a person with a mentally illness has as much right to be in the community when they are *stable* as anyone else (Lunt, 2004). A concept we can support; but a concept that is extremely difficult to operationalize using symptomatology. In particular, the term *stable* is difficult to operationalize when the influence of culture on behavior changes symptomatology that defines a diagnosis.

Although wrought with problems, the illness perspective created a climate that viewed institutional care as one of several levels of care including outpatient care. Nevertheless, one of the underlying messages to people with a mental disorder is that they are being supervised as much as treated by the clinicians who represent a rigid and intractable mental health treatment community. Services and treatment provided in this atmosphere leave the people being treated for a mental illness with little hope, power, or vision of what life will be like if their symptoms have diminished (Grenville, 2001).

Too often, one of the consequences of a therapeutic intervention for a person who is being treated for a mental disorder by paternalistic clinicians is the message it conveys. The message reinforces a belief on the part of the clinician and the person with a mental disorder that people with a mental disorder have a lifelong mental impairment that will always need care and treatment by professionals in the field of mental health. The more recent development of the 'community model,' as a way of providing mental health services outside of institutions and facilities has turned out to be merely another 'care model' that *institutionalizes* and makes *helpless* the people the system is trying to rehabilitate (Lunt, 2004). By including the concept of "recovery" as it is understood in the addiction field, in the treatment of people with a co-occurring disorder, the therapeutic message is exactly the opposite from the message conveyed by a paternal philosophy (Becker, Drake, & Naughton, 2005).

Practitioners in the field of medicine have a different view of treatment and care when it comes to physical injuries and illnesses. In the medical field, when a person has another episode or relapse with a medical problem, treatment is often required, but the person is expected to recover and continue on with their life. Similar to breaking a leg, surgery, or cancer, the expectation of practitioners and those with a co-occurring disorder should be that they will recover and resume their life as a student, an employee, an artist, an engineer, a mental health clinician, and so forth. All interactions and treatments need to be based on the expectation that the person will recover and resume or become engaged in a productive life.

Taking all this into consideration, there is little doubt that practitioners in the mental health field clearly differ from clinicians in the substance abuse treatment community on the issue of "personal responsibility" (Wing, 1995). For better or worse, at least substance abuse counselors hold their clients accountable for their behavior even if the tools that substance abuse counselors offer are often useless. Counselors in mental health have little or no expectation of their clients, even when the tools they offer can be quite helpful in reducing symptoms associated with a mental illness (Lunt, 2004).

6.2 A punitive attitude and confrontation are NOT treatment

Since the late 1950s, what is known as traditional substance abuse treatment for the indigent and chronically addicted has been residential treatment that varied far from the clinical treatment path. For instance, if you walked onto a traditional Therapeutic Community, you would likely see a resident walking around wearing a diaper over his/her clothes with an oversized pacifier around his/her neck with a sign on the person's back reading, 'I won't grow-up.' Outside in the court yard you could very well see a woman with a shaved head digging a hole three feet deep and placing a penny at the bottom of the hole, filling in the hole and then digging the penny out again. These types of degrading punishments, called *therapeutic intervention* are used to demonstrate to the addict the fruitlessness of their addictive behavior. Similar castigation is called *therapy* in hundreds of Treatment Communities in the United States. States and the Federal government pay millions of dollars each year to Treatment Community programs to provide this type of punitive *treatment*. Logically, if punishing and being callous to people who are abusing drugs was a cure for their misuse there would be no drug abuse anywhere in the world. If the punitive approach worked, there would be fewer people in prison for drug possession and use.

Modern drug treatment, for all intent and purposes, began in the 1930's with the development of Alcoholics Anonymous (AA) and AA's use of the self-help group. AA and Narcotics Anonymous (NA) type self help groups use a non-judgmental passive approach. AA and NA members extend themselves to people who want help with their addiction. They do not compel a person to quit or give up their addiction. But, they support the person who is committed to overcoming their addiction. To its credit, over the years, many addicts have been helped by AA and NA. A large percentage of addicts, however, needed and continue to need more than AA and NA can offer. Because clinical treatment was expensive and admittedly not very successful, the next major change in the treatment of addiction was residential treatment provide by addicts in "recovery." The two best known programs are the Synanon model developed in the late 1950s and the Therapeutic Community model developed in the mid 1970's (Janzen, 2001).

The Synanon program and the Therapeutic Community (both closely related in philosophy and treatment) were a clear departure from the psychiatric and therapeutic treatment in general and specifically for the treatment of addiction. The Synanon and Therapeutic Community leaders largely rejected professional psychotherapeutic treatments with the exception of self-help groups. The preferred counselor was a recovering addict.

6.3 The Synanon model

The Synanon group started in 1958 in Santa Monica, California as a drug and alcohol rehabilitation program. Charles Dederich (1914 to 1997) the founder of Synanon gained national prominence for developing a program that could cure narcotic addiction. Not as well known is the reality that this treatment approach was not very successful and graduated few people who lived productive lives outside of the Synanon community. In

1967, Synanon leadership abolished "graduation" and offered itself as an alternative-lifestyle community. Later it became the Church of Synanon (Janzen, 2001; Yates, 2003).

By 1977, Synanon was being referred to as a cult that controlled members using what was called the "Synanon Game." A pseudo *therapeutic approach*, the "Synanon Game" involved members humiliating one another and being forced to expose their innermost weaknesses and fears. This was a distortion of the encounter group process. This approach is based on the premise that when challenged, people examine themselves and learn new ways of behaving (Kaplan & Broekaert, 2003).

At its peak in the mid 1970s, Synanon women were made to shave their heads, married couples were forced to break up and take new partners, males were forced to submit to vasectomies, and a number of women who became pregnant while living in the community were required to have abortions (Yates, 2003).

What began as a highly praised drug treatment program, ended when Synanon leaders became implicated in an attempted murder. Synanon was closed in 1991 because of megalomania and financial problems brought on by lawsuits and disputes with the Internal Revenue Service over its nonprofit status (Janzen, 2001).

This was not the end, however, of Synanon's influence. Programs based on the Synanon model sprang up across the United States for adolescent drug users. First called the "Seed," this program later operated under names such as *Straight Inc., Safe Recovery, Kids Helping Kids, Growing Together of Lake Worth, and Pathway Family.* From 1976 to 1993 Straight, Inc. operated the world's largest chain of juvenile drug rehabilitation programs. They are reported to have treated as many as 50,000 adolescents. In 1974 the U.S. Senate "likened" the methods of The Seed to those used by North Korean brainwashers (ISCA, 2002).

6.4 The treatment community model

After being discredited, Synanon's concept of community treatment inexplicably became the foundation for the residential treatment approach called the Therapeutic Treatment Community model. The punitive attitude and retaliatory consequences that defined Synanon treatment were carried over in great part as treatment interventions used by Therapeutic Treatment Community counselors. The philosophy is based on the notion that if an addicted person is harshly challenged, they will examine themselves and learn new ways of coping without the substance. To paraphrase a drug counselor, "We can make life so horrible that giving up drugs is the lesser of two evils." As many working in the field of substance abuse treatment, I have witnessed people in a Therapeutic Treatment Community treated worse than people in prison. You could not legally treat people in U.S. prisons like the people in Therapeutic Treatment Community programs are treated. Such treatment would be unconstitutional.

To be fair, those who advocate for the Therapeutic Community model see the primary goal of a Therapeutic Treatment Community is to "foster personal growth." One accomplishes personal growth by "changing one's lifestyle" this is brought about through a community of concerned people working together to help themselves and each other. The Therapeutic Treatment Community is designed to be a highly structured environment "with defined boundaries, both moral and ethical." Personal growth is promoted by "community imposed sanctions and penalties, as well as earned advancement of status and privileges," which are perceived as "part of the recovery and growth process" (Charles & Eric, 2003). Hayton, (1998)defined a *therapeutic community* as a structured method and environment for changing human behavior in the context of community life and responsibility (SAMHSA, 2006b). This sounds like a helpful and benign environment, but the description can also be used to describe a prison or jail.

In spite of its history, there is a consensus among experts that using a Modified Therapeutic Community model for treating people with a co-occurring disorder can be beneficial. To be fair, those who advocate using a Modified Therapeutic Community model for people with a co-occurring disorder, do *not* recommend using confrontational approaches and provide services that allow co-occurring clients to access and take medication while in treatment (Skinner, 2005).

The behavioral literature clearly differentiates between positive reinforcement and negative reinforcement, and punishment. The *punitive approach* has no place in the treatment of a person with a co-occurring disorder. The *punitive approach* does not come up to the standards of care proposed by SAMHSA in the publication, *Co-Occurring Disorders: Integrated Dual Disorders Treatment Implementation Resource Kit* (SAMSA, 2003a). As a component of a therapeutic milieu, the punitive approach has no empirical support.

7. A third technology

7.1 Why do we need a third technology?

Why do we need a third technology? We need a third technology for at least two compelling reasons. First, research consistently finds that mental health and substance abuse treatment, as they are practiced in 2012, are marginally effective. They are not efficient. Multiple relapse is the rule. The failure rate makes current treatment cost exorbitant. Second, as the brief history presented in this chapter again reminds us, the mental health and substance abuse treatment approaches are grounded in tradition, not in science. This is not to say that many of the interventions used in mental health and substance abuse treatment have not been tested. Most of the standard therapeutic interventions used have been investigated, some using the double-bind methodology. What is not included in the calculus when testing these interventions is the difficulty involved in testing the effectiveness of a traditional treatment technique. The influence of a tradition is subtle and affects the thinking of researchers and thus the formation of the research questions asked by the researchers. Without considering the history of the development of the two traditions, investigators and clinicians are at risk for thinking that the reason why specific interventions are used in mental health and addiction treatment is because they have met some standards such as "safe and effective." This could not be farther from the truth.

Since the 1950s, we have continually tweaked these traditional approaches. And, with each tweak the traditional approach is found to be more effective. Yet, outcome studies do not confirm that these short-term treatment successes actually manifest themselves in long time successful outcomes. The research showing a lack of long-term success is particularly distressing. Especially, if you consider that success in treatment is distorted because expectations are already so low almost any outcome of treatment that is slightly above being a vegetable is considered a successful outcome by today's standards.

A final argument would be philosophical. Using an analogy, I would compare efforts to continue to tweak the two traditions to make them seem to work better is similar to patching up an old rotten and a leaky roof. At some point, the roof is going to have to be replaced. There might be parts of the old roof that can be used in the new roof, but a point will be reached when the repairs cost more than replacing the roof. In the field of mental health and

Mixing Oil and Water: Developing Integrated Treatment for People with the Co-Occurring Disorders of Mental Illness and Addiction

249

substance abuse treatment, a growing cadre of practitioners and researchers believed that we have reached the point where something needs to change.

Among the problems that I had when radically changing technology at a substance abuse treatment facility to treat people with a co-occurring disorder was changing the addiction culture. As one would expect, some staff resisted any change. They were committed to the tradition, especially those staff "in recovery" who were also counselors and clinicians. Staff, however, are at a disadvantage. Administrators and supervisors extend or withhold rewards to change behavior. This was not the case among clients who came for treatment, or for the community of AA members. Those two groups of people were as resistant, or more resistant to change than staff.

7.1.1 No new treatment model has emerged

Mixing oil and water is not a solution. A third technology needs to be developed. A new treatment model specifically designed to treat people with a co-occurring disorder is needed to replace the *Integrated Treatment* model. The contorted rationale that was used to integrate mental health and addiction treatment modalities to develop the integrated treatment model is so intellectually dishonest one has to suspend a sense of reality to even imagine that the two are compatible in practice.

The panel of experts, involved in writing SAMHSA's Tip 9 clearly recognized the incompatibility of the two treatment fields. Given their combined experience, they agreed that the conflict between the two treatment modalities was largely responsible for the failure to provide effective treatment for people with the co-occurring disorders of mental illness and substance misuse. They wrote:

> For people with dual disorders, the attempt to obtain professional help can be bewildering and confusing. They may have problems arising within themselves as a result of their psychiatric and AOD use disorders as well as problems of external origin that derive from the conflicts and clashing philosophies of the mental health and addiction treatment systems.
>
> Historically, when patients in AOD treatment exhibited vivid and acute psychiatric symptoms, the symptoms were either: 1) unrecognized, 2) observed but were described as symptoms of intoxication or "acting-out behavior," or 3) accurately identified, prompting the patients to be discharged or referred to a mental health program. Virtually the same process occurred for patients in mental health treatment who exhibited vivid and acute symptoms of AOD use disorders. (p.11)

Yet, between the publication of Tip 9 and Tip 42, there was no reported work by the committee of experts on those two panels to address the issues of incompatibility. Even so, the panel of experts involved in the identification of interventions applicable to treating people with a co-occurring disorder continued to recommend integrated treatment. Basically, the recommendation was to combine the philosophies and techniques from each field and ignore their intrinsic differences.

7.2 Selecting the best components from each field

A limited number of variations on the Integrated Model promoted by SAMHSA have been proposed but no model proposed is based on deliberately selecting and discarding components from the interventions used to treat mental illness and substance abuse. All the same, even without this level of deliberation about interventions a number of addiction treatment programs that simply modified their services to include psychotropic medication have shown improved outcomes when treating people with co-occurring disorders (SAMHSA, 2003c; Osher & Drake, 1996; Sacks et al., 1997; Sciacca & Thompson, 1996).

7.2.1 Components that seem to be compatible
- Clinicians from both fields are trained in the psychosocial model of behavior.
- Clinicians from both fields see a need for a continuum of care which embraces the value of a variety of treatment settings and program types in both public and private settings.
- Clinicians from both fields support the extremely important adjunct role played by self-help organizations in both fields.
- Clinicians from both fields accept case management and care management as an important component of treatment and care.
- Clinicians in both fields see the value of peers or professionals with lived experiences as a critical support in developing and implementing an individual's care and support plan;
- Genetic research to identify the cause of the behavioral disorder is important to both fields.
- The evolving recipient of care movements that periodically influence change in the delivery of treatment services has affected both fields, most often in mental health.
- The emerging professional perspective and training that gives a higher priority to more basic needs of food, shelter, clothing, work, friendship, etc. has affected the workforce issues in both fields;
- The ever-increasing role of pharmacologic therapy in the treatment of substance misuse, moves substance-abuse treatment closer to the mental health perspective on treatment.
- There is a growing recognition that family members and significant others, as a group may be in need of services themselves.
- There is a potential for a common, or at least a convergent treatment modality for both fields.

(SAMHSA, 1995, p. 14; Centre for Addiction and Mental Health, 2002, p. 70-71)
There is an increasing recognition of the overlap in the population needing help and the expressed needs of consumers for better continuity of care within and across the respective systems. Hopefully this recognition will motivate scrutiny of treatment failure, relapse, and less than optimal long-term treatment outcomes.

7.2.2 Components to discard
A first step that would go a long way to improving the treatment and services provided people with a co-occurring disorder would be to decriminalize mental illness and addiction. The underlying threat of arrest and confinement if one does not comply with the treatment recommendations of one's illness undermines the best intentions of the mental health and addiction treatment practitioners.

Clinicians in both fields rely too heavily on the correctional system for formal and informal social control. Forcing people into treatment, without it being absolutely necessary, results in resistance and defiance from the person designated with a mental health or substance misuse disorder. This should be replaced with a collaborative therapeutic and case management relationship.

Confrontation is never acceptable. Even using less than a confrontational approach, what some resource material refers to as "being direct" may feel like abuse to the person in treatment. Identifying and pointing out irrational thinking, based on the perspective of the clinician, can result in a conflict between the clinician and client. Insisting on random alcohol and other drug tests when working with people with a co-occurring disorder can reduce the level of trust and harm the therapeutic relationship.

Consequences and contingencies are not therapeutic modalities. They belong to corrections and social control agencies. Making a person responsible for his or her behavior sounds good but when a person is responding to delusional thoughts, is this really being defiant? Should clinicians spend time keeping records of violations of rules? Who does it benefit when clients are made to experience consequences of their behavior; the client who learns from being punished? When is developing therapeutic insight less beneficial than breaking through denial?

Stigma is often cited as a reason why individuals do not seek treatment from mental health providers or from substance abuse treatment facilities. The community at large is often cited as the source of stigma. As important as stigma in the community, is stigma among professionals in the field of mental health and substance abuse treatment. To reduce the stigma, professionals must first advocate for the rights of individuals seeking treatment in their own professional organizations. In a community context, advocates and professionals need to promote public education and understanding. As long as stigma remains high among clinicians, however, it will be nearly impossible to change the minds and attitudes of people in the community at large.

Widespread use of residential treatment for substance misuse disorders and confinement at a mental health treatment facility needs to be radically curbed. This is a relic left over from the days of the asylum. Outpatient, day treatment, and self-help groups need to be better supported and expanded.

The resistance to sharing power with the client in a therapeutic relationship by clinicians, an antiquated paternal attitude, renders treatment planning less effective and distorts therapeutic intentions.

In the field of mental health, the reluctance of clinicians to work with paraprofessional with lived experience (people in recovery after experiencing a mental illness) denies clients a major source of understanding, empathy, and a view of a positive future for themselves and others who have suffered from a mental disorder. This also denies the clinician a positive view of people who have been treated for mental illness.

Mandated treatment needs to be discarded. Treatment should be offered and available as a tool or resource to help the person reach their life goals.

This is a short list and by no means comprehensive. This list will also grow and continue and expand as clinicians and researchers began to see people with a mental health and addiction disorder as people rather than people as their disorder. Disorders that too many clinicians believe need to be controlled and managed. Instead, when clinicians become more sensitive to the needs of people seeking treatment and view clients as living in a context normalized by ethnicity, culture, language, and education, both mental health and substance abuse treatment will become more effective.

7.2.3 Components to keep

The following is proposed as a starting point in the selection of the best treatment interventions from the mental health and substance abuse treatment fields. From the Mental Health treatment field we need to keep the knowledge of "symptomology" and information about the course of a mental illness that has been developing since Moral Treatment was introduced by Philippe Pinel (1745-1826) and Jean-Baptiste Pussin (1745-1811) (Rousseau, 1990). From the Substance Abuse treatment field we need to keep the philosophy and concept of "recovery" (Lunt, 2004). In the substance abuse treatment community, people receiving treatment for substance abuse are not thought to need treatment for the rest of their lives. Although, not needing continual treatment for the rest of their lives (like a person with a mental illness), clinicians working in substance abuse treatment, Alcohol Anonymous (AA), and Narcotic Anonymous (NA) believe that a person who was once addicted will always be an addict and will need to be in recovery mode for the rest of their lives.

8. Synthesizing the two fields

In addition to using Kuhn's description of a "paradigm shift," to explain the shift in philosophical and clinical assumptions to include treatment for people with a co-occurring disorder, the emergence of treatment philosophies and interventions can be described as a process of "thesis, antithesis, and synthesis" (this construct is often incorrectly attributed to Hegelian theory) (Plant, 1999). Professional treatment by licensed clinician's could be thought of as the thesis. Treatment based on tradition derived from people who have experienced addiction could be the antithesis. The work of synthesizing the best components of the two fields can be used as an analytic tool in continuing the development of a third technology, a new model, perhaps simply called Behavioral Medicine.

The Society of Behavioral Medicine offers a beginning definition:

> Behavioral Medicine is the interdisciplinary field concerned with the development and integration of behavioral, psychosocial, and biomedical science knowledge and techniques relevant to the understanding of health and illness, and the application of this knowledge and these techniques to prevention, diagnosis, treatment and rehabilitation. (http://www.sbm.org/about/definition.html)

8.1 Consider a model using select components from both fields

In the mental health and drug addiction treatment systems that I have been associated with and that I have evaluated, all too often it is not the service needs of the individual that drive the treatment system; it is the treatment system that drives and determines the treatment services available and ultimately provided the client. In the mid 1990s, an opportunity presented itself that allowed me to redesign a traditional Treatment Community model program so as to provide services and treatment for people with a co-occurring disorder. The treatment programming we developed (for lack of a better term, called the Sapient Model) combined empirically based practices with the best consensus based practices that were thought to be effective among people with a co-occurring disorder.

Treatment started with an engagement model that included motivational intake interviewing, activities to develop and maintain a bond between the person seeking treatment and the staff, the other residents, and the program philosophy of recovery as defined by "Bill and Bob" in the "Big Book." Individual and group therapy was based on cognitive behavioral techniques. Treatment included individual and group work on developing and maintaining relationships, and developing and maintaining social supports. Services included education about co-occurring disorders, case management, outpatient treatment, and help with housing and employment.

Mixing Oil and Water: Developing Integrated Treatment for People with the Co-Occurring Disorders of Mental Illness and Addiction

253

Psychiatric services were introduced and psychotropic medications became a common component in the overall treatment plan. One practice that was extremely useful with residents was the policy of negotiating treatment with those who did not believe that they needed psychotropic medication or did not want to take it. They wanted to recover on their own. If the treatment team believed medication was needed, the psychiatrist, the clinical director, and the person's individual therapist would meet with the resident and negotiate an agreement. Typically, it was an agreement that the person would not be asked to take medication, but if they relapsed, then they would work with the team and try medication if recommended to see if it helped.

Programming policy did not allow "encounter groups," "confrontational approaches," or playing "the game" by staff or residents. The confrontation approach had been the primary form of treatment before the program was redesigned. The policy created much consternation among the Certified Addiction Counselors and the proponents of the traditional treatment community.

This treatment community model intervention also called, "getting pulled-up" or "getting called on your s**t" can be extremely harmful. These approaches tend to encourage confrontation and punishment by counselors and confrontation between residents who can also call someone on their "s**t." This form of the treatment community life experience was replaced with a community experience of self governance. The Resident's Council made and negotiated program policy with the staff and administration. They advocated for services and provided valuable community service to the neighborhood where the treatment program was located.

Residents who broke rules were apprised of the consequences of their behavior and their responsibility for their behavior. The staff would determine appropriate consequences for the resident who broke the rules. This could range from housekeeping tasks, to starting treatment over at day one. If the person chose to accept the consequences, he or she would continue their treatment in the program. If the person chose to leave the program, he or she was asked to return to our treatment program when they were ready to resume treatment.

Another program policy that was discarded because it was counterproductive was the policy of discharging people who relapsed while in treatment. Relapse was considered the same as breaking any of the rules. The staff would determine appropriate consequences for the resident who relapsed, but a relapse would not bar the person from continuing in treatment. It is difficult to treat a person who has been "kicked" out of the program.

Another valuable policy encouraged residents who were discharged as a treatment success to return to our program for additional work on their recovery efforts if they relapsed. As a staff, we knew the person and believed that we would not have to start from square one. The typical policy among treatment community programs is that a resident who is discharged (whether they succeeded or failed) is not allowed to return to the program for any reason, even for a visit for at least one year. Obviously, this would keep people who failed treatment out of sight.

A related policy gave each resident the right to belong to the Program's alumni association. Everyone was asked to come back to the Program for monthly meetings.

Another helpful policy related to facilitators who brought AA and NA meetings into the treatment center. They were required to accept people into meetings who took medication for psychiatric problems. As the clinical director, I also met with several AA and NA rooms that residents attended and asked that they to be more understanding of people from our program that were taking medication for a mental illness.

As a retention model, the success is supported by State and Medicaid data that show a retention rate of around 90% for the first 30 days over a continuous four year period. Long-term success, however, was not as impressive as the engagement model. Long-term recovery was hampered by a lack of community support services available to residents who completed treatment. In many cases, the problem was obtaining and paying for expensive atypical psychotropics after the resident left treatment. A lack of programs to provide supportive housing and employment were also problematic. Even so, the recovery rate for residents, in the first year after discharge varied around 50% for residents over a three year period.

More recently, in 2004, I had the good fortune to become the evaluator of the Oklahoma Co-Occurring State Incentive Grant from SAMHSA. The grant supports efforts at the State level to integrate the mental health and substance abuse service systems. Analogous to my experiences, over the last 30 years, the knowledge base and conceptualization of treatment for people with a co-occurring disorder has evolved and continues to evolve.

Given my experience at this point, if I were redesigning the program today, I would also incorporate knowledge about the *stages of change* in both residential and outpatient treatment. I would also promote the development of self-help groups for people with a co-occurring disorder such as Double Trouble in Recovery, Dual Recovery and other self-help groups, both at the program level and in the community.

9. Conclusion: An emerging treatment model

The role played by SAMHSA using the COSIG project as a catalyst for a process that exposed both the strength, weaknesses, and points of philosophical incompatibility of the two traditions should not be underestimated even though it was probably happenstance. In particular, endorsing the Integrated Treatment model without addressing the differences and incompatible components in these traditional models created a crisis. This crisis although disturbing and creating havoc much like any major change, does give us the opportunity to rethink and realign concepts of treatment. Based on the accumulated knowledge from mental health and the treatment of addiction, and knowledge gained since the 1990s during a major effort to develop better treatment interventions for people with co-occurring disorder, that knowledge is available to begin to develop a modern, scientifically based third technology specifically designed for people wanting treatment for a co-occurring disorder.

10. References

AIHW. (2005). National comorbidity initiative: a review of data collections relating to people with coexisting substance use and mental health disorders. Cat. No. PHE 60. (Drug Statistics Series No. 14). Canberra: Australian Institute of Health and Welfare. Retrieved from: http://www.aihw.gov.au/publication-detail/?id=6442467722.

Angell, B., Mahoney, C. A., Martinez, N. I. (2006). Promoting Treatment Adherence in Assertive Community Treatment. *Social Service Review, 80*(3), 485-526.

Becker, D. R., Drake, R. E., & Naughton, W. J. (2005). Supported Employment for People with Co-occurring Disorders, *Psychiatric Rehabilitation Journal* (Vol. 28, pp. 332-338): Center for Psychiatric Rehabilitation.

Beers, C. (1908). A Mind That Found Itself. NY: Longman.

Butler, T., Indig, D., Allnutt, S., & Mamoon, H. (2011). Co-occurring mental illness and substance use disorder among Australian prisoners. Drug and Alcohol Review, 30(2), 188-194.

Cherry, A. L., Dillon, M. E., Hellman, C. & Barney, L. D. (2007). The AC-COD Screen: Rapid Detection of People with the Co-occurring Disorders of Substance Abuse, Mental Illness, Domestic Violence, and Trauma. Journal of Dual Diagnosis, 4(1), DOI: 10.1300.

Centre for Addiction and Mental Health. (2002). Best practices: concurrent mental health and substance use disorders. Ottawa: Health Canada.

Center for Mental Health Services (CMHS). (2004). Building Bridges: Co-Occurring Mental Illness and Addiction: Consumers and Service Providers, Policymakers, and Researchers in Dialogue. DHHS Pub. No. (SMA) 04-3892. Rockville, MD. Substance Abuse and Mental Health Services Administration.

Center for Substance Abuse Treatment. (2007). The Epidemiology of Co-Occurring Substance Use and Mental Disorders. COCE Overview Paper 8. DHHS Publication No. (SMA) 07-4308. Rockville, MD: Substance Abuse and Mental Health Services Administration, and Center for Mental Health Services.

Charles, K., & Eric, B. (2003). An introduction to research on the social impact of the therapeutic community for addiction. International Journal of Social Welfare, 12(3), 204-210.

Clement, J. A., Williams, E. B., & Waters, C. (1993). The client with substance abuse/mental illness: Mandate for collaboration. Archives of Psychiatric Nursing, 7(4), 189-196.

COSIG Clinical Protocol Committee. (May, 2006). Definition of the Co-occurring Disorders Population. Retrieved on July 25, 2011 from: http://www.cahsd.org/PDFs/Publications/CoOccuringDisorders%20DEFINITIO N.pdf.

Croton G. (2004). *Co-occurring mental health and substance use disorders: an investigation of service system modifications and initiatives designed to provide an integrated treatment response*. Wangaratta Australia: Northeast Health,. Retrieved from: http://www. dualdiagnosis.org.au/Croton_Fellowship_Co-occurring%20Disorders. Pdf.

Crowley, T., Mikulich, S., MacDonald, M., Young, S., & Zerbe, G. (1998). Substance dependent, conduct disordered adolescent males; Severity of diagnosis predicts two year outcome. *Drug and Alcohol Dependence, 49*, 225 – 237.

de Leon, G. (1989). Psychopathology and substance abuse: What is being learned from research in therapeutic communities. Journal of Psychoactive Drugs, 21(2), 177-188.

Dongier, M. (2005). Integrated Treatment for Dual Disorders. A Guide to Effective Practice. *Canadian Journal of Psychiatry, 50*(5), 299-300.

Drake, R. E., & Mueser, K. T. (1996). The course, treatment, and outcome of substance disorder in persons with severe mental illness., American Journal of Orthopsychiatry (Vol. 66, pp. 42).

Drake, R. E., Osher, F. C., & Bartels, S. J. (1996). The "dually diagnosed." In W. R. Breakey (Ed.), Integrated mental health services: Modern community psychiatry. (pp. 339-352): Oxford University Press.

Drake R. E., Brunette, M. F., Mueser, K. T., & Green, A. I. (2005). Management of patients with severe mental illness and co-occurring substance use disorder. *Minerva Psichiatrica, 46*(2), 119-132.

Flynn, B. K. (2001). The consumer/case manager working alliance and its relationship to dual-disordered client outcomes in a representative payee treatment program. Univ. Microfilms International.

Grenville, R. J. (2001). Unspoken voices: The experiences and preferences of adult mental health consumers regarding housing and supports., Univ Microfilms International.

Hayton, R. (1998). *The Therapeutic Community*. Kansas City, MO: Mid-America Addiction Technology Transfer Center.

Hintz, T. & Mann, K. S. (2006). Co-occurring disorders: policy and practice in Germany. American Journal on Addictions, 15(4), 261-267.

Hoge, M. A., Morris, J. A., Daniels, A. S., Stuart, G. W., Huey, L. Y. & Adams, N. (2007). An Action Plan for Behavioral Health Workforce Development: Executive Summary. Washington, DC: Substance Abuse and Mental Health Services Administration (SAMHSA).

Hurd, H. N. (1916). The institutional care fo the insane in the United States and Canada. Baltimore: Hopkins Press.

ISCA. (2002). Stright, Inc. Tax Report. Bealeton, VA: International Survivors Action Committee.

Janzen, R. (2001). The Rise and Fall of Synanon: A California Utopia. Baltimore, MD: The John Hopkins University Press.

Kaplan, C., & Broekaert, E. (2003). An introduction to research on the social impact of the therapeutic community for addiction. International Journal of Social Welfare, 12(3), 204-210.

Kataoka, S., Zhang, L, & Wells, K. (2002). Unmet need for mental health care among U.S. children: Variation by ethnicity and insurance status. *American Journal of Psychiatry, 159*, 1548-1555.

Kessler, R., Beglund, P., Demler, O., Jin, R., & Walters, E. (2005). Lifetime prevalence and the age-of-onset distribution of DSM-IV disorders in the National Comorbidity Survey Replication. *Archives of General Psychiatry, 62*, 593-602.

Kessler, R., McGonagle, K., Zhao, S., Nelson, C., Hughes, M., Eshelman, S., Wittchen, H., & Kendler, K. (1994). Lifetime and 12-month prevalence of DSM-III-R psychiatric disorders in the United States: Results from the National Comorbidity Study. Archives of General Psychiatry, 51, 8-19.

Kessler, R., Nelson, C., McGonagle, K. A., Edlund, M. J., Frank, R. G. & Leaf, P. J. (1996). The epidemiology of co-occurring addictive and mental disorders. *American Journal of Orthopsychiatry, 66*, 17–31.

Kuhn, T. S. (1962). The structure of scientific revolutions.: University of Chicago Press: Chicago.

Lamb, H. R., & Oliphant, E. (1978). Schizophrenia through the eyes of families. *Hospital & Community Psychiatry, 29*(12), 803-806.

Landry, M. J., Smith, D. E., McDuff, D. R., & Baughman, O. L. (1991). Anxiety and substance use disorders: the treatment of high-risk patients. Journal of the American Board of Family Practice, 4: 447-456.

Lefley, H. P. (1998). Families, culture, and mental illness: Constructing new realities. *Psychiatry: Interpersonal and Biological Processes, 61*(4), 335-355.

Lehman, A. F., & Dixon, L. B. (1995). Double jeopardy: Chronic mental illness and substance use disorders.: Harwood Academic Publishers/Gordon.

Lehman, A. F., Myers, C. P., & Corty, E. (1989). Assessment and classification of patients with psychiatric and substance abuse syndromes. Hospital and Community Psychiatry, 40(10): 1019-1030.

Libby, A., Orton, H., Stover, S., & Riggs, P. (2005). What came first, major depression or substance use disorder? Clinical characteristics and substance use comparing teens in a treatment cohort. Addictive Behaviors, 30, 1649-1662.

Lunt, A. (2004). The implications for the clinician of adopting a recovery model: The role of choice in assertive treatment. Psychiatric Rehabilitation Journal, 28(1), 93-97.

Mathew, T., Shields, A., Yanov, S., Golubchikova, V., Strelis, A., Yanova, G., Mishustin, S., Fitzmaurice, G., Connery, H., Shin, S. &. Greenfield, S. F. (2010). Performance of the Alcohol Use Disorders Identification Test Among Tuberculosis Patients in Russia. Substance Use and Misuse, 45(4), 598-612.

McGovern, M. (2008). Clinical administrator's guidebook: Integrated services for substance use and mental health problems. Center City, MN: Hazelden.

McGovern, M. P., Xie, H., Segal, S. R., Siembab, L., & Drake, R. E. (2006). Addiction treatment services and co-occurring disorders: Prevalence estimates, treatment practices, and barriers. Journal of Substance Abuse Treatment, 31(3), 267-275

McLellan, A. T., & Druley, K. A. (1977). Non-random relation between drugs of abuse and psychiatric diagnosis. Journal Of Psychiatric Research, 13(3 (Print)), 179-184.

Menezes, P., Johnson, S., Thornicroft, G., Marshall, J. (1996). Drug and alcohol problems among individuals with severe mental illness in South London. British Journal of Psychiatry, 168(5), 612-619.

Meyer, R. E. (1986). How to understand the relationship between psychopathology and addictive disorders: another example of the chicken and the egg. In: Meyer, R. E., ed. Psychopathology and Addictive Disorders. New York: Guilford Press.

Minkoff, K. (1991). Program components of a comprehensive integrated care system for serious mentally ill patients with substance disorders. In New Directions for Mental Health Services (Vol. 50, pp. 13-27): Jossey-Bass Publishers, Inc.

Minkoff, K. (1993). An integrated treatment model for dual diagnosis of psychosis and addiction. In Dual diagnosis of mental illness and substance abuse: Collected articles from H&CP. (pp. 17-22): American Psychiatric Publishing, Inc.

NASMHPD--NASADAD. (1999). NASMHPD, NASADAD reach agreement on federal dual-diagnosis policy. Mental Health Weekly, 9(27), 1.

Osher, F. C., & Drake, R. E. (1996). Reversing a history of unmet needs: Approaches to care for persons with co-occurring addictive and mental disorders. American Journal of Orthopsychiatry, 66(1), 4-11.

Quinn, J. F., Bodenhamer-Davis, E., & Koch, D. S. (2004). Ideology and the stagnation of AODA treatment modalities in America. Deviant Behavior, 25(2), 109-131.

Peters, R. H., Bartoi, M. G., & Sherman, P. B. (2008). Screening and assessment of co-occurring disorders in the justice system. Delmar, NY: CMHS National GAINS Center.

Plant, R. (1999). Hegel: NY: Routledge.

Putnam, C. (2000). Integration of behavioral health care with child protection services: Weaving together practices for improved outcomes. Lansing, MI: Health Management Associates.

Reebye, P., Moretti, M., & Lessard, J. (1995). Conduct disorder and substance use disorders: Comorbidity in a clinical sample of preadolescents and adolescents. *Canadian Journal of Psychiatry, 40,* 313-319.

Regier, D. A., Farmer, M. E., Rae, D. S., Locke, B. Z., Keith, B. J., Judd, L. L. & Godwin, F. K. (1990). Comorbidity of mental disorders with alcohol and other drug abuse: Results from the Epidemiologic Catchment Area (ECA) study. *Journal of the American Medical Association, 264,* 2511–2518.

Regier, D. A., Narrow, W. E., Rae, D. S., Manderscheid, R. W., Locke, B. Z., & Goodwin, F. K. (1993). The de facto US mental and addictive disorders service system. Epidemiologic Catchment Area prospective 1-year prevalence rates of disorders and services. *Archives of General Psychiatry, 50,* 85–94.

Ritzler, B. A., Strauss, J. S., Vanord, A., & Kokes, R. F. (1977). Prognostic implications of various drinking patterns in psychiatric patients. The American Journal Of Psychiatry, 134(5 (Print)), 546-549.

Roberts, A., Corcoran, K. (2005). Adolescents growing up in stressful environments, dual diagnosis, and sources of success. *Brief Treatment and Crisis Intervention, 5,* 1-8.

Robins, R., & Regier, D. (1991). Psychiatric disorders in America: The epidemiologic catchment area study. New York: Free Press.

Rowe, C., Liddle, E., Greenbaum., P., & Henderson, C. (2004). Impact of psychiatric comorbidity on treatment of adolescent drug abusers. *Journal of Substance Abuse Treatment, 26,* 129-140.

Sacks, S., Sacks, J., De Leon, G., Bernhardt, A. I., & Staines, G. L. (1997). Modified therapeutic community for mentally ill chemical 'abusers': Background; influences; program description; preliminary findings. Substance Use & Misuse, 32(9), 1217-1259.

SAMHSA (1995). Assessment and Treatment of Patients with Coexisting Mental Illness and Alcohol and Other Drug Abuse Treatment Improvement Protocol (TIP) Series no. 9. Rockville, MD: Center for Substance Abuse Treatment.

SAMHSA (2005). Substance abuse treatment for persons with co-occurring disorders. Treatment Improvement Protocol (TIP) Series no. 42. Rockville, MD: Center for Substance Abuse Treatment.

SAMHSA Office of Applied Studies. (2005). *Results from the 2004 National Survey on Drug Use and Health: National Findings.* (www.drugabusestatistics.samhsa.gov/nsduh.htm#NSDUHinfo)

SAMHSA. (2002). Report to Congress on the Treatment and Prevention of Co-Occurring Substance Abuse and Mental Disorders. Rockville, MD: Substance Abuse and Mental Health Services Administration.

SAMHSA. (2003a). Co-Occurring Disorders: Integrated Dual Disorders Treatment: Implementation Resource Kit. Rockville, MD: Substance Abuse and Mental Health Services Administration.

SAMHSA. (2003b). President's New Freedom Commission on Mental Health--Achieving the promise: Transforming mental health care in America. Rockville, MD: Substance Abuse and Mental Health Services Administration.

SAMHSA, (2003c). Strategies for developing treatment programs for people with co-occurring substance abuse and mental disorders. Washington, D.C.: US Department of Health and Human Services. (www. samhsa.gov).

SAMHSA. (2005). Substance abuse treatment for persons with co-occurring disorders. Treatment Improvement Protocol (TIP) series no. 42. Rockville, MD: Center for Substance Abuse Treatment.

SAMHSA. (2006a). Overview Paper 3: Overarching Principles To Address the Needs of Persons With Co-Occurring Disorders. Rockville, MD: Substance Abuse and Mental Health Services Administration.

SAMHSA. (2006b). Therapeutic Community Curriculum: Trainer's Manual (No. DHHS

Sciacca, K. (1991). An integrated treatment approach for severely mentally ill individuals with substance disorders. New Directions for Mental Health Services, 50, 69-84.

Sciacca, K., & Thompson, C. M. (1996). Program development and integrated treatment across systems for dual diagnosis: mental illness, drug addiction, and alcoholism (MIDAA). Journal of mental health administration., 23(3), 288-297.

Scott, K., McGee, M. A., Schaaf, D., & Baxter, J. (2008). Mental-physical comorbidity in an ethnically diverse population. *Social Science & Medicine, 66*, 1165-1173. doi: 10.1016/j.socscimed.2007.11.022

Shaffer, D., Fisher, P., Dulcan, M. K., Davies, M., Piacentini, J., Schwab-Stone, M. E., Lahey, B. B., Bourdon, K., Jensen, P. S., Bird, H. R., Canino, G., & Regier, D. A. (1996). The NIMH Diagnostic Interview Schedule for Children Version 2.3 (DISC-2.3): Description, acceptability, prevalence rates, and performance in the MECA Study. Methods for the Epidemiology of Child and Adolescent Mental Disorders Study. *Journal of the American Academy of Child and Adolescent Psychiatry*, 35, 865-877.

Skinner, D. C. (2005). A Modified Therapeutic Community for Homeless Persons with Co-Occurring Disorders of Substance Abuse and Mental Illness in a Shelter: An Outcome Study, 40(4), 483-497.

Solomon, J., Zimberg, S., & Shollar, E. (1993). Dual diagnosis: Evaluation, treatment, training, and program development.: Plenum Medical Book Co/Plenum Publishing Corp.

Sowers, W. (2005). Transforming Systems of Care: The American Association of Community Psychiatrists Guidelines for Recovery Oriented Services. Community Mental Health Journal, 41(6), 757-774.

Tjaden, P. & Thoennes, N. (2000). Extent, Nature, and Consequences of Intimate Partner Violence, Authors. Washington, D.C.: The Centers for Disease Control and Prevention and The National Institute of Justice, the U.S. Department of Justice, Office of Justice Programs. Retrieved from:
https://www.ncjrs.gov/pdffiles1/nij/181867.pdf

Thomas, G. and Pring, R. (Eds.) (2004). Evidence-based Practice in Education. Open University Press.

Virgo, N., Bennett, G., Higgins, D., Bennett, L & Thomas, P. (2001). The prevalence and characteristics of co-occurring serious mental illness (SMI) and substance abuse or dependence in the patients of Adult Mental Health and Addictions Services in eastern Dorset. Journal of Mental Health (2001) 10, 2, 175–188, doi: 10.1080/09638230020023732.

Wing, D. M. (1995). Transcending alcoholic denial. IMAGE: Journal of Nursing Scholarship, 2(2), 121-126.

Wise, B., Cuffe, S., & Fischer, D. (2001). Dual Diagnosis and successful participation of adolescents in substance abuse treatment. *Journal of Substance Abuse Treatment, 21*, 161-165.

Yates, R. (2003). A brief moment of glory: The impact of the therapeutic community movement on the drug treatment systems in the UK. International Journal of Social Welfare, 12(3), 239-243.

Permissions

The contributors of this book come from diverse backgrounds, making this book a truly international effort. This book will bring forth new frontiers with its revolutionizing research information and detailed analysis of the nascent developments around the world.

We would like to thank Prof. Dr. Luciano L'Abate, for lending his expertise to make the book truly unique. He has played a crucial role in the development of this book. Without his invaluable contribution this book wouldn't have been possible. He has made vital efforts to compile up to date information on the varied aspects of this subject to make this book a valuable addition to the collection of many professionals and students.

This book was conceptualized with the vision of imparting up-to-date information and advanced data in this field. To ensure the same, a matchless editorial board was set up. Every individual on the board went through rigorous rounds of assessment to prove their worth. After which they invested a large part of their time researching and compiling the most relevant data for our readers. Conferences and sessions were held from time to time between the editorial board and the contributing authors to present the data in the most comprehensible form. The editorial team has worked tirelessly to provide valuable and valid information to help people across the globe.

Every chapter published in this book has been scrutinized by our experts. Their significance has been extensively debated. The topics covered herein carry significant findings which will fuel the growth of the discipline. They may even be implemented as practical applications or may be referred to as a beginning point for another development. Chapters in this book were first published by InTech; hereby published with permission under the Creative Commons Attribution License or equivalent.

The editorial board has been involved in producing this book since its inception. They have spent rigorous hours researching and exploring the diverse topics which have resulted in the successful publishing of this book. They have passed on their knowledge of decades through this book. To expedite this challenging task, the publisher supported the team at every step. A small team of assistant editors was also appointed to further simplify the editing procedure and attain best results for the readers.

Our editorial team has been hand-picked from every corner of the world. Their multi-ethnicity adds dynamic inputs to the discussions which result in innovative outcomes. These outcomes are then further discussed with the researchers and contributors who give their valuable feedback and opinion regarding the same. The feedback is then collaborated with the researches and they are edited in a comprehensive manner to aid the understanding of the subject.

Apart from the editorial board, the designing team has also invested a significant amount of their time in understanding the subject and creating the most relevant covers. They scrutinized every image to scout for the most suitable representation of the subject and create an appropriate cover for the book.

The publishing team has been involved in this book since its early stages. They were actively engaged in every process, be it collecting the data, connecting with the contributors or procuring relevant information. The team has been an ardent support to the editorial, designing and production team. Their endless efforts to recruit the best for this project, has resulted in the accomplishment of this book. They are a veteran in the field of academics and their pool of knowledge is as vast as their experience in printing. Their expertise and guidance has proved useful at every step. Their uncompromising quality standards have made this book an exceptional effort. Their encouragement from time to time has been an inspiration for everyone.

The publisher and the editorial board hope that this book will prove to be a valuable piece of knowledge for researchers, students, practitioners and scholars across the globe.

List of Contributors

Silke Wiegand-Grefe, Susanne Halverscheid, Franz Petermann and Angela Plass
University Medical Center Hamburg-Eppendorf, Center for Clinical Psychology and Rehabilitation at Bremen University, Germany

Andrew Soundy
University of Birmingham, Birmingham, England

Thomas Kingstone
Freshwinds Charity, Birmingham, England

Pete Coffee
School of Sport, University of Stirling, Scotland

Lawrence T. Lam
The School of Medicine Sydney, the University of Notre Dame Australia, Australia
Disciple of Pediatrics and Child Health, Sydney Medical School, the University of Sydney, Australia

Kenneth M. Coll and John Butgereit
Boise State University, USA

Brenda J. Freeman
Northwest Nazarene University, USA

Patti Thobro and Robin Haas
Cathedral Home for Children, USA

José A. Carmona Torres, Adolfo J. Cangas Díaz and Álvaro I. Langer Herrera
University of Almeria, Spain

Jerry L. Jennings
Liberty Healthcare Corporation, Bala Cynwyd, PA, USA

James D. Bell
Central State Hospital, Petersburg, VA, USA

Geoffrey Thompson
Saybrook University, San Francisco, CA, USA

Cecilia Hansen Löfstrand
Department of Sociology, University of Gothenburg, Sweden

Michela Gatta, Lara Dal Zotto, Lara Del Col and Pier Antonio Battistella
Neuropsychiatric Unit for Children and Adolescents and Pediatrics Department, ULSS 16 and University of Padua, Italy

Francesca Bosisio, Giannino Melotti and Roberta Biolcati
Psychology Department, University of Bologna, Italy

Ruth F.G. Williams
La Trobe School of Economics, La Trobe University, Australia

D.P. Doessel
School of History, Philosophy, Religion & Classics, the University of Queensland, Australia

Francesca Pernice-Duca, Wendy Case and Deborah Conrad-Garrisi
Wayne State University, USA

Ewa Wojtyna
University of Silesia in Katowice, Poland

Jacqueline Conway
Team 24, London, England

Andrew L. Cherry
University of Oklahoma, Anne & Henry Zarrow School of Social Work, Tulsa Campus, Tulsa, USA